HEALTH
CARE
in
2020

*PRE-MACRA &
IMPRECISE PREDICTIONS*

HEALTH CARE in 2020

Where Uncertain Reform, Bad Habits, Two Few Doctors and Skyrocketing Costs Are Taking Us

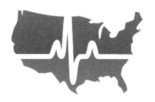

Steve Jacob

Books may be purchased by contacting
the publisher or author at:
    Dorsam Publishing
    www.DorsamPublishing.com

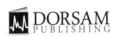

Cover Design: NZ Graphics, Inc.
Interior Design: Ronnie Moore, WESType Publishing Services, Inc.
Editor: Peter Kaufman
Index: John Maling, EditingByJohn
Book Shepherd: Judith Briles
Publisher: Dorsam Publishing

Library of Congress Catalog: #2011937977

ISBN: 978-0-9839950-0-5

1. Health Care.   2. Health Reform.   3. Health Workforce.
4. Health Costs.

First Edition: Printed in the USA

*Dedicated
to the loving memory of
Mary Jo Dorsam Yentes, 1922-2011*

Contents

Acknowledgments

Book publishing is a team effort. I want to thank the patient and professional collaboration of several people: content editor and lifelong friend Peter Kaufman; book designer Ronnie Moore; cover designer Nick Zelinger; researcher Alicia Benson; indexer John Maling, and book shepherd Judith Briles. Daughter Megan Brooks and son Ben Jacob offered valuable advice, as well as technical and editing assistance.

Although her name is not on the cover, this book would not have been written without the support of my wife, Paula. Her editing prowess, loving encouragement and patience sustained me and made this project a reality.

Finally, I want to acknowledge posthumously my late mother-in-law, Mary Jo Yentes. A life-long book reader, she was my biggest fan. Right before I began writing, she told me enthusiastically (and forcefully), "I cannot wait to get that book into my hands!" I will regret until the day I die that I could not deliver it to her before she lost her long battle with heart failure.

Part 1

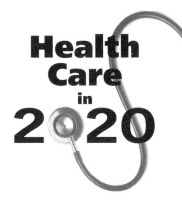

Health
Care
in
2020

Introduction

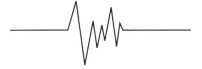

Chapter 1

Health Care in 2020

A defining decade

U.S. health care will change more in the next decade than it has in the last half-century. The health-reform law, if it survives, will be fully implemented by 2020.

Nearly 40 percent of the nation's doctors will have reached retirement age by then. The estimated physician shortage by 2020 is expected to surpass 90,000. About one-third of nurses are 50 or older, and more than half of those want to retire before 2020. Estimates of the nursing shortage by 2020 range from 600,000 to more than one million.

There is no end in sight for medical cost increases that annually surpass the growth of the nation's economy and the Consumer Price Index.

Health reform survived a raucous political debate, defied historical odds against passage and forged ahead despite the worst recession since the Great Depression. The U.S. faces financial risks that have not been confronted since World War II. When President Obama took office in 2009, the federal budget deficit was $6.3 trillion, or about $72,000 per household. The Congressional Budget Office estimates the deficit will be more than $20 trillion—or $172,000 per household—by 2020. The U.S.

debt-to-gross domestic product ratio was 55 percent in 2009. That is expected to rise to 90 percent by 2020. A significant portion of this will be driven by health-care spending.

By 2020, nearly 20 cents of every dollar spent in the U.S. will be spent on health care. The size and scope of these costs have an enormous impact on the nation's financial well-being. Whether the nation comes to grips with controlling them will be pivotal. Since the creation of Medicare and Medicaid in 1965, medical costs have grown faster than the U.S. economy and have resisted cost-control measures except for a brief period in the 1990s. If the price of gasoline had risen at the same rate as health-care spending since 1980, it would be $9 per gallon.

Donald Berwick, administrator of the Centers for Medicare and Medicaid Services, wrote an article in the journal *Health Affairs* in 2008 (before he was appointed by President Obama) outlining what he called the "triple aim," or three goals that needed to be pursued simultaneously:

- Improving the experience of patient care. He pointed to six dimensions of care from a 2001 Institute of Medicine report on quality: safety, effectiveness, patient-centeredness, timeliness, efficiency and equity.
- Improving population health by addressing "upstream" causes of disease, such as poor nutrition, physical inactivity, and tobacco and alcohol abuse.
- Reducing per-capita costs.

When Berwick assumed his role in the Obama administration in 2010, he reaffirmed that the triple aim was "my main focus" in his new job.

Declaring a full-scale revamping of health-care quality and population health while lowering costs is a daunting task. That tension is highlighted by what Yale University professor William Kissick calls "the iron triangle" of health care: quality, cost and access. Each component competes for resources at the expense of the others. Costs can be cut but, if that is done incorrectly, quality and access suffer. Access can be broadened, but it inevitably will cost more and may harm quality. Improving quality also likely will cost more and may restrict access.

Nowhere does this conflict play out more often than in the Medicare program. More than one-quarter of Medicare outlays are spent on beneficiaries in their last year of life. Sharon Kaufman and Wendy Max, professors at the Institute for Health & Aging at the University of California, San Francisco, note the "societal tension" between the program's cost control and "the value of open-ended technology" to extend life. As the baby boomers join the program's ranks in record numbers, an increasing number of patients and their families will find it difficult to resist physicians who recommend potentially beneficial, but expensive, treatments.

Cost-effectiveness and value are important to Medicare's solvency, but are certainly not considerations in individual treatment decisions. Bioethicists Daniel Callahan and Sherwin Nuland call chronic disease "the front line" of U.S. medicine in the near-future. They point out that the medical system has not made much headway in conquering specific diseases but its "main achievements today consist of devising ways to marginally extend the lives of the very sick ... for a relatively short period of time— at considerable expense and often causing serious suffering to (the patient)."

Callahan and Nuland acknowledge that the views of most Americans regarding the medical system are much more optimistic: belief in limitless medical advances; the notion that major lethal diseases, in theory, can be cured, and that scientific progress is affordable if well-managed.

A 1994 Harvard study found that more than one-third of Americans believed that modern medicine could cure almost any illness suffered by those with access to the most advanced technology. Americans generally are happy with their own individual health care. It is the broader system that upsets them. A 2010 Gallup poll found more than 8 out of 10 consider their health care excellent or good, which is the highest percentage in a decade.

However, in another 2010 Gallup poll, only 40 percent expressed "a great deal" or "quite a lot" of confidence in the health-care system. Gallup conducted a worldwide poll on national confidence in health-care systems in 2006. The U.S. ranked 88th in confidence level out of 120 nations, scoring lower than countries such as India, Iran, Malawi, Afghanistan and Angola.

Paul Keckley, executive director of the Deloitte Center for Health Solutions, wrote in a foreword to that group's 2010 health consumer survey: "They (Americans) are neither patient nor patients; they are consumers ... 'They' want more value from the system, more transparency in pricing and quality, better use of technology and better service ... And 'they' do not want to pay more than they currently pay out-of-pocket, if at all."

The lack of confidence in the health-care system stems in part from insecurity about the future availability of health benefits. A 2010 Employee Benefit Research Institute survey, taken after health reform was signed into law, reflected that the federal legislation did not instill much confidence. Only half of respondents were confident that they would have job-based insurance in the future. About 59 percent were confident just one year earlier, and 68 percent were confident in 2000.

Patient engagement is lacking

The most effective way to cut health-care costs is to use less health care. And many Americans have control over this. A significant percentage of disease—especially chronic conditions—is self-inflicted. For example, a 2004 study found that lifestyle changes could prevent at least 90 percent of heart-disease cases. Nearly 4 out of 10 U.S. deaths are attributable to four behaviors: tobacco use, diet, physical inactivity and alcohol abuse. Declines in tobacco use have slowed in the past decade. Obesity has been increasing slowly but steadily. The rates of physical activity and binge drinking have barely improved since 2000.

And when they do need treatment, patients are not holding up their end of the bargain. Only half take medication in the prescribed doses. About half do not take referral advice, three-quarters do not keep follow-up appointments, and about half of those with chronic illnesses abandon medical care within a year.

About this book

Chapter 2, *Health Reform: Big achievement, limited results,* reviews the creation and impact of The Patient Protection and Affordable Care Act of 2010 (referred to in this book generically as "health reform"), the most far-reaching health-policy development since Medicare and Medicaid were created in the 1960s. A detailed account of legislation that encompassed more than 2,000 pages is well beyond the scope of this book. Several chapters include brief synopses of how the law affects several key players in the health-care sector.

The second section of the book examines American health behavior and its consequences. A 2003 *Health Affairs* journal article attempted to quantify the most important factors in determining health and premature death. The authors concluded that controllable factors—health behavior, environmental exposures and social disadvantages—made up a majority of causes. Medical care, which accounts for 95 percent of U.S. health-care spending, affected only 10 percent of premature deaths.

That research provides the framework for this section's chapters. Chapter 3, *Life Expectancy: Going in the wrong direction,* explores why there was a surprising dip in U.S. life expectancy in 2008. Many suspect that rising rates of obesity and poverty are beginning to overwhelm the positive effects of decreased cigarette smoking and medical advances.

Chapter 4, *Health Behavior: The four habits that count most,* discusses how crucial but difficult it is to change destructive habits and replace them with healthy practices.

Chapters 5 through 8 cover the four most important behaviors that raise—or lower—the risk of disease and death. Chapter 5, *Nutrition: Taste, convenience and price rule,* notes that the average American consumed 500 calories more per day in 2000 than in 1970. The price of many processed foods has decreased in the past 20 years, while the cost of fruits and vegetables has risen significantly.

In Chapter 6, *Physical Activity: No medicine like it,* the overwhelming evidence of physical activity's benefits contrasts starkly with how few Americans are meeting recommended guidelines. Only about 5 percent of U.S. adults exercise vigorously on any given day. The No. 1 self-reported "moderate activity" was food and drink preparation. Chapter 7, *Weight Control: The U.S. as an "obesogenic" society,* explores how overweight is the "new normal" in the United States and how obese people have to absorb society's scorn. Ten years ago, the percentage of people considered clinically obese was less than 20 percent in 28 states. That is the case now in only one state—Colorado. Moreover, in nine states, more than 30 percent of the residents are now obese. Obesity is the fastest-growing public-health issue the U.S. has ever faced. Obesity is expected to account for more than 20 percent of health-care spending by 2018.

Chapter 8, *Tobacco and Alcohol: Progress has stalled,* examines what are considered vices. One of the greatest public-health achievements of the last century was cutting the smoking rate in half from its peak in the 1960s. However, it remains the No. 1 preventable cause of death. Half of all smokers can expect to die of tobacco use. Americans are drinking more than they have in the last 25 years. It is not clear whether, on the whole, that is good or bad. Temperance has long been considered a virtue. Nevertheless, an onslaught of research has found that moderate drinking extends life and combats a number of health risks.

Chapter 9, *Personalized Medicine: Its promise remains elusive,* discusses the impact of genes on health and the elusive promise of personalized medicine. Genetics is important to health, but is often given far too much credit or blame for health outcomes. Genes load the gun, but environment pulls the trigger. Genes affect how a body will react to its environment. They are either suppressed or expressed because of health behavior or environmental factors. Personalized medicine, or tailoring medical treatment to an individual's genetic profile, represents an important frontier in combating disease.

Chapter 10, *Health-Care Disparities: "Causes of causes" of death and disease,* explores the social determinants of health. Ironically, rapidly rising health-care costs are crowding out funding for federal and state programs that have a greater effect on health than medical interventions do. Public and preschool education, nutrition programs, environmental controls, public health and public housing are being cut because of rapidly growing government insurance programs. Medical care is a contributor to only 10 percent of premature deaths. Social circumstances—where people are born, live, work and play—and environmental factors determine 20 percent of disease and death. People with low income and education are more exposed to environmental harm. Disadvantaged circumstances also help drive health behavior and gene expression.

As Chapter 11 *Prevention: What's too much and what's too little* points out, prevention has a reputation that it cannot live up to. Most believe more preventive care saves money. However, less than 20 percent of preventive services do so. Prevention advocates correctly argue that holding prevention to a different standard is unfair. After all, most curative care does not save money. The larger issue, proponents say, is to determine the best way to allocate health-care dollars to improve Americans' health. Other experts believe preventive care is often overused, leading to overtreatment either by finding "pseudo-disease" that never would harm the patient or through false-positive test results.

Workplace wellness programs, the subject of Chapter 12 *Workplace Wellness: Health as a tangible asset*, have surged in larger American companies. Forward-thinking businesses believe employee health is too important to rely on the broader health-care system. They create healthy environments that reward individual effort and build self-esteem. They help pay for the treatment of illness, but they place equal emphasis on keeping employees' health from deteriorating.

Chapter 13, *Patient Engagement: Paying attention pays off,* points out that patients who are actively engaged in their health have better outcomes and more years of healthy life. They are not deterred by the complexity and fragmentation of the health-care system. They practice good health habits. They manage over-the-counter medications, minor wounds, illnesses and injuries on their own. They collaborate with their providers and participate in making treatment decisions. They seek out reliable information on their own. Health reform and the growth of high-deductible health plans will require patients to become better health consumers.

Chapter 14, *Chronic Disease: Health care's big-ticket item,* covers chronic disease, which accounted for 85 percent of health-care spending in 2004. Viewed optimistically, the prevalence of chronic disease is a testament to medical and public-health advances in the 20th century. In 1900, life expectancy was 47 years. Most people died of infectious disease, accidents and childbirth, at a point in life well before today's chronic conditions could develop. Chronic disease is increasing. It is closely tied to the aging of the U.S. population and to the rising obesity rate, which contributes to diabetes, high blood pressure and heart disease. Successful chronic-disease management is tricky but, if successful, could take a huge bite out of the nation's health-care costs.

The third section of the book examines rapidly increasing health-care costs and their consequences. Chapter 15, *National Health Costs: Technology and market power drive increases,* approaches spending from a national perspective. The current trend is sobering. Health-care spending is on track to consume 119 to 142 percent of current U.S. per-capita spending over the next 75 years. That means health care would crowd out other valuable areas of the budget, such as national defense and education. Medical technology accounts for an estimated one-half to two-thirds of spending growth. Another major factor is the market power of dominant health-care organizations, which can dictate steep annual prices increases.

Chapter 16, *Consumer Health Costs: Struggling with bills and higher deductibles,* looks at the impact of rising medical expenses on households. About 40 percent of Americans had trouble paying medical bills in 2010, up from 34 percent in 2005. More than one-quarter of insured households reported problems with medical debt. The disturbing result is widespread self-rationing. Nearly 6 out of 10 adults say they have delayed care because of cost. About 40 percent of those in fair or poor health did not fill at least one prescription in the past year. People with chronic conditions who fail to take medication are flirting with disastrous consequences.

Chapter 17, *Waste and Overtreatment: No incentive for efficiency,* considers what the Institute of Medicine (IOM) calls health-care system's "overuse, underuse, misuse, duplication, system failures, unnecessary repetition, poor communication, and inefficiency." The IOM estimates that 30 to 40 percent of health-care spending is of no benefit. The FBI estimates an additional 3 to 10 percent of spending is fraudulent.

Chapter 18, *Private Insurance: Heart and soul of reform,* covers individual and employer insurance. The new law will help put small businesses and individual health-insurance buyers on a more equal footing with large employers. Health-insurance exchanges, scheduled to begin in 2014, will lower administrative costs and provide a more orderly insurance market. Insurance coverage will be more comprehensive, and plans will be more transparent in their offerings. However, it remains to be seen whether employers will continue to offer insurance to their employees or shift them to the exchanges.

Chapter 19, *Government Insurance: Here comes reform*—and *baby boomers,* details the expansion of government insurance programs. Medicare and Medicaid, government's health-insurance programs for elderly and low-income Americans, are going to expand significantly by the end of the decade. The number of Medicare recipients is expected to grow from 47 million to 64 million, as more baby boomers enter its ranks. Medicaid will nearly double by 2021 to 100 million recipients, as health reform expands eligibility. More than half of Americans will be enrolled in at least one of these two programs or the Children's Health Insurance Program (CHIP) by the beginning of the next decade.

The fourth section of the book deals with health-care delivery.

Chapter 20, *The Doctor: Overworked and underappreciated,* considers the plight of the beleaguered family physician, the most revered member of the health-care system. These primary-care physicians are the front line of medicine. Their income essentially has stayed the same since the 1990s, while their practice expenses have steadily increased. Their workdays are brutal. They have to fight to collect every dollar. Primary-care physicians' share of the U.S. health-care dollar is only 7 cents. However, primary-care doctors *control* 80 cents of the health-care dollar by sending their patients to hospitals, referring them to specialists and handing out prescriptions.

Chapter 21, *The Hospital: Reinventing itself by necessity,* explores how hospitals are attempting to remake themselves. A key goal for new health-care delivery models is to provide care that results in fewer hospitalizations and emergency-room visits. Hospitals are buying physician practices at a rapid pace to enhance their bargaining power and to strengthen their referral networks.

Chapter 22, *Pharmaceuticals: Industry at a crossroads,* points out that the pharmaceutical industry is facing major near-term challenges. Worldwide sales of brand-name prescription drugs could be cut in half by 2015 as lucrative brands lose patent protection. For decades, it lived off what it called "blockbuster" drugs: patented medications aimed at broad populations with chronic conditions. Cheaper generics now account for more than 3 out of 4 U.S. prescriptions.

Chapter 23, *End-of-Life Care: Quality of death,* deals with end-of-life care, shamelessly smeared by headline-seeking politicians braying about nonexistent "death panels." The most important issues to any patient are how to live and die. The U.S. health-care system does a good job enabling the former, and an awful job with the latter.

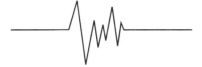

Chapter 2

Health Reform
Big achievement, limited results

The Patient Protection and Affordable Care Act of 2010 (referred to in this book generically as "health reform") unquestionably is the most far-reaching health-policy development since Medicare and Medicaid were created in the 1960s.

The law is audaciously ambitious. It is expected to reduce the number of uninsured Americans under age 65 by 32 million, and an estimated 94 percent of legal U.S. residents are expected to have *Access* health insurance by the end of the decade. It attempts to make health care more affordable through subsidies and competitive health-insurance exchanges. It establishes a framework for slowing *cost* health-care spending. It strives to coordinate traditionally fragmented U.S. health care. It expands clinical research to determine which treatments work best, and seeks to hasten the adoption of *quality* health-information technology by hospitals and physicians.

For all of its aspirations, many policymakers and health-care leaders believe the reform law did not go far enough to control costs, offer a government-sponsored insurance option and expand the health-care workforce. Yet reformers were laboring in a hostile economic environment. The legislation was crafted during the worst recession since the Great Depression. Congress had just signed off on financial-bailout and economic-stimulus packages. The nation was fighting wars in Iraq and Afghanistan.

The health-care industry was less than enthusiastic about the prospect of more government regulation and possible reimbursement cuts. Most Americans understood health care needed reform, but largely were content with their health insurance and doctors.

Given this political climate, reformers went about as far as they could—especially in the face of virulent and often-irrational opposition. Even if it fails in its attempts to corral escalating costs and improve health-care delivery, reform was, essentially, spackling to fill unjust gaps in a fragmented system. People no longer can be turned down for insurance because of pre-existing conditions. Health-insurance exchanges should level the playing field for individual Americans by offering affordable insurance comparable to that enjoyed by large companies.

The $1 trillion price tag largely will be financed by taxes on a small slice of Americans, as well as fees and reimbursement reductions borne by major health-care industry players. Higher-income workers will pay more in Medicare payroll taxes, and excise taxes will be levied on high-cost health-insurance policies. Payment cuts and fees will affect hospitals, pharmaceutical companies and medical-device makers. Payments to Medicare Advantage, Medicare's private insurance alternative for the elderly, will be reduced.

An unlikely political achievement

The Obama administration's strategy was to create a coalition of health-care industry groups that supported reform. With the exception of Lyndon Johnson's creation of Medicare and Medicaid, every president from Franklin Roosevelt on failed at health reform. Most of those efforts were defeated by powerful health-care lobbies that outspent and outflanked one administration after another.

- Most Americans will be required to have health insurance by 2014.
- Those without access to affordable employer coverage can purchase coverage through a health-insurance exchange. Premium and cost-sharing credits will be available to some exchange participants, depending on income. Small businesses also will be able to purchase insurance through a separate exchange.

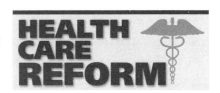

Major provisions

- Health insurers will be prohibited from denying coverage based on health, and from charging higher premiums based on gender or health status.
- Employers with 50 or more workers will be charged penalties for employees who receive tax credits for health insurance through the exchanges.
- Medicaid will be expanded to cover non-elderly adults up to 133 percent of the federal poverty level ($29,327 for a family of four).
- Health reform will reduce the number of uninsured by 32 million.

This time, health-industry groups climbed aboard the bandwagon for a number of reasons. As administration allies, they could cut the best possible deal for their constituents. Health-reform insurance expansion would create more customers. Most conceded they were part of a dysfunctional system in need of repair.

Health-care lobbyists spared no expense. The Center for Public Integrity (CPI), a nonprofit investigative journalism organization, examined Senate lobbying-disclosure forms for 2009. It found that more than 1,750 companies and organizations deployed more than 4,500 advocates to influence health-reform legislation. That is about eight for each member of Congress.

The disclosure forms revealed an odd collection of lobbyists, such as the National Rifle Association, the Golf Course Superintendents Association of America and the League of American Orchestras. It was not clear why these groups cared about health reform.

CPI quoted an Association of Art Museum Directors official as saying dozens of arts centers had asked the Senate leadership to add "creative arts therapists ... to the definition of mental-health service professionals."

Ten key health-care groups—including the American Medical Association, the American Hospital Association and a number of pharmaceutical organizations—spent nearly $139 million in 2009 and nearly $126 million in 2010 on lobbying.

Even with such persuasive financial heft, health reform was in doubt until the end. Obama took a hands-off approach in 2009, hoping congressional leadership could create a package that could garner bipartisan support. Instead, negotiators became bogged down in details and allowed momentum to slip away. Obama's decision to intervene in 2010, when the outcome was in doubt, was pivotal to success. Almost as important was the ability of Senate Majority Leader Harry Reid, D-Nev., to get 60 senators to vote for the legislation before newly elected Sen. Scott Brown, R-Mass, was seated in January to replace the late Edward Kennedy. Democrats needed the 60 votes to avoid a Republican filibuster that could have defeated the effort. The steely determination of Speaker Nancy Pelosi, D-Calif., rammed the bill through the House.

Americans like the pieces, wary of the whole

Several elements of health reform consistently polled well during the congressional debate and since the law's passage. In a February 2010 Kaiser Health tracking poll, about 45 percent favored the health reform law and about 50 percent opposed it. However, about three-quarters of respondents considered the law's health-insurance reforms and subsidies, tax credits for small business and closing the Medicare prescription-drug funding gap (also known as the "doughnut hole") as "extremely" or "very" important.

Both sides claimed to represent American public opinion. Reform's opponents pointed to the overall opposition. Supporters emphasized broad support for the law's individual elements.

The individual mandate, which was the least-popular component of the law, was supported by an average of 53 percent of poll respondents. Its support differed wildly—from 26 percent to 73 percent—depending upon how pollsters described it.

A January 2011 Kaiser/Harvard poll reflected how split the American people remained on the law: 28 percent wanted to expand it; 19 percent wanted it unchanged; 23 percent wanted to repeal and replace it with a Republican-sponsored alternative, and 20 percent wanted to repeal and not replace it.

Reform dominated news coverage for several months. According to the Pew Research Center for the People & the Press, the health-care battle was the No. 1 story in the mainstream media from June 2009 to March 2010. It accounted for an average of about 14 percent of the news coverage during that period across all media. Reform consumed about one-third of the airtime on ideological talk shows.

Health reform pop quiz

Take this true/false quiz to test your knowledge of health reform. More than 1,200 U.S. adults answered these questions in a December 2010 survey. About one quarter answered 7-10 questions correctly. About one-third answered 0-4 questions correctly. Less than 1 percent got all 10 correct.

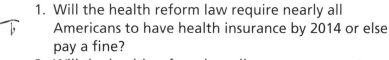

T   1. Will the health reform law require nearly all Americans to have health insurance by 2014 or else pay a fine?

F   2. Will the health reform law allow a government panel to make decisions about end-of-life care for people on Medicare?

F   3. Will the health reform law cut benefits that were previously provided to all people on Medicare?

T   4. Will the health reform law expand the existing Medicaid program to cover low-income, uninsured adults regardless of whether they have children?

T   5. Will the health reform law provide financial help to low and moderate income Americans who don't get insurance through their jobs to help them purchase coverage?

T   6. Will the health reform law prohibit insurance companies from denying coverage because of a person's medical history or health condition?

F   7. Will the health reform law require all businesses, even the smallest ones, to provide health insurance for their employees?

T   8. Will the health reform law provide tax credits to small businesses that offer coverage to their employees?

F   9. Will the health reform law create a new government run insurance plan to be offered along with private plans?

10. Will the health reform law allow undocumented
    immigrants to receive financial help from the
    government to buy health insurance?

Answers: 1. T; 2. F; 3. F; 4. T; 5. T; 6. T; 7. F; 8. T; 9. F; 10. F.

Source: Pop Quiz: Assessing Americans' Familiarity With the Health Care Law"
(#8148) The Henry J. Kaiser Family Foundation, February 2011. This information
was reprinted with permission from the Henry J. Kaiser Family Foundation. The
Kaiser Family Foundation is a non-profit private operating foundation, based in Menlo
Park, California, dedicated to producing and communicating the best possible analysis
and information on health issues.

———

As the debate progressed, people became more confused. In July 2009, 63 percent said they had trouble understanding the bill. Six months later, the percentage was 69 percent.

In March 2011, 53 percent admitted they still did not understand the law, a figure only slightly changed from 55 percent the year before.

Many wanted government to take a more radical approach to health care. A September 2010 Associated Press poll asked about the proper role of government in health care, regardless of whether respondents supported or opposed the reform law. The survey found that 4 of 10 U.S. adults believed the new law did not go far enough to change the health-care system, compared with 2 of 10 who said the government should stay out of the health-care arena.

More broadly, Americans have favored rebuilding or making major changes to the health-care system since the mid-1980s. In 1986, two-thirds favored an overhaul. By 1991, that number had risen to 90 percent. In 2009, during the reform debate, it stood at 84 percent.

Health care is an easy issue to demagogue because it stirs very personal insecurities. Opponents successfully created anxiety and fear about reform's potential consequences. The percentage of people who believed reform would affect them negatively doubled, from 21 to 40 percent, during the latter part of 2009.

Republican pollster Frank Luntz instructed Fox News host Sean Hannity on how to refer to a proposal to offer a government-sponsored health plan on the insurance exchange, according to the website The Daily Beast. "If you call it a public option," Luntz counseled Hannity, "the American people are split. If you call it the government option, the public is overwhelmingly against it."

Despite the fact that the law did not include the public option, opponents continued to describe the law as "a government takeover of health care." PolitiFact, the Pulitzer Prize-winning truth-in-politics reporting project sponsored by the *St. Petersburg Times*, named that phrase the 2010 "Lie of the Year."

However, the "government takeover" rhetoric is mild compared with some of the myths that persisted in the wake of the debate. National Public Radio spotlighted some of the more outlandish claims—that the law would:

- Require people who received government health insurance to be implanted with a microchip.
- Create a "private army" for President Obama.
- Require the hiring of 16,500 new IRS agents.
- Dictate what you could eat.
- Allow hospitals to fire obese employees.

As University of North Carolina professor Jonathan Oberlander pointed out, Democrats continually will have to resell the reform law because it was not initially sold convincingly. He said people are more likely to believe it contains imaginary provisions, such as "death panels," rather than real benefits such as preventive services without deductibles.

What reform will and will not do

Perhaps the biggest disappointment about reform is that it did not address more forcefully health care's biggest problem: relentlessly rising costs.

Short-term cost savings, such as reduced payments to Medicare Advantage plans and lower annual increases in rates paid to hospitals, will help fund the expansion of Medicaid and subsidies for people buying insurance on the exchanges beginning in 2014.

Long-term cost savings require changes to the delivery of and payment for medical services. Policy experts estimate that about 30 percent of health-care spending can be eliminated without harming patient care. Rooting out those excess expenditures is what true reform needed to address.

Medical costs are expected to rise more than 6 percent annually and consume nearly 20 percent of the nation's economy by 2020, according to the Centers for Medicare and Medicaid Services.

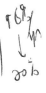

Stakeholders, especially private employers and insurance plans, worry that the law's cost-containment efforts will wilt under the pressure of medical inflation's momentum. It does not require patients or physicians to use treatments or tests that have been proven effective, or to strive for the most cost-effective alternative. It does not fundamentally change the fee-for-service model that rewards service volume rather than results.

If health-care spending growth is not corralled, government, businesses and individuals will not be able to deliver on the law's requirements and reforms.

The Obama administration and reform proponents are optimistic that the pilot projects and demonstration programs that test delivery and payment reforms will lead to long-term savings. According to one health blogger, the law contains 312 mentions of demonstrations and 80 mentions of pilot projects. These experiments generally test providing coordinated care among primary-care physicians, specialists and hospitals. They pay a single price for treatment of injury or illness, to be shared by providers who have formed accountable care organizations. The goal is to pay physicians and hospitals bonuses or shared savings for delivering better care at a lower cost.

The newly created Independent Payment Advisory Board will have some authority to reduce Medicare spending, but it is handcuffed initially by a number of restrictions. The law also encourages the adoption of health information technology and of comparative-effectiveness studies to test the performance of various treatments. However, the Congressional Budget Office (CBO) did not count any of these savings through 2020 when it forecast the financial impact of the law because they are unproven, hard to quantify and too far in the future.

Success hinges on implementation

Wilbur Cohen, a high-ranking Johnson administration health-policy official and principal architect of the Medicare program, once said that health policy is 10 percent legislation and 90 percent implementation.

Any law that seeks to revamp one-sixth of the economy is bound to be complicated, unwieldy and ripe for unintended consequences. Health reform carries the added burden of being implemented by many players who oppose it. Every congressional Republican voted against it. More than half of the states are suing to test its constitutionality. Despite the American Medical Association's support of the law, a majority of the nation's physicians are against it.

Reformers will have to push harder in this poisoned environment because unmet expectations inevitably will weaken the law's already shaky support. Public support will rise or fall based on how the law affects individuals, as well as their friends and families. That support, if it gathers momentum, also may create political capital to allow reformers to strengthen the law as its effects become known and conditions change.

The ultimate fears are that the insurance companies will choose not to participate in the exchanges and businesses will decide to abandon their traditional role of sponsoring insurance for their employees.

Republicans have threatened not to fund the bill if they cannot repeal it. That could result in understaffing of health exchanges and spotty enforcement of the individual mandate. Both could undermine public confidence.

Some programs already have failed to receive funding that was authorized, but not mandated, by the law. These funding problems have more to do with the budget deficit than Republican retribution. In 2011, a $50 million program to test alternative ways of resolving medical-malpractice disputes received no funding. A $50 million program for nurse-run clinics received just $15 million. A $24 million effort to regionalize emergency care to overcome staff shortages was not funded.

Another significant threat to implementation is the potential demise, either judicially or legislatively, of the individual mandate. Republicans have said they oppose the mandate and subsidies for insurance purchased on the exchanges. However, they promised to retain the most popular portions of the law, such as those prohibiting insurance companies from canceling coverage because of pre-existing conditions and limiting the variation of insurance-premium prices.

Health reform is supported by what experts call a three-legged stool to spread risk and costs more evenly. Leg one: Everyone must buy insurance, which ensures that the young and healthy are included. Leg two: Insurers cannot deny people health insurance, which spreads the insurance-premium costs for the healthy and sick more evenly. Leg three: Government subsidies bring premium costs to within reach of every household.

Repealing the individual mandate would enable healthy people to wait until they got sick to buy health insurance. Repealing the subsidies as well as the individual mandate would further erode the incentive to buy health insurance when one is healthy. Insurance premiums would be higher because there would be a greater percentage of sick people in the risk pool.

Massachusetts offers a good example. In 1996, it prohibited insurers from charging premiums based on the condition of a person's health. However, it did not require people to buy insurance. Premiums soared. When an individual mandate went into effect in 2006, the number of uninsured dropped 60 percent and premiums decreased an average of 40 percent.

The CBO estimated that the lack of an individual mandate would reduce the number of uninsured who gain coverage from 32 million to 16 million. It also estimated that individual and small-business premiums would rise by 15 to 20 percent because fewer healthy people would buy insurance. The CBO also projected, however, that the lack of a mandate would lower the cost of health reform by $49 billion by 2019, or about 25 percent of the cost of the entire legislation. The reason costs would decrease by one-quarter despite covering half as many uninsured: the sickest, and therefore the costliest, uninsured would become the most likely to get coverage.

According to an Urban Institute computer simulation, health reform would reduce the uninsured rate from more than 18 percent to about 8 percent. Without the individual mandate, the uninsured rate would be about 15 percent.

Even if the individual mandate is upheld in court and in Congress, it might be ineffective if the penalty for not buying insurance proves to be too low or loosely enforced.

Another implementation danger is that the federal government may overreach in its zeal to ensure that employer-based insurance is generous and secure. Regulatory burden could encourage businesses already struggling to sponsor health insurance to walk away and send employees to the exchanges instead.

Effects on the states

Many state governments, struggling to balance their budgets, are dreading the rollout of health reform. Their Medicaid-related spending undoubtedly will rise. The individual mandate is expected to increase enrollment among the estimated 40 percent of low-income people who already qualify but have not signed up. The federal government will not subsidize those enrollees beyond the share it traditionally pays, which on average is about 60 percent. Reform requires Medicaid to cover all adults with incomes at or below 133 percent of the federal poverty level (FPL). That is an annual income of $14,484 for individuals, or $29,726 for a family of four. The federal government will pay 100 percent of the health-care costs for the newly eligible from 2014 to 2016, with the states' share rising gradually to 10 percent from 2017 to 2020 and thereafter.

According to an Urban Institute computer simulation, state governments collectively will save between $92 billion and $129 billion from 2014 to 2019. The law eliminates states' optional Medicaid coverage for those above 133 percent of FPL and shifts them to federally funded subsidies on the exchanges. Medicaid expansion helps reduce state and local spending on uncompensated care for the uninsured. It will also replace state and local spending on mental-health services with federally funded Medicaid coverage. The amount each state will save depends on its current Medicaid eligibility rules and the characteristics of its Medicaid population.

Federal Medicaid dollars will provide economic-development stimulus for each state's health-care sectors and local economies. The exchange subsidies also will contribute to state economies to the extent that households are able to shift their spending from health care to other goods and services.

States either may run their own exchanges or allow their residents to participate in a federally run exchange. For states that want to set up exchanges, there are several issues to consider. They must decide whether to have one exchange or separate ones for individuals and small businesses. They may split their states, or operate collaboratively with nearby states.

States may opt out of setting up exchanges, either for political or financial reasons. That would ensure that health reform becomes a largely federal program.

Prior to the invasion of Iraq, Colin Powell, U.S. Secretary of State under George W. Bush, was quoted as citing what was called the Pottery Barn rule: "You break it, you own it."

That rule will apply to President Obama and health reform. The new law feeds the perception that government controls what happens in health care. Fairly or not, his administration will be blamed for soaring medical costs, despite the fact that they have persisted for decades. Moreover, health reform ushers 32 million new people into a dysfunctional system plagued by overuse of services and testing, misaligned incentives and fragmented care. Health reform contains a tentative foundation for addressing these problems. Nonetheless, poor implementation of the law can overwhelm those efforts and put us in a bigger financial fix than we are in today.

Part 2

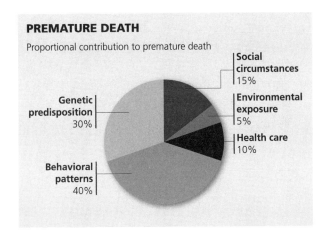

PREMATURE DEATH

Proportional contribution to premature death

Social circumstances 15%

Environmental exposure 5%

Health care 10%

Genetic predisposition 30%

Behavioral patterns 40%

Health Behavior and Its Consequences

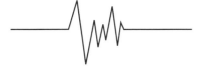

Chapter 3

Life Expectancy
Going in the wrong direction

Live the longest life possible. Live it free of chronic disease and disability. Those are the federal government's top goals for Americans and, on some level, the aspirations of everyone. Everything else about the health-care system, health policy and medical science is just details. Health, then health care. Those are the priorities.

Life expectancy is the average number of years that an infant born today is expected to live. It currently is about 75 years for men and 80 years for women. Mathematician Benjamin Gompertz proposed a "law of mortality" in 1825 that applies today: The death rate increases exponentially with age, doubling every eight years.

Life expectancy has been rising about three months each year since 1840. However, it won't necessarily keep going up. Life expectancy actually fell by a month in 2008, the last year for which there are official statistics. It remains to be seen whether that was a statistical blip or the beginning of a trend.

The three largest, most controllable factors in health and premature death are health behavior, the social determinants of health and the health-care system. Of these, health care gets far too much credit—and blame—for the state of the nation's health.

Of the 30-year increase in U.S. average life expectancy in the last century, only five years can be credited to advances in medical care. The other 25 years are credited to public-health measures, yet less than 1 percent of Americans can specify the mission of public health.

Public-health measures virtually eliminated the scourge of infectious diseases by providing safeguards such as clean and fluoridated drinking water, improved sanitation, widespread immunization, motor-vehicle and occupational safety, family planning and smoke-free public places.

What controls health and premature death

A 2002 *Health Affairs* journal article calculated the contribution of factors that determined health and premature death. Those influences were personal behavior, life circumstances, environmental toxins, medical care and genes.

Behavior accounts for 40 percent of premature deaths. The leading causes in this category are smoking, obesity and physical inactivity. While Americans place great faith in medical technology to extend life, simple changes in health habits would have far more impact.

Life circumstances cause 15 percent of premature death, but may contribute significantly to the other factors. People with lower income, less education and lower social status die sooner and are more likely to be disabled. People in lower classes are more likely to have poor health behavior: They smoke more, and have riskier lifestyles.

Environmental exposures account for 5 percent of premature deaths. Occupational products, pollution, lead paint and chemical contaminants are unpleasant facts in dangerous jobs and substandard living conditions.

Medical care affects only 10 percent of premature deaths, yet it accounts for 95 percent of U.S. health-care spending. The big

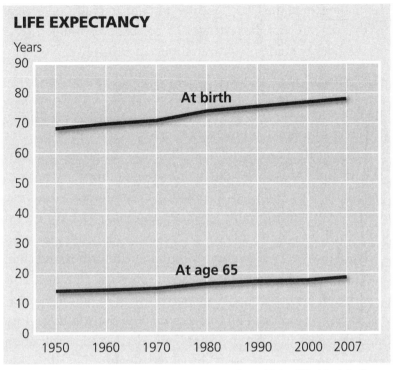

LIFE EXPECTANCY

Years

Source: National Vital Statistics System.

Since 1950, life expectancy at birth has risen more sharply than life expectancy at age 65. The primary reason is a reduction in infant mortality. The increase in 65-and-over life expectancy is an important factor in projecting Medicare and Social Security obligations.

contributors in this category are lack of access and medical errors, which the Institute of Medicine estimates kill as many as 98,000 people annually. Lack of health insurance, which affects 16 percent of the U.S. population, also contributes to premature death.

Genes, which are considered an uncontrollable factor, cause 30 percent of premature deaths. Yet genetic predisposition is not destiny. About two-thirds of obesity risk is genetic, but the condition does not happen without poor health habits. Dr. David

Heber, director of the UCLA Center for Human Nutrition, points out that the human DNA changes 0.5 percent every million years but the obesity epidemic is only about 30 years old.

The epidemiological threat: Obesity

Epidemiology seeks to explain how death and disease are distributed among groups of people. Epidemiologists study these patterns to determine their causes and head off their consequences. Patterns of death and disease have undergone several transitions, most of them in the past 100 years. Population health does not improve in a linear fashion. Health advances and setbacks have waxed and waned.

Until the late 19th century, infections, malnutrition and child mortality kept life expectancy to about 30 years. (Infant deaths skew overall life expectancy figures downward significantly.) Advances in sanitation and immunization in the early 20th century led to tremendous progress against early death. Industrialization and urbanization increased household wealth and education attainment. The biggest contributor to life expectancy was a significant decrease in infant and childhood death rates.

After World War II, infectious disease receded as a lethal threat, replaced by chronic disease. More than 40 percent of Americans smoked cigarettes, they ate an increasingly fat-laden diet of processed food and labored at increasingly sedentary occupations. Death from cardiovascular disease and cancer soared.

By the mid-1960s, the tide turned. The U.S. surgeon general's office released its landmark report on the perils of smoking in 1964. Tobacco users quit in droves. Advances in treating heart disease and high blood pressure slowed cardiovascular death rates. Medicare and Medicaid were established in 1964, providing a medical safety net for the elderly and the poor. More people began to die of degenerative disease later in life. The probability of a 65-year-old surviving to age 85 doubled from 1970 to 2005, rising from 20 percent to about 40 percent.

At the turn of the 20th century, life expectancy rose primarily because more children survived. After 1960, life expectancy rose because death rates dropped for those over 60 years old. The leading causes of death at the turn of the century—tuberculosis, pneumonia and diarrhea—have virtually disappeared as lethal threats. They have been replaced by cardiovascular disease, cancer, diabetes and high blood pressure.

Smoking rates have been halved and medical advances have increased longevity and lessened disability. However, obesity threatens to undo the progress. In the early 1960s, about 1 out of 3 U.S. adults were overweight and less than 1 out of 7 were obese. By 2008, 68 percent of Americans were overweight, and half of those were obese.

Excess weight increases the risk of several debilitating and expensive chronic conditions: diabetes, high blood pressure, stroke, heart disease, arthritis, cancer and several others. Obesity accounted for about 10 percent of U.S. medical spending in 2008.

There is some evidence that the rate of increase in obesity has reached a plateau. Some cynics suggest that everyone with the genetic propensity to become obese has now done so. Nevertheless, child obesity has sown the seeds for the next generation's struggle with weight. About 32 percent of school-age children are overweight, and half of those are obese. Eighty percent of children who are overweight at ages 10 to 15 will be obese at age 25.

Obesity may overtake smoking as the greatest U.S. population health risk threat if it persists. It has the potential to undo the progress made by declining smoking rates in the past half-century.

An estimated 25 percent of men and 43 percent of women in the United States attempt to lose weight each year. Nearly all of them fail. Excess weight is arguably the greatest public-health challenge now. Medical science continues to search for an answer. So far, there isn't one.

So, what causes preventable death now?

The four leading causes of premature death: smoking, high blood pressure, elevated blood glucose and being overweight or obese, according to a Harvard School of Public Health study. Those factors reduced life expectancy about five years for men and four years for women.

Health disparities exist on every health measure in the U.S. However, they are particularly pronounced in life expectancy. For example, a black man living in Washington, D.C., on average will die 17 years sooner than a white man in adjacent Montgomery County, MD.

Ralph Keeney, a Duke University professor, bluntly declares that nearly half the people who die before age 65 have only themselves to blame. The list of poor decisions is a familiar one: smoking; binge drinking; overeating; not exercising; unprotected sex; not wearing a seat belt; using drugs; suicide and homicide. By comparison, only 5 percent of deaths in 1900 and 25 percent in 1950 were self-inflicted.

Nearly one-quarter of American women and one-third of American men die before age 75 of causes that potentially could have been prevented by timely and effective health care. They either chose not to seek care or could not afford it. The U.S. ranked 15th out of 19 industrialized nations on regular use of health-care facilities. If the U.S. had performed as well as the top three nations—France, Japan and Australia—it would have averted more than 100,000 deaths a year.

In 1975, Americans who reached 50 years old could expect to live slightly longer than Europeans did. By 2005, the U.S. had fallen significantly behind Europe in life expectancy, primarily

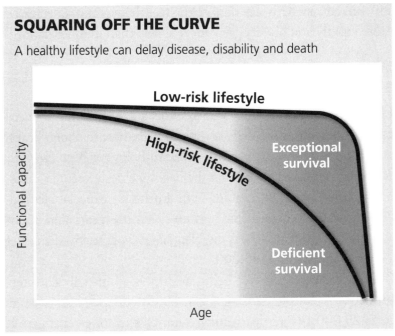

SQUARING OFF THE CURVE

A healthy lifestyle can delay disease, disability and death

Low-risk lifestyle

High-risk lifestyle

Exceptional survival

Deficient survival

Functional capacity

Age

Source: Cooper Wellness

This graphic illustrates the ideal "compression of morbidity" scenario—a long, healthy life that ends abruptly, or "squaring off the curve." Alternatively, poor health behaviors often result in a premature decline in well-being and a gradual lingering early death.

because of chronic disease among the near-elderly. Americans are twice as likely to have high blood pressure, be obese or have diabetes. Economists calculated that the U.S. could save up to $1.1 trillion by 2050 if its health status were comparable to that of its peers.

A *Health Affairs* study measured survival rates in 12 other industrialized nations and compared them with national health-care costs. In 1975, the U.S. was close to the average per-capita cost and ranked last. By 2005, health-care costs had tripled and were twice as much per capita than any other nation—and the U.S.

still ranked last. This was despite the fact that smoking decreased more rapidly and obesity grew more slowly than in other nations.

Which is cheaper: A long healthy life or a shorter disabled life?

Health economists and policy analysts debate the national financial burden of the healthy elderly compared with those in poorer health who die earlier. An often-cited 2003 study in *The New England Journal of Medicine* found that the healthy elderly spent as much on medical care as the disabled with shorter life expectancies did. A healthy 70-year-old lived about 14 more years and spent $136,000 in 1998 dollars. A disabled 70-year-old survived another 11 years and spent $145,000.

The excess expense of being healthy is admittedly counter-intuitive. A couple turning 65 in 2009 will spend an average of $220,000 before death for insurance and long-term care if one or both have chronic conditions. A couple with no chronic conditions will spend $260,000. The reason: At age 80, a healthy person will live, on average, 29 percent longer than one in an unhealthy household will.

According to the Employee Benefit Research Institute, a man retiring in 2010 at age 65 would need savings of $65,000 to $109,000 to have a 50-50 chance of covering health insurance premiums and out-of-pocket medical expenses. To improve the odds to 90 percent, the projection rose to $124,000 to $211,000. The estimates are even higher for women because of their longer life expectancy. Expenses of long-term care were not included.

A 2008 Dutch study compared the lifetime medical costs of groups of healthy-living people, smokers and the obese. The healthy had the highest lifetime expenditures because they lived the longest. Smokers cost the least because they died younger.

The obese were in between. However, among the three groups, more health-care dollars were spent on obese people until the age of 56. The estimated medical cost of treating obesity in 2008 in the U.S. was $147 billion.

The underweight or the extremely obese are more likely to die earlier worldwide. The impact of being obese on dying has decreased over the years, perhaps because of improved chronic-disease management. However, obesity unquestionably hastens the onset of disease and disability, as well as increasing medical costs. One study estimated that an obese 70-year-old would spend $39,000 more on health care in a lifetime than someone of normal weight would. The researchers estimated that Medicare spends 34 percent more on an obese person because, unlike other chronic diseases, the higher costs are not offset by earlier death.

'Compression of morbidity'

A long life is one thing. A healthy life free of disease and disability is another. The evidence suggests that life overall is lengthening, but that disease and disability may be increasing. The result: More months and years spent in poor health. It has been dubbed a "failure of success."

It is also a failure of "compression of morbidity," a concept developed by Stanford professor James Fries 30 years ago. He believed the same forces that lengthened life expectancy would also decrease—or compress—the number of years of disease and disability prior to death. In other words, the ideal healthy life would be one spent without impaired functioning right up until the moment of death.

People over 50 generally do not fear death as much as disability. When questioned, they express a dread of potential chronic illness, pain and immobility. They fear senility, loss of memory and dependence on others.

Disease trends are mixed. People are acquiring chronic disease at earlier ages, but disability generally is being delayed because of medical technology. For example, a 20-year-old today can expect to live one less healthy year than a 20-year-old did a decade ago—even though life expectancy has grown. A typical 20-year-old man today can expect to spend nearly six years of his life without basic mobility, two more years than a decade ago. For a 20-year-old woman, it will be nearly 10 years of being unable to walk up 10 steps or sit for two hours.

Despite medical progress, the age of a first heart attack has remained relatively constant since the 1960s and the incidence of several forms of cancer continued to increase until recently. High cholesterol and high blood pressure have decreased only because of successful pharmaceutical treatments.

These trends certainly shatter the illusion that each successive generation would live longer and healthier lives. They also do not bode well for the extra burden placed on age-based entitlement programs such as Medicare and Social Security.

Physical decline is not inevitable. Fries and his colleagues followed more than 400 people for 12 years and categorized them based on lifestyle risk factors: cigarette smoking; physical inactivity, and being under- or overweight. Those with no risk factors had almost no disability 10 to 12 years before death, and the incidence of disability rose slowly until the end. Those with two or more risk factors had more disability, which rose significantly 18 months before death. Those with moderate risk declined swiftly three months before death.

Disability can be delayed relatively late in life by lifestyle choices. Mental and physical facilities can be improved at any age. It has been called the "plasticity of aging," a phenomenon that can significantly diminish the effects of aging. This plasticity is why some 80-year-olds can run marathons and 90-year-olds can substantially increase strength by weightlifting. Age-related decline in maximum athletic performance is only 1 percent a year beginning at age 25. Training to achieve one's athletic potential is far more important than one's age. The body tends to rust out rather than wear out. Several studies show that improving one's lifestyle and health behaviors reduces late-life disability more than it lengthens life expectancy—thus decreasing the amount of time spent with illness.

The rate of disability has been declining steadily since the early 1980s, although it is unclear why. It could be a number of factors: declining smoking rates; assistive medical devices; rising educational levels, and improved cardiovascular treatment. However, obesity may reverse that trend. Researchers estimate disability will begin to increase 1 percent a year by 2020 because of the excess weight carried by people 50 to 70 years old—and that's assuming they gain no more weight.

Future life expectancy: Which way will it go?

Predicting life expectancy is far from an exact science. Statistical modeling may be mathematically precise, but assumptions are far more subjective. A 2009 study confidently stated that most babies born in the U.S. and Western Europe today should live to 100. Another group of scientists predicts life expectancy at birth will be 100 years by 2060, based on current trends. A more modest projection by the United Nations arrived at the same figure by the year 2300.

On the other hand, an influential article in the *New England Journal of Medicine* estimated that the effect of obesity could trim as much as five years of life by the middle of this century.

Other research echoes this. Researchers used a forecasting method that accounts for the delayed effects of accumulated health risks among younger adults. The results suggested the effects of rising obesity on future life expectancy and health-care costs could be far worse than currently anticipated.

Projecting life expectancy is much more than an academic exercise. If it is underestimated by just one year, that would mean an extra 53 million years lived by Americans 65 and older between 2000 and 2050. That would have enormous implications for Medicare and Social Security costs.

If life expectancy continues to grow and disease is kept at bay, life stages—education, work, retirement—will continue to be blurred. Young people are taking longer to complete higher education because of steeply rising costs and dim career prospects. Meanwhile, the elderly are delaying retirement because of eroded stock portfolios, the security of health-insurance benefits in the workplace or self-fulfillment—especially if they are in robust health.

One trend is clear: The world is going gray. The number of people 65 and older will double to 1.3 billion globally by 2040. The elderly will outnumber children under age 5 for the first time in history.

At this point, there is no technology to extend the human life-span. Dr. Nortin Hadler, in his book *Worried Sick: A Prescription for Health in an Overtreated America,* contends that the best we can hope for is 85 disease-free years—at which point life's warranty expires. Any time beyond that is a bonus. He argues that medicine has little impact on longevity because it saves the lives of only a small percentage of the population.

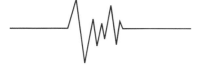

Chapter 4

Health Behavior

The four habits that count most

The daily avalanche of health news too often focuses on minutiae: Nutrient X will lower the risk of Y, or toxin A raises the risk of cancer B. It is safe to ignore most of it.

Four behaviors determine most chronic disease and premature death—cigarette smoking, physical inactivity, excess weight and binge drinking of alcohol. If people made the right decisions about those four, health-care costs would recede as a public-policy ticking time bomb and Americans' quality of life would soar.

Do not smoke. Eat at least five daily servings of fruits and vegetables. Drink moderately at most. Exercise at least 30 minutes a day. Sounds easy enough. But only 3 percent of Americans do all four. That, more than anything in the rest of this book, may explain the health-care fix we are in.

Those with the American Heart Association ideal cardiovascular profile are even rarer. According to University of Pittsburgh researchers, there are seven factors: body mass index of less than 25; untreated cholesterol under 200; blood pressure below 120/80; fasting blood sugar level below 100; exceeds the government-recommended physical activity guidelines, and follows a heart-healthy diet. Of 1,933 people between the ages of 45 and 75, only one met all seven conditions. Less than 10 percent met five or more of the criteria.

The opposite—smoking, drinking too much, inactivity and poor nutrition—can age a body as much as 12 years. An English study found that practicing the four health habits could add 14 years to life expectancy.

In the United States, these four behaviors are responsible for 4 out of every 10 deaths. Nearly two-thirds of the annual growth in U.S. health spending comes from Americans' worsening health habits, especially the rising tide of obesity.

Exercising, eating right and maintaining a normal weight would cut the odds of heart disease, cancer and diabetes by about 80 percent. It is the difference between life and death, and health and illness. In a study of nearly 80,000 U.S. women ages 34 to 59, it was calculated that more than half of the deaths from cancer and heart disease would not have occurred if the three practices had been adopted.

Psychological factors also seem to have an impact. People who believe they are in control of their lives and have positive social relationships—and who remain physically active—can delay declining health by up to a decade.

(Not so) Healthy People

In the late 1990s, the U.S. government gathered experts to study Americans' physical condition and health behavior and to set goals for improvement by 2010. The initiative, called Healthy People 2010, established 635 targets. As of mid-2009, Americans had achieved 117 of them—or fewer than 1 out of 5. There was important progress on heart disease, but obesity and diabetes went in the wrong direction. Healthy eating and smoking rates essentially stayed the same.

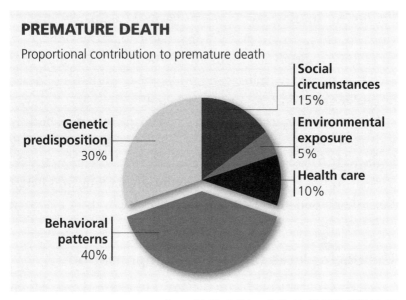

PREMATURE DEATH

Proportional contribution to premature death

Social circumstances 15%

Environmental exposure 5%

Health care 10%

Genetic predisposition 30%

Behavioral patterns 40%

Source: McGinnis JM, et al. *Health Aff.* 2002; 21(2):78-93.

Health care in reaction to an illness or condition has a small influence in determining health and premature death. Health behavior has the greatest influence. The four major behavioral factors are obesity, physical inactivity, tobacco use and alcohol abuse.

One disturbing trend is that the lifestyles of older Americans have become increasingly unhealthy in the past 20 years. The number of those ages 40 to 74 who say they have five daily servings of fruits and vegetables declined by nearly half. The percentage who worked out 12 times a month was 43 percent, compared with 53 percent in 1988. Even those who had acquired heart disease, high blood pressure or diabetes were no more likely to change their habits than those without the conditions.

This group is the most at risk for developing chronic conditions that can bring premature death or ruin post-retirement quality of life. They have the knowledge and experience to understand the consequences, and changing behavior is ultimately an individual pursuit. Physicians and pharmaceuticals can only go so far to forestall death and disability. Those in this age group who made the necessary changes in middle age cut the risk of death or cardiovascular disease by as much as 40 percent.

Some say Americans are actually behaving in a more healthy way. Despite large increases in obesity, the probability of dying in the next 10 years dropped for adults 55 to 74, from nearly 26 percent to less than 22 percent. Reduced smoking and better control of blood pressure offset the negative effects of increased obesity.

The doctor lacks faith—and compensation

Counseling of patients by physicians could have an impact on health behaviors, but it rarely happens. Physicians are paid by insurance companies and government health programs to perform tests and procedures, not to talk to patients. The average 18-minute doctor-patient encounter does not leave much time for lectures. Doctors also do not think they are very good at it. According to a survey of 620 physicians, less than half felt competent prescribing weight-loss programs because they believed they had been inadequately trained.

This lack of reimbursement and confidence yields predictable results. Doctors advise only about one-third of their obese patients to lose weight. That proportion rises to about one-half only if the obesity has created some other medical conditions. Physicians offer to help about 1 out of 4 smokers quit.

Doctors also do not have faith that patients will change their habits. Who could blame them? Barely 1 in 10 diabetics follow dietary guidelines limiting saturated fat. About 18 percent of heart-disease patients continue to smoke, which is not much better than the smoking rate for everyone.

A doctor's pep talk at the end of the visit does not do much. Success requires a joint action plan and a commitment to follow up. In one study, physicians counseled inactive patients to exercise and had a staff member call later to monitor progress. Those patients walked five times more than those who had standard care.

The American Heart Association advises physicians to use this sort of approach to lower the risk of heart disease. The organization reviewed a decade of research to determine what works best. Joint goal-setting, physician feedback and monitoring topped the list. Self-monitoring, such as food diaries, also helps. However, clinical initiatives are employed infrequently because they are time-consuming and insurance companies will not pay for them.

Change is hard, even for the motivated

Changing health behavior is difficult, especially when there does not seem to be an immediate need to do so. The majority do not die of their bad habits, so it is more convenient to ignore the risks.

That makes healthier people angry. They resent having to pay for the consequences of others' unhealthy lifestyles. An extreme example is a Melbourne, Australia, hospital that refused to perform heart and lung transplants on smokers. Hospital surgeon Greg Snell said it was a waste of taxpayer money to attempt to heal patients who were killing themselves.

"It's about rationing medical resources," Snell said. "There is obviously a morality and ethics base to all of this."

The Australian Medical Association called the hospital's policy "unconscionable."

Change is difficult even after life-altering chronic conditions. At least 40 percent of smokers who survive a heart attack continue to smoke a year later. In a group of more than 1,200 overweight heart-attack survivors, the average weight loss was .2 percent. That is less than a one-pound loss for a 220-pound man.

In another study, 884 of 2,500 heart-attack patients had eaten fast food at least once a week a month before the attack. Nearly all receive dietary advice before leaving the hospital. Three months later, 503 were still eating fast food at least once a week.

One out of 5 diagnosed lung-cancer patients continue to smoke. A study of 9,000 cancer survivors found that only 1 out of 20 were not smoking, consuming at least five fruits and vegetables daily and engaging in regular physical activity. However, their physicians do not give cancer survivors much guidance. Less than one-third received dietary guidance or exercise advice, and less than half had been asked whether they smoked.

According to the Stanford University psychologist Albert Bandura, behavior change requires a situation-specific form of self-confidence called self-efficacy. Confidence comes from these factors:

- You previously have been successful doing something similar.
- You have a successful role model.
- You are getting positive reinforcement from family, friends or your doctor.
- You can anticipate what will happen while engaging in the new behavior.

Health habits are only part of the disease and death equation. Lack of education, low income, dangerous neighborhoods and genetics arguably play a larger role (see Chapter 10). Assessing blame for poor lifestyle choices becomes a very complex issue.

A World Health Organization report noted, "It's the context of people's lives that determines their health. So blaming in-dividuals for poor health or crediting them for good health is inappropriate."

Reality check: Optimism bias

The doctor-patient disconnect

A 2009 poll of 2,000 Americans in New Orleans is an elegant example of optimism bias at work. More than half the respondents said other people's health "was going in the wrong direction," compared with 17 percent who characterized their own health that way.

Only one-quarter to one-third knew their personal basic health numbers—body-mass index, blood pressure, cholesterol, blood-glucose level—yet the most said keeping those numbers in a good range was important to health.

About 95 percent said regular physician checkups were important, but 70 percent admitted avoiding their doctors by hoping health problems would go away or asking a friend for medical advice.

Pollsters asked respondents to grade their health behaviors, and asked doctors to do the same. One out of 3 gave themselves an "A" for nutrition, exercise and personal health management. More than 90 percent of the doctors, however, graded patients "C" or worse on these.

Another survey reflected Americans' strong sense of personal control over their health, but also their reluctance to accept financial responsibility for it.

The Vitality Group surveyed more than 1,000 U.S. adults in 2008. About 82 percent said they alone were responsible for their health. However, 44 percent said they should bear no responsibility for paying for their health care, while 56 percent thought they should pick up part of the cost. Six out of 10 thought their employer should be partially responsible, and about one-half believed the government should pick up the tab.

Optimism bias

What cripples Americans' health as much as anything is a misguided tendency known as optimism bias. People tend to believe they are invincible. They expect misfortune to befall others rather than themselves. It is a judgment error, not to be mistaken for an optimistic outlook on life.

Rutgers psychology professor Neil Weinstein stumbled across this when he discovered that his students had unrealistic expectations about their performance on tests. He studied the bias extensively and found it exists in many facets of life, but especially in health.

Most people believe their skills are "above average," a statistical impossibility like Garrison Keillor's assertion about the children in mythical Lake Wobegon. They overestimate how swiftly they will accomplish tasks and usually reach optimistic conclusions based on little or no evidence.

A good example of optimism bias was found in a survey of about 1 million high school seniors in the 1970s. About 70 percent believed they had above-average leadership skills, compared with 2 percent who said they were below average. About 60 percent rated themselves in the top 10 percent in ability to get along with others, and 25 percent said they were in the top 1 percent.

Health research is full of optimism bias. Patients guide themselves with half-baked medical theories and misinformation, often with dire consequences for their health and longevity. People tend to predict the future based on experience: If there were no consequences to behavior before, there will be none in the future. They consider themselves somehow exempt from risk.

This self-confidence can be fatal. People with heart-attack symptoms delay seeking medical attention because the signals do not match their notions of what they think a heart attack should feel like. Likewise, a majority of patients with high blood pressure believe they can tell whether it is elevated, according to one study—even though the condition has no symptoms. People in the blood-pressure "symptom" group acknowledged that most people cannot detect when their blood pressure rises—but said they themselves could. (This actually made them more compliant patients. This false notion led them to follow doctors' orders to take medication, watch their diet and exercise to control the mythical symptoms.)

Weinstein surveyed adults with risky lifestyles to see how they rate their chances of acquiring health conditions such as cancer or alcoholism, or encountering other negative events such as auto accidents or getting divorced. The response: Somewhere between average and lower than average. The bias occurred regardless of age, gender, income or education level.

People take this notion of self-control even farther by over-rating the effectiveness of their actions. That inflates the self-delusion even more. On the other hand, people are reluctant to take responsibility for poor performance. They tend to blame factors outside their control, such as the difficulty of the task.

Optimism bias is fairly immune to intervention. It is difficult for those who have it to believe otherwise. They rarely alter their behavior even after being shown that their chances of early death and disease are no better than average. The reason: They still believe their own risk is relatively low.

In international studies, Americans show a stronger association of optimism bias and personal control than non-Americans. The sense of control over events and the concept of personal responsibility are deeply embedded in capitalist nations such as the United States. Such notions tend to result in faulty risk estimations, leading to a disconnect between misinformed judgment and reality.

However, optimism bias is not without its merits. The outlook reflects a high level of self-esteem, which itself is beneficial to good health. An attitude of invincibility has a way of reducing anxiety. People who are optimistic about their futures place a higher value on their health because they expect good things ahead. They are better at building social networks, which help protect health, and probably are less likely to have had their health compromised by life's tragedies.

In personal health, fear is good but pessimism is not

Caution about health hazards leads to doing the right things. A wealth of research shows that the degree to which people feel vulnerable to health problems predicts how likely they are to engage in healthy behavior. Optimism bias leads to ignoring information about what promotes health, and a tendency toward riskier behavior. In short, there is not enough fear.

However, unrealistic pessimism can be as bad as optimism bias. People with fatalistic beliefs, consumed by hopelessness, think nothing they do will alter their destiny.

The onslaught of everything-causes-cancer news contributes to this. Indeed, a national survey of more than 6,000 U.S. adults found that about half agreed with the statement: "It seems like almost everything causes cancer." Three-fourths agreed that "there are so many recommendations about preventing cancer that it's hard to know which ones to follow."

Remarkably, about 1 out of 4 agreed with this: "There's not much people can do to lower their chances of getting cancer." Those with the strongest fatalistic beliefs were less likely to eat fruits and vegetables and more likely to continue to smoke.

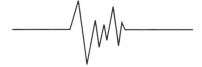

Chapter 5

Nutrition

Taste, convenience and price rule

Regardless of good intentions, people choose their food based mainly on convenience, taste and cost. And they usually eat too much of the wrong things.

Americans have abundant food choices, making it too easy to select the least nutritious food available. Animals, too, will pick food high in fat and sugar even if they have equal access to healthy alternatives. Like humans, they eat too much, gain weight and ruin their health.

David Kessler, the former commissioner of the U.S. Food and Drug Administration and author of *The End of Overeating: Taking Control of the Insatiable American Appetite*, interviewed food designers and manufacturers, several of whom refused to be named, on how they intentionally use the unholy trinity of fat, sugar and salt to hook consumers. The food industry spends lavishly for research on how to combine these substances to produce cravings that can be satisfied only by consuming more. They concentrate on creating anticipation, aroma, visual appeal, and pleasing taste and texture.

Food cues chemically cause the brain to release dopamine, which drives eaters to seek the food they crave. Eating that food releases stress-easing opioids that provide temporary emotional relief. Those two chemicals conspire to drive the desire to repeat the cycle.

Eating is strongly associated with emotions, so food marketers attempt to associate their products with celebration, fun and love rather than nutrition. According to Kessler, the three major contributing factors in overeating are available portion size, the density of sugar and fat, and variety (think chocolate chips added to ice cream).

Inflation-adjusted food prices have been falling over the past two decades—with fruits and vegetables being notable exceptions. Between 1990 and 2007, for example, the cost of a 2-liter bottle of Coca-Cola fell by more than a third and the price of a McDonald's Quarter Pounder with Cheese dropped more than 5 percent. One study claims that falling fast-food prices account for more than 40 percent of the rise in young adults' body-mass index in the 1980s and 1990s. In contrast, the cost of produce rose 17 percent between 1997 and 2003.

The average American's daily calorie consumption increased by one-quarter, or about 530 calories, between 1970 and 2000. The number of servings provided by recipes for desserts, cookies and waffles in *The Joy of Cooking* shrank from its 1964 to 1997 editions, and shrank again in its 2006 edition—even though the amounts of ingredients in the recipes did not change. That means portion sizes in home-cooked meals have grown to adjust to expanding appetites and waistlines. Perhaps not coincidentally, the obesity rate began its ascent in the 1970s.

Almost 90 percent of Americans have no clue how many calories they should eat per day. Calories consistently rank toward the bottom of consumer eating priorities. According to a Food

An unhealthy diet can contribute to or aggravate many chronic diseases and conditions, including type 2 diabetes, hypertension, heart disease, stroke, and some cancers.

These are among the major federal government nutritional goals for the year 2020. The starting points were based on nutritional data in 2001-2004 for people aged 2 years and older.

Fruit dietary contribution

Starting point: 0.5 cups/1000 calories consumed
Goal: 0.9 cups/1000 calories consumed
Government recommendation: 2-3 cups, depending upon age, gender and weight

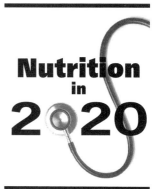

Vegetable dietary contribution

Starting point: 0.8 cups/1000 calories consumed
Goal: 1.1 cups/1000 calories consumed
Government recommendation: 1.5-2 cups, depending upon age, gender and weight

Whole grain dietary contribution

Starting point: 0.3 oz./1000 calories consumed
Goal: 0.6 oz./1000 calories consumed
Government recommendation: 3-4 oz., depending upon age, gender and weight

Reduction in added sugars

Starting point: 15.7 percent
Goal: 10.8 percent
Government recommendation: Minimize

Marketing Institute study in 2002, only 13 percent said they were concerned about calories. Annual per-person meat consumption rose by 57 pounds and cheese intake quadrupled from 1950 to 2000.

Do not necessarily count on your doctor to dispense authoritative nutrition advice. Diet and nutrition education is given short shrift in medical school. During the 2008-09 academic year, only 27 percent of medical schools met the 25-hour classroom minimum for the topic set by the National Academy of Sciences. About 38 percent of schools met the standard four years earlier, meaning the trend is going in the wrong direction. The doctors most likely to know much about nutrition have made a personal commitment to follow a healthy lifestyle themselves.

The American diet

Americans are eating more from all of the major food groups—even fruits and vegetables—at the same time that the obesity rate has doubled since 1970. However, many are not meeting dietary recommendations. To do so, they would have to cut back significantly on added fats, refined grains and added sweeteners while increasing consumption of fruits, vegetables, whole grains and low-fat dairy products.

The typical Western diet—fried foods, salty snacks and generous portions of fat-laden meat—accounts for nearly a third of the heart-disease risk worldwide, according to a study of dietary patterns in 52 nations.

What constitutes an ideal diet continues to be elusive. Diets rich in lean meat, poultry and beans keep weight off best, according to a November 2010 *New England Journal of Medicine* study.

An analysis of 21 studies involving 350,000 people found "no significant evidence" that long-maligned saturated fat increases heart risk. But refined carbohydrates—white bread, white pasta and processed baked goods—do.

The health-reform law's nod toward fighting obesity is the requirement that chain restaurants with 20 or more locations, and owners of 20 or more vending machines, will have to display the calories in their menu items. The information will have to be on menus, menu boards and drive-through signs. Vending machines will have to post calorie information on the food they sell unless it is already visible on individual packages inside the machine. Restaurants also must display brochures that include detailed nutritional

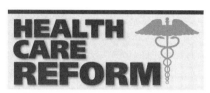

Nutrition

information, such as the fat content of their dishes. Movie theaters were exempted.

Although the evidence is mixed, menu labeling generally has had little impact on diners' eating habits. But experts suspect the transparency of information will force restaurants to slim down the caloric content of their offerings to avoid embarrassment—or diner sticker shock.

Another study compared the effectiveness of low-fat vs. low-carbohydrate diets. The verdict: Either works. Both groups lost about 7 percent of their body weight. A 2009 study was even more detailed, creating four groups with diets of varying amounts of fats and carbohydrates. For example, one diet consisted of 40 percent fat and 35 percent carbohydrates. Another had 20 percent fat and 65 percent carbohydrates. The same result: They also lost equal amounts of weight.

The safest way of eating for nutrition and weight control is what is known as the Mediterranean diet. It is more of a dietary

Reality check: Nutrition

Lying about produce

In medical research, people routinely underestimate their weight. However, they apparently overestimate how many servings of fruits and vegetables they eat.

According to a 2008 study in *Nutrition Journal*, women goosed up their estimates because of something called "approval bias." They knew they were supposed to eat five or more servings, so that is what they told interviewers.

In this study, University of Colorado researchers recruited a random sample of 163 women. Half were informed by letter that the survey would be about consumption of fruits and vegetables. The mailing included information about the benefits of eating fresh produce, a Five-a-Day sticker and Five-a-Day magnet. The other half received a generic letter without mentioning the survey's topic.

Because the group was selected randomly, fruit and vegetable consumption should have been similar. However, the group that received the promotional material reported eating an average of 5.2 servings a day, compared with 3.7 per day for the control group.

What I eat is someone else's fault

Americans usually believe they exert a high level of personal control over their health habits. A survey by Foodminds showed otherwise. A surprising 38 percent said others were responsible for what they put in their mouths. About 14 percent blamed food companies, 12 percent pointed to the government, 9 percent said the health-care system was somehow responsible and 3 percent blamed the educational system.

I don't have a crummy diet. You do

A GlaxoSmithKline Consumer Healthcare survey showed a disconnect between beliefs and actions about personal nutrition. About two-thirds of Americans are overweight. Despite that, nearly 8 out of 10 said they were satisfied with their personal eating habits. However, about two-thirds admitted poor eating practices such as skipping meals and eating when they were not hungry.

They were also quick to criticize others. Three-quarters said most Americans have an unhealthy relationship with food (apparently excluding themselves). More than half placed an immediate family member in that group, including 44 percent who were concerned about their spouse's eating habits.

Define 'eating healthy'

Nearly 90 percent of Americans said they were eating a healthy diet, according to a Consumer Reports telephone survey in November 2010.

What did they eat? Only 30 percent said they eat five servings of fruits and vegetables a day, 43 percent drank at least one sugared drink daily and only about half attempted to limit consumption of sweets and dietary fat.

Nancy Metcalf, senior editor at Consumer Reports Health, said in a statement: "Americans have a tendency to give themselves high marks for healthy eating. However, when we asked how many sugary drinks, fatty foods, and fruits and veggies they consumed, we found that their definition of healthy eating was somewhat questionable.

"We were surprised that very few Americans weigh themselves and count calories, two strategies that can help dieters stay on track. Americans seem to rely instead on their own internal compasses to slim their girths."

About 13 percent weigh themselves every morning and 8 percent monitor daily calories.   *continued*

Define 'eating healthy' (*continued*)

There was a similar disconnect on physical activity. Some seem to conflate being busy with being active. About 8 out of 10 said they were somewhat or very active. Yet most said they spent an average of five hours a day sitting.

About one-third who said their weight was in a healthy range had a body-mass index that qualified as overweight or obese.

Let's call it aspirational eating

In health surveys, respondents often reflect what people *think* they should be doing rather than what they *are* doing.

A September 2010 Harris Poll analyzed results based on the respondents' body mass index. Most said they were changing what they consumed based on what experts say is a healthy diet. They said they were eating more fruits, vegetables and whole grains while avoiding sugary drinks, white bread and processed food.

About three-fourths said they eat healthier at home compared with when they eat out, drink water at meals, eat healthy snacks and eat a balanced diet. About two-thirds said they examine nutritional information on packaged foods before buying, try to eat smaller food portions and exercise regularly.

However, only about 1 out of 5 ate a full breakfast or well-balanced lunch, and about one-third ate a well-balanced dinner at least five times a week.

Those who were obese—and even morbidly obese—claimed to be practicing the same healthy habits as normal-weight people.

pattern than a specific list of foods. Its key elements: fruits and vegetables, whole grains, nuts, olive oil and beans; moderate amounts of red wine, low-fat dairy, poultry and fish, and not much meat or added unhealthy fats. Experts say the diet contains thousands of vitamins, minerals and micronutrients that guard against heart disease and cancer, protect mental health and lengthen life. The diet even has the ability to change the genes that influence heart disease.

Going hungry in the Land of Plenty

The U.S. produces nearly twice as many calories as its citizens can consume. Yet 15 percent of the nation's households are "food insecure"—meaning they lack a steady and dependable food supply for active, healthy lives. The cruel irony is that women and children in food-insecure households are more likely to be obese. Low-income households spend less on food, and the least expensive food is high in calories and low in nutrients.

America wastes far more food than it would take to feed the hungry a nutritious diet. According to Jonathan Bloom in the book *American Wasteland*, the nation has an unhealthy relationship with food. It wastes nearly half of what it produces, yet two-thirds of its citizens are overweight. There is clearly a food-distribution problem.

Tainted produce is common in low-income neighborhoods. Compared with stores in more affluent areas, these shops' produce have higher levels of microorganisms, yeasts and mold. Food is of poorer quality and spoils more quickly because of improper storage.

About 85 percent of food-insecure households include a working adult, of whom 70 percent have a full-time job. Fewer than half have an adult with more than a high-school education.

About half are headed by single women. In about half of the households, adults deprive themselves to feed their children.

People with more income and education spend more for food that has fewer calories but more nutrition. Healthier diets are more strongly associated with higher education than income. The suggestion is that educated people are willing to spend more for good nutrition, regardless of income. This explains, in part, why people who are more educated have lower rates of obesity, diabetes, heart disease and cancer.

Spending more on food can mean a healthier diet, but some of the best dietary choices are inexpensive. Nuts, soy, beans and whole grains are low-cost and pack plenty of nutrition. Another trick: Pay cash. Paying with credit or debit cards for groceries encourages impulsive and often-unhealthy purchases.

Restaurants and fast food

Nearly half of every U.S. food dollar is spent in restaurants, where jumbo portions have become the norm. People consume an average of 800 calories in one fast-food meal, with one-third eating more than 1,000 calories at a sitting. Full-service restaurant meals contain even more calories. Super-sized meals remain a compelling marketing weapon. Serving portions at many popular chain restaurants are at least twice as large as the government's definition of a serving.

Beth Mansfield, spokeswoman for CKE Restaurants Inc., which owns the Carl's Jr. and Hardee's chains, defended the practice. She told *The Los Angeles Times*, "The bottom line is we're in business to make money ... If we wanted to listen to the food police and sell nuts and berries and tofu burgers ... we'd be out of business."

Full-service and fast-food meals are larger and have more calories than those cooked at home. A typical restaurant meal

Dumping the pyramid for a plate

After nearly 20 years, the U.S. Department of Agriculture (USDA) finally retired the food pyramid and put its recommendations on a plate.

Most nutritionists praised the move. They said the new icon recognized that people eat off a plate rather than a pyramid. They called the pyramid confusing and ineffective.

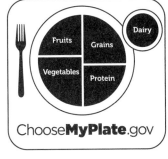

The USDA joined other organizations that use plates to convey nutritional information, such as the American Diabetes Association, the American Institute for Cancer Research, and the Physicians Committee for Responsible Medicine.

Fruits and vegetables should take up half of the plate. The icon attempts to illustrate proportions and supplements the government's revised guidelines released in January 2010. Those guidelines urge Americans to switch to fat-free or low-fat milk; make at least half of the grains they eat whole grains; minimize sodium and avoid sugary drinks.

Dr. David Kessler, a former commissioner of the Food and Drug Administration, told *The New York Times*, "The reality is that very few of us eat like what has been suggested" in government guidelines. "There's a world of difference between what's being served and what's on that plate."

has 60 percent more calories than the average home-cooked meal. Fast-food meals are smaller than those at full-service restaurants and consequently have fewer calories. But full-service restaurant diners are more likely to reduce what they eat later in the day, thus consuming fewer total calories than fast-food eaters do.

People who live in neighborhoods with a high concentration of fast-food restaurants weigh more than those living in areas with abundant full-service restaurants. Fast-food restaurants are up to one-third more common than full-service eateries in urban black and racially mixed neighborhoods. Mobility is also a factor. Researchers found that adults without a car and in areas where fast food was readily available weighed 12 pounds more than those not in those circumstances. What is less clear is whether convenient fast food contributes to excess weight, or whether full-service restaurants are more available in high-income areas where people tend to weigh less.

The appeal of fast food is undeniable. The most frequently cited reasons for eating fast food include quick service, convenience and taste. But families who consistently eat fast food are likelier to have unhealthy eating habits and are more likely to be obese. Families who eat fast food for dinner three or more times a week also have more salty snacks and sweetened soft drinks in their cupboards, and fewer fruits and vegetables in their refrigerators. More than half of U.S. families eat fast food together once or twice a week, and 7 percent have fast food for dinner three or four times a week.

An alarmed group of British scientists suggested that fast-food restaurants should offer free cholesterol-lowering statin drugs like condiments to counter the dietary effects of their food. (Statins are available over-the-counter in low doses in Great Britain.) They calculated that the drug's reduction in cardiovascular risk would help offset the increase in heart-attack risk from eating a cheeseburger and milkshake.

Will transparent menus help?

The battle against expanding waistlines increasingly has focused on greater consumer awareness of the calories packed into a typical food emporium's menu.

The federal health-reform law requires chain restaurants with more than 20 outlets to give prominent display to calorie counts for menu items. But a handful of states did that prior to the law's passage, and the results were disappointing. For example, a review of sales in fast-food outlets after New York City required calorie labeling found that diners consumed *more* calories, even though they said they believed they had ordered healthier items. However, a separate New York City study found that 1 out of 6 fast-food customers used the provided calorie information and ordered lower-calorie items.

This phenomenon, often called the American obesity paradox, reflects the fact that Americans continue to gain weight even as the popularity of healthy food rises. Diners overestimate food's nutritional value and underestimate calories to the point of ultimately consuming more calories than they would have with "unhealthy" choices.

Labeling at least can take the guesswork out of the caloric value of menu items. About 200 diners were asked to estimate the calories and fat in nine restaurant entrees. They guessed 642 calories. The actual amount was more than 1,300. They especially had difficulty with the unhealthy items. They guessed a 3,000-calorie serving of cheese fries only had 1,000 calories.

People can be deeply influenced by marketing. Researchers found that McDonald's customers were more accurate at estimating calories than Subway customers. Subway has relentlessly advertised that its sandwiches have one-third the fat of a Big Mac, creating what researchers called a "health halo." Researchers gave participants coupons for a 900-calorie sandwich or a 600-calorie Big Mac. Subway customers were more likely to add a large non-diet soda and cookies to their meal, even though Subway's 12-inch Italian sandwich had more calories than a Big Mac. The result: Subway diners ate 56 percent more calories than McDonald's diners.

Jane Hurley, nutritionist at the Center for Science in the Public Interest, expressed the irony to *The Los Angeles Times*: "Remember when the Big Mac was considered the bad burger? And now it's the diet alternative to some of these items."

The restaurant-labeling effort is further complicated by the unreliability of posted calorie counts. An analysis of food in 29 Boston chain restaurants and 10 supermarket frozen meals showed that the food items had 18 percent more calories than what was stated.

Labeling can matter if people understand the information. However, only 20 percent know how to interpret how much a single food item contributes to a day's recommended caloric allowance. The food-labeling effort assumes that restaurant overeating is a result of a lack of information. However, it is more likely a willful desire to indulge in something other than a home-cooked meal.

Fruits and vegetables: The nutritional bellwether

A balanced diet includes a variety of foods. But fruit and vegetable consumption has become the proxy for good nutrition. Less than 1 in 10 Americans eat the recommended amount. The government and advocacy groups have ongoing campaigns to change that, but per-person average consumption actually declined between 2000 and 2005 to 687 pounds a year. However, fruit and vegetable consumption exceeds that of 1970.

The National Fruit and Vegetable Alliance, a coalition of public and private health-advocacy groups, developed a national action plan in 2005 to boost consumption. Five years later, it issued a report card on the results of its campaign. The overall grade: D-. Adult consumption held steady during the five years while teenage consumption actually dropped. The average American eats 1.13 servings of vegetables and 0.68 servings of fruit a day. Only about 7 percent of Americans eat at least five servings of produce daily, as recommended by the U.S. Centers for Disease Control. Orange juice is the top source of fruit and potatoes are the favorite vegetable, especially fried potatoes for adolescents.

The Dietary Guidelines for Americans, released in January 2005, changed the fruit and vegetable recommendations. Previous guidelines recommended 5 to 9 daily servings of fruits and vegetables. The new guidelines recommend 2 to 6.5 cups of fruits and vegetables, or the equivalent of about 5 to 13 servings. Government research found that people could more easily visualize what they should eat based on cups rather than servings.

The advantages of fruit and vegetable consumption are well-known. They provide essential vitamins and minerals, fiber and other nutrients important to good health. Those who eat generous amounts are more likely to reduce their risk of chronic disease, especially stroke, diabetes, heart disease and high blood pressure.

"Sin taxes" for unhealthy food?

Whether to impose excise taxes on unhealthy food—much like those on tobacco and alcohol—is a matter of continual debate in health-policy circles and state governments. Advocates assert that the increased cost of food with dubious nutritional value would reduce consumption of it. They have an attentive audience in state legislators, who legally must balance their budgets. Opponents argue that such a tax would be regressive, unduly penalizing low-income residents who spend a greater percentage of their household budgets on food.

Most states already tax soda sold in grocery stores and vending machines, but not at a level that significantly affects sales. A study of North Carolina young adults showed that a 10 percent increase in the price of pizza and soda was associated with a 7 percent decrease in calories consumed in soda and 12 percent decrease in pizza.

A U.S. Department of Agriculture analysis estimated that a 20 percent price increase in sugar-sweetened beverages—including some fruit juices—would decrease average consumption by 37 calories a day, lowering the adult incidence of obesity and being overweight by 10 percent each.

Scientists tested the effectiveness of "sin taxes" compared with price discounts for healthier food. A group of volunteers—all mothers—shopped at a simulated grocery store. First, they bought groceries at regular prices. Researchers then imposed taxes of 12.5 percent, then 25 percent on unhealthy items, or they decreased the prices of healthy food comparably. The result: Sin taxes were more effective than discounts in raising the nutritional value of the shopping basket.

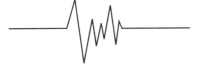

Chapter 6

Physical Activity
No medicine like it

The convenience of technology continues to engineer physical activity out of daily life. However, this inactivity has helped usher in obesity and chronic disease.

Humans hunted and gathered food for most of the past 100 centuries, ensuring a certain level of fitness. Tools and simple mechanization enabled an agrarian lifestyle through most of the 1800s. Machinery that was more sophisticated developed around the turn of the 20th century, allowing industrialization to flourish. Blue-collar work increasingly gave way to office-bound work.

With each transition, less movement was needed to perform daily tasks. At home, chores and entertainment have become equally sedentary. Much of life's activity has devolved into pushing buttons and typing on keyboards.

Trips from home by automobile became 10 times more frequent from 1969 to 2001. Self-reported physical activity began to decrease measurably in 1996, the year the Surgeon General released its first report on physical activity and exercise.

Exercise is the fountain of youth. Even people in their 90s can increase their strength and endurance. Consistent physical activity produces long-term benefits and reduces the risk of chronic conditions such as heart disease and diabetes. It can also increase the chance of living longer, help control weight, boost self-confidence and improve sleep. Generally the more one does, the larger the benefits. If it were a vaccine or medication, everyone would take it regardless of cost.

A review of more than 40 studies found regular exercise was associated with the prevention of more than two dozen physical and mental health problems. They included some cancers, type 2 diabetes, hypertension, stroke, dementia and depression.

Physical activity is in dire need of rebranding. For many of the inactive, exercise represents drudgery, boredom, sweat and the inability to overcome real or imagined barriers.

Eyes rolled when a large-scale 2010 study found that normal-weight women who want to prevent weight gain had to do an hour a day of moderately intense activity, such as brisk walking. The study essentially reaffirmed a 2002 recommendation by the Institute of Medicine to do at least one hour of exercise daily to reach optimum health and maintain weight.

Other studies have shown short bouts of exercise can have powerful effects. According to one, vigorous activity for 14 minutes three times a week can reduce the impact of stress on aging.

Exercise must be a ritual, and an enjoyable one, to be consistent. Some prefer to work out in groups. Others prefer to do it alone. Many believe they need to travel to a gym because being at home somehow saps their willpower. Others like the convenience and privacy of exercising at home, which requires no membership fees.

Regardless, it is easy to find excuses not to exercise, and difficult to resume after a layoff because the habit and momentum are broken.

Physical activity is one of the most important behaviors in maintaining health. It reduces the risk of dozens of diseases, improves life expectancy, helps control weight, strengthens bones and muscles, and boosts mental health and mood.

These are among the federal government's major physical-activity goals for the year 2020. The goals are based on federal guidelines.

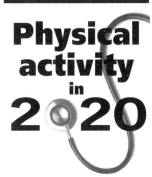

Increase the percentage of adults who engage in moderate physical activity for 150 minutes weekly, or vigorous physical activity for 75 minutes

Starting point: In 2008, 43.5 percent of adults engaged in aerobic physical activity of at least moderate intensity for at least 150 minutes a week, or 75 minutes a week of vigorous intensity, or an equivalent combination

Goal: 47.9 percent (10 percent improvement)

Increase the percentage of adults who engage in moderate physical activity for 300 minutes weekly, or vigorous physical activity for 150 minutes

Starting point: In 2008, 28.4 percent of adults engaged in aerobic physical activity of at least moderate intensity for at least 300 minutes a week, or 150 minutes a week of vigorous intensity, or an equivalent combination

Goal: 31.3 percent (10 percent improvement)

continued

Increase the proportion of adults who perform muscle-strengthening activity two or more days a week

Starting point: In 2008, 21.9 percent of adults performed muscle-strengthening activities on two or more days of the week in 2008
Goal: 24.1 percent (10 percent improvement)

U.S. government guidelines: What you're supposed to do, and how many do it

The federal government released its latest exercise guidelines in 2008. The basic guideline was simple: 30 minutes of moderate exercise a day, five days a week, for basic health or 75 minutes of vigorous exercise. For greater health benefits, double that amount or make it more intense. The guidelines endorsed the concept of accumulated exercise, such as splitting the 30 minutes in as many as three 10-minute segments throughout the day. They also recommended muscle-strengthening activity for major muscle groups two or more days a week. The guidelines advise children to get 60 minutes of physical activity daily.

The federal government's 2010 goal was for 50 percent of adults to meet the guidelines. In 2008, less than 44 percent met the goals for moderate exercise, 28 percent reached the vigorous-exercise guidelines and 22 percent achieved the weight-training goal. About 18 percent met both the aerobic and weight-training goals. Those figures have barely budged in the past decade.

Only about 5 percent of U.S. adults exercise vigorously on any given day, according to the American Time Use Survey. The most frequently reported "moderate activities" were food and drink preparation (26 percent), and lawn and garden care (11 percent), which may be a hint why self-reported physical-activity surveys grossly overestimate what people consider exercise.

However, even self-reported physical activity has been declining over the past several decades. This coincides with a steep decline in the number of people who use walking to get about, a steady increase in the number of vehicle miles the average person travels annually, and population growth in suburban areas where foot traffic is nearly impossible.

The average U.S. adult takes 5,117 steps a day, compared with 9,695 for Australians and a similar number for the Swiss. The American obesity rate is 34 percent, compared with 16 percent for Australians and 8 percent in Switzerland.

Exercise may be the most popular New Year's resolution, but January is one of the months when Americans exercise the least. Exercise peaks in the summer and is the lowest in the winter. Those who are most likely to say they exercise: those making more than $90,000 or young adults ages 18 to 29. In fact, the most educated overcome the "I don't have time to exercise" excuse by sleeping much less than others and using the extra time to exercise and work more.

Any kind of exercise helps

Exercise does not necessarily have to involve a gym or equipment. Dr. James Levine, a physician at the Mayo Clinic, contends people can lose weight simply by incorporating more activity into daily routines.

The scientific term behind what he advocates is a mouthful: non-exercise activity thermogenesis (NEAT). The principle is simple: Move. Do not sit when you can stand, and do not stand when you can walk.

Levine, director of the clinic's Active Life Research Team, equipped a Minneapolis law firm with Walkstations so that workers could work while on treadmills. Workers burned at least 100 calories an hour by walking at a very slow pace.

Levine, in his book *Move a Little, Lose a Lot: How N.E.A.T. Science Reveals How to Be Thinner, Happier, and Smarter,* suggests tactics on how to reintroduce into life the movement that was expunged slowly by technologically enabled conveniences. He urges working up to 135 minutes of movement into a day.

Doing so may depend on attitude. There is a direct correlation between a positive attitude toward exercise and unintentional physical activity. People who like exercise also are more likely to take the steps rather than the elevator, or not to be so intent on finding the closest parking space to the store's front door.

Fifty years ago, Americans were a mostly lean bunch living in a land with few gyms. Almost no one allocated time to "work out." Even those who exercise regularly now have difficulty keeping weight off because most of their non-exercising time is spent in a chair, behind a steering wheel or lying in bed.

Americans spend an average of nine hours a day in "sedentary activities," meaning almost no movement. That has consequences. Men who spend more than 23 hours a week watching television or driving their cars have a 64 percent greater chance of dying from heart disease, compared with men who spend half as much time doing those things, according to a 2010 study. What was surprising was that heart problems developed regardless of whether the men exercised. In other words, hours spent on the treadmill cannot undo many more hours being immobile in a chair. An Australian study found that each hour spent in front of a television daily increases the general risk of death by 11 percent, cancer death by 9 percent and cardiovascular-disease death by 18 percent.

Reality check: Physical activity

How much do you exercise *really*?

Of all health behaviors, people are least aware of how physically active they are. After all, the scale does not lie about weight and it is easier to see what you are eating.

Exercise's version of a weight scale is an accelerometer. It can measure vertical movement as well as the number of steps the wearer takes. The technology is similar to what NASA uses to monitor the movements of astronauts.

In one study, about 40 percent of adults said they got enough physical activity in a day to have a positive impact on their health. They wore accelerometers to track what percentage actually met the government guideline. The result: about 4 percent.

The researchers also measured how many children ages 6 to 11 and adolescents met the government's guideline of 60 minutes a day of physical activity for those 18 and under. About 42 percent of the younger group met this goal, compared with 8 percent of adolescents.

After more than a decade of health-promotion campaigns and news stories, most Americans are still clueless about how much they are supposed to exercise.

Since 1995, the U.S. government has mounted multiple campaigns to exhort people to get at least 30 minutes of moderate physical activity a day.

Only one-third of Americans know the guidelines, according to the 2005 Health Information National Trends Survey. Men, the unemployed and those born in the U.S. were the least aware. Researchers speculated that Americans are so inundated by health recommendations that they tune them out.

The effects of exercise

Physical activity has a powerful effect on other health behaviors. People who exercise are less likely to smoke, more likely to eat nutritious food and generally have habits that maximize the length and quality of life. They are less likely to acquire chronic conditions such as heart disease or cancer. They also have higher levels of education and income. It is difficult to determine whether it is the exercise that prevents disease or that people who exercise are less likely to develop those conditions for other reasons.

About half of adults are dissatisfied with their bodies. But, research shows that exercising improves self-image regardless of whether people lose weight, increase muscle strength or improve cardiovascular fitness. The amount of exercise does not seem to matter. Exercise lessens anxiety and depression, which may translate into a better body image.

The Gallup organization has what it calls a Well-Being Index that measures, among other things, physical and emotional health and health behavior, based on daily surveys. Its index reflects a strong emotional benefit to frequent physical activity. Those who exercise at least two days a week are happier and less stressed than those who do not. The benefits increase with each additional day of exercise up to six days.

In fact, exercise is as potent as an antidepressant in fighting depression. Duke University researchers showed that depressed adults who participated in an aerobics program improved as much as those who took sertraline, a drug more commonly known as Zoloft before its patent expired in 2006. Although physical activity cannot replace medication or psychotherapy, it lacks the stigma of those regimes and gives exercisers an immediate mood lift.

Physical activity also has a powerful effect on the immune system. People who walked for 45 minutes five days a week and did so for several weeks had fewer and less severe cases of colds and flu, reducing sick days by 25 to 50 percent compared with sedentary people.

Appalachian State University professor David Nieman, who conducted that study, told *The Wall Street Journal* that exercise enables two types of immune cells to neutralize pathogens more effectively. The immune system returns to normal after three hours, but exercise has cumulative effect to ward off illness. He likened the process to "a cleaner who comes in for an hour a day, so by the end of the month, your house looks much better."

Metabolic syndrome is a group of risk factors that occur together and increase the risk of cardiovascular disease and diabetes. According to the American Heart Association and the National Heart, Lung, and Blood Institute, a patient has the condition if there are three or more of these signs: high blood pressure; high blood sugar; excess weight around the waist; low good cholesterol, or high triglycerides. About 36 percent have the syndrome.

Exercise combats the symptoms, and the risk factors decrease with greater doses of activity. People who take at least 5,000 steps a day have a 40 percent lower risk, and those who exceed 10,000 steps have a 72 percent lower risk, compared with sedentary people.

Dr. Paul Williams, a researcher and avid runner, has been encouraging Americans to go way beyond the federal guidelines for even greater benefits. He has found progressively better health for runners who exceed 30, 40 and 49 miles a week. Williams calculated that people who ran more than 25 miles a week had up to 80 percent lower incidence of high blood pressure—depending upon age—than those who ran less than five miles a week.

It is easy to overdo it. Weight-training-related injuries treated in U.S. hospital emergency rooms have increased 50 percent since 1990. Males ages 13 to 24 represent the bulk of those injuries. However, the largest increase is among those 45 or older. Female injuries also increased faster than those of males during that period.

Unfortunately, exercise won't make you thin: Myth vs. reality

An enduring myth ties exercise to weight loss. What is often ignored is that physical activity generally stimulates appetite. People who exercise strenuously are also less active afterward than they would have been otherwise. Therefore, the tendency is to eat more and move less after exercising.

According to a 2000 study, willpower is a muscle. It paradoxically weakens with use. So the self-discipline that propels people onto a treadmill can be extinguished with the effort, making that post-workout beer much more inviting.

Another dubious claim is that greater muscle mass burns more calories at rest. A pound of muscle burns about six calories a day, compared with two calories for a pound of fat. Packing on 10 pounds of muscle, which is extremely difficult, would burn an extra 40 calories a day. That is the equivalent of six baby carrots.

What exercise can do is play a supporting role in weight control. The National Weight Control Registry chronicles the lives of those who have shed pounds and kept them off. About 90 percent of the people on the registry exercise in addition to eating less food.

Obesity is highly genetic. British researchers examined 20,000 people to determine the effects of 12 genes associated with a higher risk of obesity. They determined that an hour of daily exercise cut the genetic obesity risk by 40 percent.

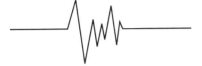

Chapter 7

Weight Control
The U.S. as an 'obesogenic' society

Ten years ago, the percentage of people considered clinically obese was less than 20 percent in 28 states. That is the case now in only one state—Colorado. Moreover, in nine states, more than 30 percent of the residents are now obese.

The Centers for Disease Control (CDC), which now reports the nation's obesity rate at nearly 27 percent, indicated that it is probably much higher because people often underestimate their weight in surveys. A previous CDC study based on actual measurements of height and weight found that almost 34 percent of Americans were obese.

Obesity is based on a body-mass index (BMI) determined by height and weight. A BMI above 30—or about 210 pounds for a 5-foot, 10-inch person—is what places a person in this category. A BMI of 18.5 to 24.9 is considered a healthy weight, and 25-29.9 is considered overweight. (The National Institute of Health's online BMI calculator is at *www.nhlbisupport.com/bmi.*)

Obesity is a factor in several causes of death, including stroke, diabetes and heart disease. Obese people have average annual medical costs of $1,429 more than healthy-weight people do. Obesity is the fastest-growing public-health issue the U.S. has ever faced. Obesity is expected to account for more than 20 percent of health-care spending by 2018.

The U.S. is the fattest of 33 affluent nations, and shares the fastest-growing rate obesity with Australia and Great Britain. Two out of 3 Americans are overweight or obese, and that rate is expected to rise to 3 out of 4 by 2020.

America is adjusting its environment to accommodate the excess weight. Bathroom scales, which used to stop at 300 pounds, now go as high as 500 pounds. Buses are now built stronger to handle bigger passengers. Commercial boats have had to decrease passenger headcount.

The statistics clearly indicate that Americans are getting heavier younger and are more likely to carry the weight throughout life. University of Michigan researchers calculated at what point age groups reached an obesity rate of 20 percent. For those born from 1966 to 1985, it was in their 20s. For those born from 1946 to 1955, it was in their 30s. For those born from 1936 to 1945, it was in their 40s. Those born from 1926 to 1935 were in their 50s before 20 percent of them became obese.

Men are more likely to be overweight or obese—72 percent, compared with 64 percent of women. However, women have a slight edge in obesity over men—35.5 versus 32.2 percent.

Why are we so fat?

There is no shortage of theories about why American waistlines continue to expand. There certainly is no single answer. The United States frequently is characterized as an "obesogenic" society. The term refers to abundant and unhealthy food choices, sedentary jobs, inactive leisure pursuits and personal technology that continues to engineer movement out of even the simplest daily tasks.

BMI AND OBESITY IN 2020

Calculated for a 5'9"man

	1999-2004	Projected 2020	Minimum BMI	Minimum weight
Median BMI	27.1	28.9		
Overweight	65.5%	77.7%	25	169
Obese	31.5%	42.1%	30	203
Obese: Class 2	13%	18%	35	237
Obese: Class 3	6.9%	9.9%	40	271
Obese: Class 4	2.1%	2.8%	45	305

Source: Ruhm CJ. Current and future prevalence of obesity and severe obesity in the United States. NBER. June 2007.

Obesity arguably is the most pressing U.S. public-health problem. Proportionally, severe obesity is expected to grow faster than obesity by 2020.

Excess weight is a politically charged issue, with complex causes and few solutions. Some are quick to label obesity a result of irresponsible personal behavior. The "personal responsibility" argument is asserted often by food companies that are trying to avoid government regulation. Cynically, this corporate approach is used to "protect personal freedoms" from "government intrusion." This twisted logic creates the apparent contradiction that although overweight people may be irresponsible, any consumer protections against that behavior help foster a "nanny state."

Others are more likely to blame an obesogenic environment. They argue that people are simply responding to the forces in their daily lives. Societal forces exert constant pressure on people to overeat, and some are better able than others to resist.

Who is to blame?

American public opinion blames the obesity epidemic on both personal and collective factors. In a Center for Consumer Freedom survey, respondents called constant presence of food the main culprit. Lack of willpower was mentioned the least. Other causes mentioned were time pressures, food advertising and addiction to certain foods. Two out of 3 selected three or more reasons.

Such nuanced opinions do not square with the widespread weight-based stereotyping and discrimination, which people may not admit in a survey. Many believe obese and overweight people are lazy, unintelligent, weak-willed and unmotivated.

There is a misguided belief by some that scorn somehow will shame people into losing weight. Ironically, it may make the problem worse. In a study of more than 2,400 overweight women in a weight-loss support organization, 3 out of 4 said they coped with the stigma against being overweight by defiantly eating more food and refusing to diet.

Examples of weight bias do not get worse than this: A proposed 2008 bill in the Mississippi House of Representatives would have prohibited restaurants from serving anyone who was obese.

Remarkably, discrimination against excess weight appears to be rampant in health-care settings. Some studies have found that it is worse than in the general population. Many health-care providers consider obese patients annoying and unwilling to follow treatment advice. They also tend to spend less time with such patients during an appointment, compared with thinner patients.

A Fort Lauderdale (FL) *Sun-Sentinel* survey found that 15 of 105 South Florida obstetrics-gynecology practices polled refused to see otherwise healthy women because they were overweight. The physicians said obese patients have a higher risk of complications

Obesity is often called an epidemic. While it is not contagious, it has spread across the nation swiftly. Consider this: The thinnest state in 2010 would have been the fattest in 1995. In 1995, Indiana had the highest obesity rate at 20.1 percent. By 2010, Colorado, the thinnest state, had an obesity rate of 21.4 percent.

Emory University professor Kenneth Thorpe developed an econometric model projecting that about 43 percent of U.S. adults will be obese by 2018. At that rate, obesity would account for more than 20 percent of all health-care spending by the end of the decade. The per-capita cost of treating obesity was $361 in 2008. That is expected to rise to $1,425 in 2018.

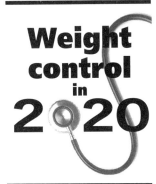

Being overweight or obese elevates the risk for several diseases and conditions, including heart disease, stroke, diabetes, some cancers, osteoarthritis and sleep apnea.

These are among the federal government's major weight-control goals for the year 2020:

Increase the percentage of adults at a healthy weight

Starting point: 30.8 percent of persons ages 20 years and over were at a healthy weight in 2005–08
Goal: 33.9 percent (10 percent improvement)

Reduce the proportion of adults who are obese

Starting point: 34.0 percent of persons ages 20 and over were obese in 2005–08
Goal: 30.6 percent (10 percent improvement)

continued

Reduce the proportion of children ages 2 to 19 who are obese

Starting point: 16.2 percent of persons 2 to 19 were obese in 2005–08
   Goal: 14.6 percent (10 percent improvement)

---

and their exam tables and other equipment could not handle people over a certain weight.

Obese patients feel the scorn. More than two-thirds of obese women say they have been discriminated against by health providers. Many feel disrespected and not taken seriously. They often report that their excess weight is blamed for all their medical problems and that they are self-conscious about discussing weight concerns with their physicians.

Many overweight people decline to seek medical attention for treatable yet risky conditions because they do not want to be harassed about their weight.

One of the reasons for the apparent discrimination could be that medical schools seem to ignore the fact that a significant portion of their students' patients will be overweight. Medical textbooks almost always display normal-sized models. Obesity calls for special diagnostic skills and altered physical examinations. For example, obesity is a risk factor for breast cancer. However, obese women are less likely to get regular mammograms and need to be encouraged to do so by their health-care providers.

People yearn to be thin, sometimes above all else. A 2010 Harris poll asked: If you could change one thing about yourself, what would it be? While 43 percent predictably picked being richer, 21 percent selected being thinner. Slimness actually out-polled being smarter (14 percent) and younger (12 percent).

There is no federal law protecting obese people from discrimination. A survey by the Rudd Center for Food Policy and Obesity at Yale University found that about 3 out of 4 people favored adopting laws that stopped employers from discriminating against obese people. They were less likely to favor considering obesity a disability under the Americans with Disabilities Act, or enacting similar protections to those granted to disabled people.

How fat happens

Conventional wisdom is that weight gain is a mathematical phenomenon. It requires 3,500 excess calories to produce a pound of fat. One's metabolism supposedly is dictated by weight and activity. For example, an active 150-pound man should consume 2,250 calories. If he consumes an average of 1,750 calories a day for a week, he would lose one pound. If he eats a daily average of 2,750 calories for a week, he would gain a pound.

If only it were that easy. Weight gain and loss is highly individual and is the result of a complex set of factors.

One theory is that everyone has a genetically determined weight set point that can fall within a range of 20 to 30 pounds, depending upon nutritional and exercise habits. If a person attempts to go below that range, the body rebels by slowing its rate of metabolism and signaling its hunger. The familiar lament of the yo-yo dieter—"I gained all my weight back, and then some!"—is a result of the metabolic change.

Some experts speculate the obesity rate is going to increase more slowly because the nation is reaching a sort of obesity saturation point. That implies that nearly everyone who is genetically meant to be obese is now there.

If one parent is obese, the child has a 50 percent likelihood of also being obese. With two obese parents, the risk rises to 80 percent. Obese children almost inevitably become obese adults.

Reality check: Weight control

Mirror, mirror...

Two-thirds of Americans are overweight or obese, so the qualitative lines blur on what is considered normal weight.

An August 2010 Harris Interactive/HealthyDay poll found that 30 percent of overweight people believed they were normal size. Moreover, 70 percent of obese people felt they were merely overweight, including 39 percent who were morbidly obese. Interviewers asked respondents for their height and weight to calculate an accurate body mass index (BMI). Interviewers then asked them to describe whether they were obese, overweight or normal size.

"While there are some people who have body images in line with their actual BMI, for many people they are not, and this may be where part of the problem lies," said Regina Corso, vice president of Harris Poll Solutions. "If they don't recognize the problem or don't recognize the severity of the problem, they are less likely to do something about it."

More said excess weight is an exercise problem, rather than a food problem. Even though exercise has little impact on weight loss, 6 of 10 respondents believed their excess weight is a result of lack of exercise. About half that many—including only 27 percent of the morbidly obese—said they ate more than they should "in general."

'Body size misperception'

A group of Dallas researchers wanted to see if one of the reasons for the swift rise in obesity was people did not realize they were overweight.

The research subjects, all of whom were obese, were shown pictures of nine figures—from very thin to morbidly obese—and asked to select an ideal body size. If they picked an image the same or bigger than themselves, they had what researchers called "body size misperception." About 8 percent fell into this category. It was more common among blacks and Latinos than among whites.

"Misperception" can be a blessing and a curse. Those in that group were happier with their health than those who acknowledged they were obese. However, they also were more likely to believe they were at low risk of developing high blood pressure or diabetes.

Of the more than 2,000 obese participants surveyed, only 14 percent of blacks, 11 percent of Hispanics and 2 percent of whites believed they needed to lose weight.

Researchers pointed out that the study is a cautionary note for physicians, who may need to establish whether their obese patients consider excess weight a health problem and actually want to lose it.

How men and women view weight as a risk ... or not

The "health belief model" is a theory of psychology that attempts to explain and predict health behavior. According to the model, people will change behavior if they feel threatened. Nevertheless, they have to believe they are at risk of getting a disease and feel the consequences will be severe if they do nothing.

People have to believe that having excess weight is a health threat before they are likely to do anything about it.

Overweight men are more likely than women (62 percent versus 43 percent) to believe weight is not a health threat. Likewise, 20 percent of obese men and 14 percent of obese women have the same belief.

continued

Predictably, they are unlikely to do anything about their weight.

In a study of more than 300 black women, more than 80 percent were either overweight or obese. Of the women who were obese, about 3 out of 4 said they were merely overweight. Even though all of the women agreed extra weight was "very serious," the overweight women thought they had the same risk of weight-related disease as normal-weight women.

In other words, the health-belief model predicts the overweight women will make no behavior changes. They feel no threat because they believe they are normal.

They're just growing children...

Parents can be blind to their child's weight. According to a Dutch study, half of the mothers of obese children ages 4 or 5 thought their offspring were normal weight. Four out of 10 fathers thought so, too.

That normal-size judgment grew to 3 out of 4 if their children were just overweight.

Predictably, mothers and fathers of overweight and obese children were significantly heavier than the parents of normal-sized children. Researchers also asked the parents to assess their own weight. They were far more aware of their own condition. About 8 out of 10 overweight parents admitted to being too heavy, as did nearly all of the obese parents. The more accurate self-assessments may reflect the fact that excess weight is not as prevalent in the Netherlands as in the U.S.

The link is likely to be cultural as well as genetic, because family members have similar eating and physical activity habits.

Genes clearly dictate who is the most vulnerable to excessive weight gain, but other factors determine whether weight gain actually happens. For example, the Pima Indians were originally from Mexico, where they were poor farmers without weight problems and the resulting chronic conditions. Those who moved to the United States adopted a different lifestyle. One-half of the Pima Indians in the U.S. now have diabetes and 95 percent of those are overweight.

Despite obesity's complex causes, researchers continue to attempt to pin the epidemic on one cause.

An Australian researcher declared in 2009 that obesity has doubled in the past 30 years exclusively because of increased calorie consumption. Physical activity had a minor role, he declared, because physical activity levels had not changed much during that time. Children are consuming 350 more calories a day than children of three decades ago, and adults are taking in 500 more.

A Canadian researcher, however, blamed office-based jobs. According to his research, people are eating better and exercising more than they did three decades ago, so sedentary work must be the culprit.

In 1960, about 50 percent of the U.S. jobs required moderate physical activity. That has fallen to 20 percent. That translates to about 120-140 fewer calories expended daily per capita. That lack of activity closely tracks the nation's weight gain over the past five decades.

A health hazard? It depends

Obesity is often called the "chronic disease gateway." Nearly 80 percent of obese adults suffer from diabetes, high blood pressure, high cholesterol, arthritis, coronary artery disease, or more than one of these conditions. Some researchers have concluded that obesity is more hazardous to health and quality of life than cigarette smoking. They also concluded that the burden on the population's physical and mental health has more than doubled in just 15 years.

Others say that if the obesity rate stays the same, U.S. life expectancy will be reduced by nine months.

North Carolina economists analyzed 366,000 Americans and drew these conclusions about the effect of weight:

- Extremely obese people—those 80 pounds or more overweight—live 3 to 12 fewer years than those who are of normal weight.
- Obese people—those 30 pounds or more overweight—live about one year less.
- Overweight people—those up to 29 pounds over normal weight—do not have shortened lives.
- Excess weight was responsible for the loss of about 95 million years of life in the U.S. in 2008.

One of the reasons moderate excess weight may not affect life expectancy is that there are many effective treatments to manage associated risk factors, such as high blood pressure and high cholesterol.

Another study involving about 1.5 million people concluded that healthy obese white adults were 13 percent more likely to die during a given time period than those of normal weight.

Regarding cardiovascular disease, obesity can be a curse and a blessing. It certainly is a strong risk factor for heart disease. But once a heart ailment is acquired, obese patients have better outcomes. Evidence indicates that being overweight increases survival from heart failure, high blood pressure and coronary artery disease, compared with people of normal or lower weight. The reason for this apparent contradiction may be that heart disease is different for the obese than it is for lean people, for whom genetics may play a larger and more lethal role.

Being overweight is not a harbinger of infirmity. One in 3 obese people have no cardiovascular risk factors, while 1 out of 4 normal-weight people do. A study that tracked 2,600 people age 60 and older for 12 years found that overweight people who exercised moderately or vigorously 30 minutes on most days out-lived their sedentary normal-weight counterparts.

Being overweight and obese is the product of government definition. In 1998, the National Heart, Lung, and Blood Institute changed the BMI benchmarks. The overweight cutoff was lowered from 27.8 to 25, and for obesity from 32 to 30. So millions of people acquired these chronic conditions overnight. BMI is a crude tool that can do a poor job of reliably predicting health.

The diet struggle continues

Anyone who struggles to maintain an ideal weight understands the uphill battle. Only about 1 in 6 overweight Americans lose weight and keep it off. Women are better at it than men. However, being married makes it more difficult to keep an ideal for both sexes.

A review of 31 long-term studies involving tens of thousands of dieters offers grim news. More than 80 percent of dieters gain all of the lost weight back within two years, and very few kept it off for five years.

One of the biggest barriers to weight loss is striving for an un-realistic body weight. The scientific community believes diets and medications realistically cannot produce more than a 10 percent weight loss. Some of the most respected health organizations— the Institute of Medicine, the World Health Organization, the

U.S. Preventive Services Task Force, the National Heart, Lung, and Blood Institute—recommend that health-care providers ask patients to lose no more than that amount.

Linda Bacon, a professor of nutrition at City College of San Francisco and author of *Health at Every Size: The Surprising Truth About Your Weight,* runs a program to teach overweight people about healthy eating habits and the merits of physical activity.

Bacon tracked 78 obese women aged 30 to 45 for two years. Half the group participated in her program and the other half were in a traditional weight-loss program. At the end, both groups essentially weighed the same. But the group in Bacon's program lowered cholesterol and blood-pressure levels and had higher self-esteem.

Bacon contends that the body will do what it is supposed to do if people learn to enjoy physical activity and to stop eating when they are full.

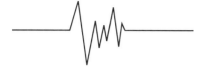

Chapter 8

Tobacco and Alcohol

Progress has stalled

The reduction in cigarette smoking is arguably the most successful achievement in U.S. public health in the last 50 years. However, smoking remains the most common cause of preventable death.

The adult smoking rate has declined by half, to about 20 percent, since the early 1960s. If the trend continues, the smoking rate will be less than 17 percent by 2020 and stabilize at about 13.5 percent by 2050, according to an Institute of Medicine computer simulation. Nevertheless, the rate essentially has hovered around 20 percent since 2004.

The U.S. government had set a goal to reduce it to 12 percent by 2010, but efforts have failed to budge the number. Nearly half of current smokers tried to quit in the previous year. Most who try do not succeed.

The percentage of people who smoke a pack or more a day has declined significantly. About 23 percent of U.S. adults smoked 20 or more cigarettes daily in 1965. By 2007, approximately 7 percent did so. In California, that rate has fallen below 3 percent.

Less than 6 percent of people with graduate degrees smoke, compared with more than 27 percent of those without a high school diploma. Nearly 1 out of 3 adults with household incomes below the federal poverty line smoke.

Experts cannot agree on the direction of smoking's impact on public health. Some see the progress of the past century and expect smoking ultimately to be a distant memory. Others see a continuing devastating death toll.

University of Wisconsin researchers boldly predicted the end of tobacco use in the United States by 2047. They mapped out a battle plan for the coming decades to extinguish smoking with taxes increases, along with the elimination of nicotine from tobacco, stepped-up anti-smoking advertising campaigns and aggressive use of individual counseling and medication.

On the other hand, the World Lung Foundation predicts that tobacco use, which killed 100 million people worldwide in the 20th century, will kill 1 billion in the current century. Of the 6 million who died of smoking-related causes last year, nearly three-quarters were in low- and middle-income nations.

Smoking's death toll is devastating by any measure. Nearly 3 out of 4 cancer deaths are attributable to smoking. Half of all smokers, especially those who started as adolescents, can expect to die of tobacco use and lose 20 to 25 years of life expectancy.

However, tobacco consumption is the lowest per capita since recordkeeping began in 1880. At that time, manufactured cigarettes accounted for only 1 percent of tobacco products. That rose to 80 percent by 1950, when Americans consumed about 13 pounds per person. That amount fell to less than four pounds per person by 2006.

Recent anti-tobacco developments

Two significant recent steps should bolster the anti-tobacco effort. First, the federal cigarette excise tax increased from 39 cents to

The nation's bars, restaurants and workplaces may be smoke-free by 2020, according to a Centers for Disease Control and Prevention (CDC) official. About half of the 50 states have banned smoking in those venues since 2000, when none of the states had such bans.

Dr. Tim McAfee, director of the CDC's Office on Smoking and Health, told the Associated Press, "It is by no means a foregone conclusion that we'll get there by 2020. I'm relatively bullish we'll at least get close to that number."

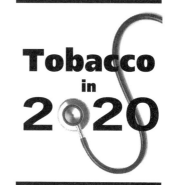

These are among the federal government's major tobacco-use goals for the year 2020:

Reduce cigarette smoking by adults

Starting point: In 2008, 20.6 percent of adults ages 18 years and older were cigarette smokers
    Goal: 12 percent (same as 2010 goal)

Reduce tobacco use by adolescents

Starting point: In 2009, 26 percent of adolescents in grades 9 through 12 said they had used cigarettes, chewing tobacco, snuff or cigars in the past 30 days
    Goal: 21 percent (same as 2010 goal)

Increase smoking-cessation attempts by adult smokers

Starting point: In 2008, 48.3 percent of adult smokers said they had attempted to stop smoking in the past 12 months
    Goal: 80 percent (same as 2010 goal)

$1.01 in April 2009. Despite that price increase, U.S. cigarettes are among the most affordable in the world.

Second, the U.S. Food and Drug Administration (FDA) can now regulate the manufacturing and marketing of cigarettes and other tobacco products. The U.S. surgeon general declared tobacco a health hazard in 1964. However, over the next 45 years, the No. 1 preventable cause of death remained virtually the last un-regulated consumable U.S. product. The regulation likely will have more impact than the 1971 ban against tobacco advertising on radio and television. It probably will eclipse the industry's $206 billion settlement with the states in 1998.

The regulation bans the use of the terms "light" and "low tar," as well as the use of fruit and candy flavorings to make products more palatable to children. Advertising and store displays will be restricted to stark black-and-white text. However, the bigger impact is the disclosure and regulation of the estimated 60 carcino-gens and 4,000 toxins emitted by cigarette smoke. The FDA will have the ability to make the products less deadly for current users.

The Congressional Budget Office predicted the law would decrease youth smoking by 11 percent and adult smoking by 2 percent, independent of the effects of higher excise taxes and public smoking restrictions.

A 2009 Gallup poll indicated that more than half of Amer-icans disapproved of the FDA regulation. The reasons for lack of support are unclear. However, even many nonsmokers oppose public smoking bans because they place a higher value on freedom of choice than on combating health risks.

Smoking's effect: The evidence continues to mount

Research on tobacco's effect on health continues to be popular, even though the results rarely surprise.

The surgeon general's office issued its 30th report on tobacco in December 2010. The 704-page document describes in detail how tobacco damages every organ in the body, resulting in disease and death. It noted that tobacco smoke contains more than 7,000 chemicals, of which hundreds are toxic and at least 70 cause cancer.

Cigarettes alter a smoker's DNA within 30 minutes of the first puff. The immediate genetic damage raises the short-term risk for cancer. Smokers' arteries stiffen with age twice as fast as those of nonsmokers. Stiff arteries are more prone to blockages that promote stroke, heart attacks and other cardiovascular disease.

A 55-year-old smoker has the same chance of dying in the next 10 years as a 65-year-old nonsmoker. The number of cigarettes smoked dictates how swiftly health-related quality of life deteriorates, even in those who eventually quit the habit.

Pipes and cigars have an impact on health similar to that of cigarettes, especially on lung function. While cigarette smoking has decreased in the past four decades, pipe and cigar smoking have increased in popularity.

A return on investment, but in what way?

For every $1 spent on treatment, state governments get back $1.26. Researchers compared the cost of treatment and counseling with the cost of premature death, productivity loss and health-care expenses. Nationally, each $5.61 pack of cigarettes costs society the equivalent of $18.05 in lost lives and productivity.

However, others have calculated that the lifetime health costs of smokers are less than those of nonsmokers because cigarettes end lives swiftly and efficiently. According to a Vanderbilt University economist, the nation saves 32 cents a pack because of shorter lives. A 2008 Dutch study said health-care costs for adult smokers were $326,000, compared with $417,000 for the thin and healthy people who inevitably lived longer.

Most employer insurance plans pay for tobacco cessation because nonsmoking employees are more productive and less likely to develop costly chronic conditions. Under health reform, even Medicare is paying for counseling for the 4.5 million elderly who continue to light up. Medicare officials estimate the program will have spent an estimated $800 billion on smoking-related illness from 1995 to 2015.

What anti-tobacco policies work best

Four proven strategies, if pursued aggressively, could nearly wipe out cigarette smoking. The only barrier is political will. The policies with documented success: increasing tobacco taxes, expansion of public smoking bans, anti-smoking advertising campaigns, and banning methods of cigarette marketing.

State excise taxes on a pack of cigarettes range from 17 cents in Missouri to $4.35 in New York. By comparison, Norway taxes cigarettes by more than $11. Tobacco has long been a significant contributor to U.S. government coffers. Alexander Hamilton first proposed tobacco excise taxes in 1794, and they were eventually implemented in the 1860s. By 1880, the taxes accounted for nearly one-third of federal tax receipts.

Steep tax increases would hit two groups especially hard: low-income households and people with chronic mental illness or substance-abuse disorders. Both groups have a disproportionate share of heavy smokers, despite the fact that it has become a very expensive habit. For example, more than 40 percent of U.S. smokers also have alcohol, drug or mental disorders. More than 60 percent of alcohol abusers are smokers. People with these disorders consume 44 percent of the cigarettes sold in the U.S.

Of the 22 million Americans who struggle with alcohol and drug abuse, nearly 95 percent say they are unaware they have a problem. However, most people who binge-drink are not alcoholics or alcohol-dependent.

The federal government defines binge drinking as four or more drinks for a woman, or five or more for a man, on a single occasion. It defines heavy drinking as more than one drink for a woman, or more than two drinks for a man, on a given day. Excessive drinking is considered binge drinking, heavy drinking or both.

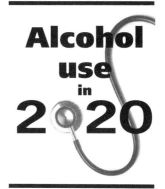

These are among the federal government's major alcohol-use goals for the year 2020:

Reduce the proportion of adults who drank excessively in the past 30 days

Starting point: In 2008, 28.1 percent of adults ages 18 years and older reported that they drank excessively in the previous 30 days

Goal: 25.3 percent (10 percent improvement)

Decrease the rate of alcohol-impaired driving (blood alcohol content [BAC] of .08 or higher)

Starting point: In 2008, 0.40 deaths per 100 million vehicle miles traveled involved a driver or motorcycle rider with a BAC of .08 or greater

Goal: 0.38 deaths per 100 million vehicle miles traveled (5 percent improvement)

However, a 10 percent increase in cigarette prices would cut their smoking by an estimated 18 percent.

Cigarette tax increases would be a double victory for cash-strapped states. An analysis by a coalition of several anti-tobacco organizations concluded that a $1 tax increase per pack would:

- Increase state revenues by more than $9 billion annually.
- Prompt 1.2 million adult smokers to quit.
- Prevent more than 2.3 million adolescents from acquiring the habit.
- Forestall more than 1 million premature deaths; and
- Save nearly $53 billion in health-care costs.

Two-thirds of voters would support the $1 increase, according to a national poll released in conjunction with the report.

However, cigarette manufacturers would fight back. They use coupons and discounts to neutralize tax increases. In 2009, tobacco companies spent nearly three-quarters of their marketing and promotion budgets on retail-price reduction.

Smoking bans continue their relentless advance nationwide. Nearly two-thirds of Americans are subject to comprehensive smoke-free laws. At one time, it was common that states would not allow local governments to enact anti-smoking laws that were more stringent—known as state pre-emption laws. The number of states that pre-empt local action against smoking melted from 19 in 2005 to 12 in 2010.

The bans have measured effects on public health. Fatal heart attacks decreased 7 percent in Massachusetts after the state outlawed smoking in workplaces. Studies in other states and nations that have imposed bans reaffirm that effect.

Bars and restaurants frequently oppose smoke-free laws, fearing that cigarette-smoking customers will go elsewhere. However, research consistently has shown that the bans do not harm sales and, in many cases, actually increase business.

An Oklahoma study found that the average particulate level in bars and restaurant smoking rooms was beyond the "hazardous" level established by the U.S. Environmental Protection Agency (EPA) for outdoor air. Tobacco smoke levels were tested based on very fine particulate matter. The EPA considers air containing 250 micrograms per cubic meter or more to be hazardous outdoor air pollution, labeling it as emergency conditions. Restaurant rooms contained an average of 380 micrograms. Bars averaged 655.

Secondhand smoke annually kills 600,000 people worldwide. More than 1 in 4 of those deaths is a child under 5 years old. Smokers are at additional risk of their own secondhand smoke. For someone who smokes 14 cigarettes a day, his or her own secondhand smoke yields the risk of having smoked 2.6 more cigarettes.

The residue from secondhand smoke—called thirdhand smoke—can leave cancer-causing toxins on furniture, carpets, walls and drapes. The chemical, called tobacco-specific nitrosamines, can mix with dust or stick to the fingers of children or infants.

It is not surprising that nearly all children—98 percent—who live with a smoker have measurable tobacco toxins in their bodies.

Anti-smoking campaigns are effective, but the recession and more pressing financial needs have decimated state tobacco-control programs. States spent $517 million on anti-tobacco programs in 2011, which is 28 percent less than in 2008 and just 14 percent of the $3.7 billion recommended by the Centers for Disease Control. Tobacco companies spend about $25 on marketing for every $1 the states spend to fight tobacco use.

Countries that have completely outlawed tobacco advertising have been effective in reducing tobacco use. Nations with limited policies, such as the United States, have not had much impact.

The FDA will require graphic images to cover the top half of cigarette packages beginning September 2012. They include photos of rotting teeth, the corpse of a smoker and a man exhaling smoke through a tracheotomy opening in his neck.

Alcohol: Mixing the good with the bad

Americans are drinking more than they have in the last 25 years. Two out of 3 adults imbibe. Beer leads the way, followed by wine and then liquor. About 37 percent drink moderately. About 28 percent drink heavily—a number that has grown in the last two decades.

A national survey of 43,000 people revealed that about 30 percent of U.S. adults have either abused alcohol or become dependent on it. However, about 70 percent of those either quit or cut back to more moderate drinking without treatment. Only 1 percent fit the definition of severe, uncontrolled alcohol addiction.

Temperance has long been considered a virtue by many Americans. Nevertheless, an onslaught of research is rehabilitating alcohol's reputation. Moderate, regular drinking—about one drink a day for women and two drinks a day for men—raises HDL (good) cholesterol and cuts the risk of heart disease by 25 percent. It may also help prevent Type 2 diabetes and the kind of stroke caused by blood clots. Even people ages 45 to 64 who began drinking wine lowered their chance of developing heart disease by more than one-third.

But it could be that people who drink are already healthier. Moderate drinkers generally have higher incomes, more education and less depression than heavier drinkers or those who abstain. They also are slimmer, have lower blood pressure, triglycerides and blood glucose—all markers for heart-disease risk.

About those binge drinkers...

Unlike moderate drinking, binge drinking is unequivocally bad. It is a leading preventable cause of death, killing about 79,000 Americans annually and shortening lives by about 30 years.

Binge drinkers consume an average of eight drinks at a time. They tend to be men younger than 35 who earn more than $50,000 a year. They drink heavily about once a week. Even binge drinkers over 65 years old consume more than six drinks at a time.

Certainly heavy drinking is a health hazard, raising the risk of liver disease, heart disease, depression, stroke and several types of cancer. But it also leads to injury and accidental death. Alcohol is a factor in about 60 percent of fatal burn injuries, drowning and homicides; 50 percent of trauma injuries and sexual assaults, and 40 percent of fatal motor-vehicle crashes, suicides and fatal falls.

The economic impact of alcohol-impaired driving is estimated at $51 billion, of which about 15 percent represents medical costs. Almost 1 out of 8 binge drinkers drive within two hours of drinking. More than half of those consume the alcohol in a bar, restaurant or club.

Professional sports events are also hotbeds of binge drinking. One out of every 12 fans leaving a game is legally intoxicated. Those who tailgated were 14 times more likely to leave the stadium with an illegal blood-alcohol level of .08 or higher. One out of 4 tailgaters had five or more drinks.

Alcohol is the lubricant of many social occasions. And drinkers are heavily influenced by how much is consumed by those around them. A study of social networks shows that people are 50 percent more likely to drink heavily if someone they are connected to does so. The network's influence has a ripple effect. If a friend of a friend drinks heavily, the effect is 36 percent. Even a third-degree separation—a friend of a friend of a friend—raises the risk by 15 percent.

The effect also works in reverse. People are 29 percent more likely to abstain if they are surrounded by nondrinkers.

The degree of social influence is dependent on the relationship. A heavy-drinking wife boosts the husband's chance of similar consumption by 196 percent. Heavy drinking by a husband boosts the wife's risk of the same by 126 percent.

The biggest alcohol deterrent? Price

A bar in a college town during "happy hour" is a perfect laboratory to gauge the effect of price on alcohol consumption. Cash-strapped young adults jam these establishments where binge drinking is acceptable, even encouraged.

University of Florida researchers analyzed more than 100 studies spanning four decades on price elasticity of alcohol. The results were consistent: When prices go down, people drink more. When they go up, people drink less.

In fact, price decreases alcohol consumption more effectively than law enforcement, media campaigns and school health classes. And price is most efficiently manipulated by taxes.

Doubling alcohol taxes would reduce alcohol-related deaths by more than one-third, traffic accidents by 11 percent and sexually transmitted disease by 6 percent, according to one study. For example, a fifth of gin in New York State had a tax of $.55 in 2010. It also estimated that a 10 percent increase in retail price would reduce drinking by 5 percent.

But alcohol prices are going in the other direction. Federal and state alcohol taxes have declined significantly since the 1950s when adjusted for inflation, as has the overall price of alcohol. That is likely a result of high profit margins on alcohol and the industry's powerful lobbying presence in state capitals and Washington.

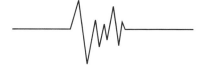

Chapter 9

Personalized Medicine
Its promise remains elusive

Genetics is important to health. However, it is easy to over-estimate its impact. An often-quoted phrase captures it: Genes load the gun, but environment pulls the trigger. Genes affect how a body will react to its environment.

People differ vastly in what they eat, the stress they experience, the toxins they absorb. DNA influences, but does not determine, whether they will develop certain diseases and how severe those ailments might be.

Swedish scientists followed 855 men born in 1913 and examined them at various ages, starting at age 50. The assumption was that men with parents who lived to a ripe old age would do so also. Not so. Those who did not smoke, drank a moderate amount of coffee, were reasonably fit at age 54 and had an adequate income and education had the best chance to reach 90 years old. By 2008, researchers were clearly able to prove that quitting smoking and lowering cholesterol and blood pressure between 1963 and 2003 explained a significant decrease in heart attacks among the men.

However, an important study of exceptional longevity identified about 70 separate genes that were important factors in life expectancy. The genome-wide study of 1,000 people ages 100 or older determined that genes controlled 20 to 30 percent of the variation in survival to age 85.

In 2000, then-President Bill Clinton grandly announced the sequencing, or "first draft," of the human genome, which is all the DNA a person possesses. Clinton said the development, which involved several federal agencies, would "lead to a new era of molecular medicine, an era that will bring new ways to prevent, diagnose, treat and cure disease." Scientists have discovered hundreds of genetic variants, with risk associations ranging from heart disease to restless-leg syndrome.

There have been significant advances in DNA processing and basic scientific knowledge. However, research clearly points out that disease has enormously complex causes, and genes cannot be sifted yet to pinpoint the handful of offending mutations.

After more than 10 years, the promise of translating the genome into clinical reality remains elusive. Drug development takes 10 to 15 years after an important genetic target is identified. Genetic tests continue to mystify physicians and their patients. The Food and Drug Administration (FDA) has blocked direct-to-consumer tests of dubious quality.

The new pharmaceutical playing field

Personalized medicine, or tailoring medical treatment to an individual's genetic profile, is the Holy Grail for medical futurists. It is often described as the right treatment for the right person at the right time in the right amount. A team of doctors, pharmacists and other health-care providers would customize treatment based on an individual's medical history, genetic profile and the result of shared decision-making with the patient.

Some physicians might argue that they already practice personalized medicine. They take into account a patient's age, family

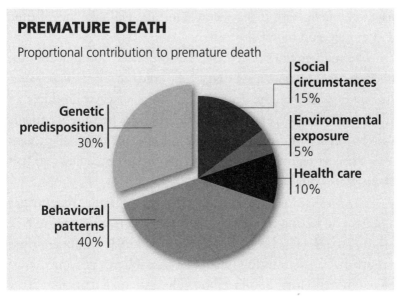

PREMATURE DEATH

Proportional contribution to premature death

Social circumstances 15%

Environmental exposure 5%

Health care 10%

Genetic predisposition 30%

Behavioral patterns 40%

Source: McGinnis JM, et al. *Health Aff.* 2002; 21(2):78-93.

Genetic predisposition is a major determinant of health. Whether those genes are activated depends strongly on other determinants in this chart – behavior patterns, socioeconomic circumstances and environmental exposures.

history and lifestyle when planning treatment or writing prescriptions. But time constraints and crude assessment techniques can limit effectiveness. The harsh reality is that the most commonly prescribed U.S. medicines are effective in fewer than 60 percent of patients. Benefits and risks vary significantly for individual patients.

Ideally, a genetic test would identify susceptibility to disease, predict response to a particular drug and match the right formulary to the right patient. The result: Fewer adverse drug reactions, less unnecessary treatment and better health outcomes. This science is called pharmacogenomics. The difficulty is that there may be millions of genetic variations that affect a patient's reaction to a drug. And it may be a complex mix of genes that produces that reaction. Navigating that genetic landscape will take lots of time and money, and high failure rates.

The mathematics of research has produced addition by subtraction. According to a February 2008 study in *The New England Journal of Medicine*, the generic HIV drug Abacavir produces an adverse reaction 99 percent of the time in the 6 percent of patients who have a specific gene. Paradoxically, sales increased 28 percent over the next eight months because physicians became confident about who would benefit.

The market for targeted therapeutics, molecular diagnostics and genetic testing is expected to grow 10 percent a year, to $42 billion, by 2015. However, the price of DNA sequencing has dropped at an astounding rate. The first human genome, completed in 2003, cost $500 million. The anticipated price in 2011 is $5,000 to $10,000.

Personalized medicine represents a paradigm shift for pharmaceutical companies. Creating drugs for large populations with chronic conditions has been the prevailing strategy for the past three decades. As the patents for those drugs expire, the drugmakers may be able to turn to high-priced targeted therapeutics for small populations.

According to one estimate, up to one-half of drug companies are using a personalized-medicine approach to pharmaceutical development.

Molecular diagnostics help identify a patient's disease susceptibility, or likelihood of having an adverse reaction to a drug. The process, which includes lab tests and imaging, can help physicians decide whether a particular drug will help a certain patient.

Genetic testing

Legitimate genetic testing often is lumped with over-the-counter drugstore tests.

Medical-device manufacturers market genetic testing kits to facilties such as hospitals, clinics and laboratories. The FDA is responsible for regulating these products, whose results are interpreted by trained health-care providers. Laboratories also develop their own genetic tests, which are overseen by the Centers for Medicare and Medicaid Services.

By contrast, Walgreens delayed the sale of Pathway Genomics genetic test in May 2010 after the FDA challenged its legality. The government appears to be deciding whether the retail products are medical devices, which would require regulation, or simply consumer information.

Direct-to-consumer (DTC) genetic tests are about probability, not certainty. Environment, behavior and luck conspire to determine whether genes will express themselves. In other words, someone who eats right and exercises may well offset a genetic propensity to gain weight.

At its best, in-home genetic testing empowers patients to manage their health and assess personal risks. However, DTC testing is predictive, not diagnostic. It attempts to assess susceptibility to, and probability of, disease—not its presence. The worst-case scenario: Consumers can easily conclude that a disease mentioned in the DTC profile will occur in the future—regardless of its statistical probability.

A Government Accountability Office (GAO) investigation of four companies found misleading test results and "egregious examples of deceptive marketing." Federal officials sent real donors' samples to four companies and posed as fictitious customers to inquire about results. According to the GAO, the companies produced different results for identical samples and told customers they had low risks for diseases they already had.

A 2006 report argued that "the potential harms (of DTC genetic tests) outweigh the potential benefits." A Federal Trade

Commission "facts for consumers" bulletin cautions that "having a particular gene doesn't necessarily mean that a disease will develop; not having a particular gene doesn't necessarily mean the disease will not."

Australian journalist Ray Moynihan was far blunter in an article titled: "Beware the fortune tellers peddling genetic tests."

He said, "For anyone concerned about the creeping medical-isation of life, the marketplace for genetic testing is one of the last frontiers, where apparently harmless technology can help mutate healthy people into fearful patients, their personhood redefined by multiple genetic predispositions for disease and early death."

The market for genetic information

Regardless of their validity, personal-health blueprints are in great demand.

In a poll taken right after the Walgreens recall, nearly 3 out of 4 said drugstores should sell genetic testing kits, compared with only about 1 in 4 doctors.

People appear willing to pay a lot of money even for imperfect or marginal genetic information about themselves. Tufts Medical Center researchers posed scenarios to about 1,500 people based on disease, risk of getting the disease and test accuracy. Most said they would be tested—from about 70 percent for a flawed test for Alzheimer's disease and 10 percent average risk, to nearly 9 out of 10 for a perfectly accurate prostate-cancer test and a 25 percent average risk. People were willing to pay an average of $320 for an imperfect arthritis test, $622 for a hypothetically accurate prostate test.

Four of 5 Americans support a national study of how genes are affected by health behavior and the environment. About 60 percent said they would supply their DNA.

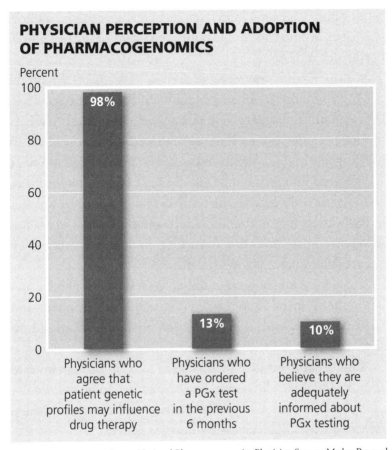

PHYSICIAN PERCEPTION AND ADOPTION OF PHARMACOGENOMICS

Source: National Pharmacogenomics Physician Survey: Medco Research.

Nearly all physicians believe genetics can influence a patient's response to a medication. However, few physicians believe they are adequately informed enough to use genetic testing to potentially improve drug therapy.

Younger adults are especially interested in genetic information. About half believe that genes play an equal role in health to lifestyle habits. Those with riskier health behavior tend to say genetics has a more pronounced effect, perhaps as a rationalization for bad habits. Those with a family history of disease also place a greater value on genetic information. In reality, genetic markers, on average, account for only about 10 percent of the overall risk of acquiring a disease.

A study in the *New England Journal of Medicine* attempted to determine how spooked people would be by the results of DTC genetic tests. Researchers assessed the anxiety levels of more than 2,000 who used the tests to analyze their probability of getting any of 22 different diseases. The result: Nine out of 10 were unfazed. Another result: Hardly any of them changed their health habits after getting the results. The implication was that the test was harmless psychologically and ineffective in making a difference in anyone's life. According to the researchers, DTC tests are "underpowered" with data.

A separate study of genetic-test takers found that about 1 in 4 slightly altered their lifestyles based on the results. About one-third shared the results with their physicians, many of whom did not know what to make of the information.

With genetic tests, consumers seem to be in one of two categories: the fatalists who consider inherited risk to be destiny that cannot be altered by changes in behavior, and those who believe they can make a difference with lifestyle changes.

Family history: The forgotten wallflower

Genetic tests have the aura of being scientific. But the old-fashioned family history appears to be more accurate and much less expensive.

A Cleveland Clinic researcher recruited 44 people to assess their risk of cancer by either preparing a family history or relying on a genetic test. Both indicated that about 40 percent had above-average risk—but picked the same people half the time. The genetic test did not identify the nine people who had a significant family history of colon cancer.

Likewise, researchers collected 101 genetic variants that had been tied statistically to heart disease in genome studies. They assessed and followed 19,000 women for 12 years to attempt to forecast disease. They concluded that the family history was a better predictor.

One reason family histories can be more accurate is that environment is a powerful influence on health. Family members generally share a common background, so the history reflects how shared genes expressed themselves in a given situation.

Family members often take important genetic information to their graves inadvertently without sharing it with relatives. According to one study, about 1 in 5 dying cancer patients could have shared important information with relatives through genetic counselors regarding the heritability of their conditions. In some instances, they could have left behind blood and tissue samples for future DNA testing. That would be a valuable legacy. (Genetic counselors help people understand their risk for genetic conditions. The National Society of Genetic Counselors website, *www.nsge. org*, lists them by zip code.)

Less than one-third of U.S. families have documented a health history, and many physicians are not particularly insistent that they have one. The U.S. surgeon general has established a website—*www.familyhistory.hhs.gov*—to help families create a history and share it with other relatives.

Many scientists have concluded that DTC genetic tests offer very little value. They say the increased risk posed by any given gene is so small that it is not information worth acting on. The best predictors of disease and death are already well known: age, gender, family history, health behavior and biomarkers such as blood pressure, blood glucose and cholesterol.

An international research consortium identified 18 new gene sites associated with obesity and 13 others tied to fat distribution in the body in 2010. The two studies, which one of the researchers called "exciting," will not have much immediate clinical impact.

Michael Jensen, an obesity expert at the Mayo Clinic, told *The Wall Street Journal*, "If you just ask people whether their parents were obese or not, the ability to predict whether a person is going to be obese is better" than by examining the identified genes.

A brighter future?

Such pessimism does not stop others from reaching for the genetic sky. Enthusiasts consider genetic knowledge an important building block to patient engagement. They see genetic profiling, advance directives, personal health records and shared medical decision-making by patients and doctors as important ways for all to seize the reins of their personal health. Health-care providers would become more like health coaches or advisers.

Dr. Robert Marion, chief of genetics and director of the Center for Congenital Disorders at Children's Hospital at Montefiore Medical Center in New York City, told HealthDay news service: "Medicine is going to change from waiting for symptoms to develop to knowing what this person is at risk for and being able to stop that from happening. Eventually, we're talking about prevention."

Marion said a doctor someday would be able to screen a newborn's 20,000 to 25,000 genes to predict specific genetic disorders, for about $5,000. The current cost is about $50,000.

However, significant challenges remain. Privacy remains a concern for many. Congress passed the Genetic Information Nondiscrimination Act (GINA) in 2008 to protect patients from discrimination by employers and insurance companies if tests reflect an elevated risk of disease. In fact, some characterize GINA as the genomics civil-rights bill.

Another barrier is that overloaded clinicians struggle to keep up with scientific and medical knowledge. Most are clueless about how to act on genetic information. When asked whom they trust most with their genomic data, patients invariably mention their physicians. However, according to a survey by Medco Health Solutions and the American Medical Association, only 10 percent of physicians said they were adequately informed about genetic testing to be able to write prescriptions based on that information.

A Baylor College of Medicine geneticist surveyed 225 Texas physicians about whether they would recommend genetic testing based on hypothetical cases. Most recommended tests that were unnecessary, and chose more comprehensive and expensive tests than were necessary. The difference in cost was $3,340, compared with $475 for the simpler test.

In many ways, technology is outrunning biology. A genetic test may be capable of detecting thousands of genetic variations for various conditions. However, they are unlikely to affect clinical decision-making if there is no practical treatment to counteract the perceived threat.

Patients clearly are misinterpreting what genetic tests are telling them and making poor decisions based on faulty conclusions. Physicians are not much better. Hank Greely, director of Stanford University's Center for Law and the Biosciences, called DTC genetic tests "reckless." He told *The Washington Post*, "Information is powerful, but misunderstood information can be powerfully bad."

Four genetic-policy experts, writing in the journal *Science*, encouraged everyone to slow down and take a deep breath. They said unrealistic expectations have created a "bubble" that is putting genomic science at risk. The authors encouraged scientists to be clearer about how scientific research works "by making responsible claims and by advocating that reporters and editors do the same."

Among their points:

- Despite the advances in pharmacogenetics, the most powerful predictor of whether a drug works is whether the patient takes it. That only happens about half the time.
- Diseases can be influenced by a large number of complex genes, making generalizations difficult for individuals as well as large populations.
- There is little evidence that genetic information affects health behavior.
- Genomic research will improve diagnostics and clinical treatment, but not for decades.

Businessweek chief economist Michael Mandel, commenting on research findings that only 1 out of 7 treatment recommendations by the Infectious Diseases Society of America were based on high-quality data, wrote: "The conventional wisdom was that breakthroughs in understanding the human genome would provide better treatments within the existing structure of medicine—like putting better windows or a new floor or more comfortable furniture into an existing house. But what if the main lesson of the past 10 years is that the house itself has rotten foundations and needs to be rebuilt completely?"

Francis Collins, director of the National Institutes of Health, said genomics "obeys the First Law of Technology: we invariably overestimate the short-term impacts of new technologies and underestimate the long-term effects."

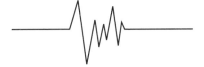

Chapter 10

Health-Care Disparities

'Causes of causes' of death and disease

Rapidly rising health-care costs are crowding out federal and state programs that have a greater effect on health than medical interventions do.

Public and preschool education, nutrition programs, environmental controls, public health and public housing are being cut back because of suffocatingly expensive government medical-insurance programs.

Medical care is a contributor to only 10 percent of premature deaths. Social circumstances—where people are born, live, work and play—and environmental factors determine 20 percent of disease and death. People with low income and education are more exposed to environmental harm. Disadvantaged circumstances also help drive health behavior and gene expression, which account for 40 and 30 percent of health respectively.

Some health-policy analysts believe these social determinants of health—low income, too little education, income inequality, discrimination and social exclusion—are the "cause of causes" of disease and death. Using a river analogy, these are considered the "upstream" factors of health. Health behavior and medical care are the "downstream" results. Advocates for social programs believe addressing upstream problems will significantly—and positively—affect downstream consequences.

Columbia University researchers recently reviewed research examining the social causes of death in 2000. The results were startling. They found that about 245,000 U.S. deaths were attributable to low levels of education; 176,000 to racial segregation; 162,000 to low social support; 133,000 to individual poverty, and 119,000 to income inequality. The 245,000 deaths attributed to low education far exceeded the 193,000 caused by heart attacks—the leading cause of death in 2000. The deaths attributed to racial segregation surpassed those caused by strokes—the No. 3 cause of death in 2000.

Health-promoting activity largely takes place outside medical settings. How people go about their daily lives determines individual—and ultimately, overall population—health. Daily choices on what to eat, whether to be physically active, whether to smoke and how to raise children are the most powerful influences. Individuals need to take responsibility for the choices that affect their health. Society's broader responsibility is to create conditions that will encourage healthier choices. Many Americans live and work in circumstances that make it extremely difficult to lead a healthy life.

The health effects of income, education, occupation, the environment, health behavior and access tend to operate jointly, confounding efforts to isolate and combat individual problems.

The key drivers are the components of socioeconomic status (SES)—income, education and occupation. Education creates opportunities for better health. It provides better odds of higher-paying employment with health benefits. Higher income affords the resources to buy foods that are more nutritious, stress-relieving leisure activities and housing in safe neighborhoods.

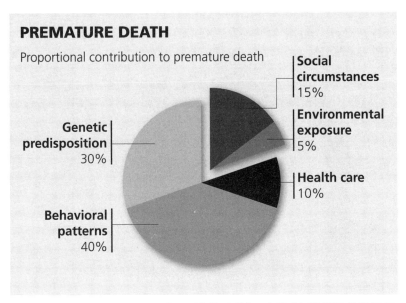

PREMATURE DEATH

Proportional contribution to premature death

Social circumstances 15%

Environmental exposure 5%

Genetic predisposition 30%

Health care 10%

Behavioral patterns 40%

Source: McGinnis JM, et al. *Health Aff.* 2002; 21(2):78-93.

Socio-economic circumstances and adverse environmental exposures are combined here as joint health determinants. Research shows that low-income people have the greatest exposure to air pollution, toxic chemicals and live in housing that does not meet local health and safety requirements.

Many Americans are unaware of SES-based health disparities. According to a recent survey, nearly three-quarters were aware of disparities between the poor and middle class. However, less than half were aware of racial health disparities, or that those in the middle class had poorer health than the rich. Barely more than one-third was aware of the link between education and health.

Education and income have what are known as gradient effects. This means there is a gradual improvement in health measures as each increases. Low-SES Americans have levels of illness in their 30s and 40s that are not seen in groups with higher SES, even three decades of age later.

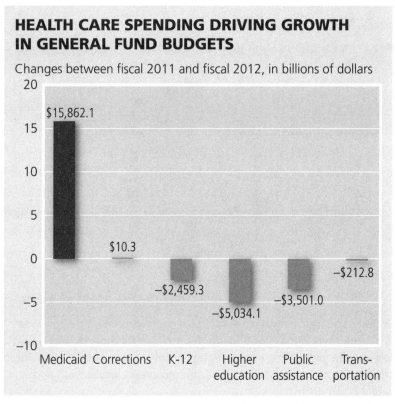

HEALTH CARE SPENDING DRIVING GROWTH IN GENERAL FUND BUDGETS

Changes between fiscal 2011 and fiscal 2012, in billions of dollars

Source: National Association of State Budget Officers.

The combined state budgets offer a one-year snapshot of the impact of Medicaid increases on other programs that also affect health. The fiscal 2011 data is based on enacted budgets and the fiscal 2012 data is based on governors' proposed budgets.

SES strongly reflects race and ethnicity, to the point that SES largely accounts for race-based health differences. Health differences by SES within each racial group often are larger than the overall racial differences in health. In other words, the health profile of low-income blacks looks more like that of low-income whites than of middle- or upper-income blacks.

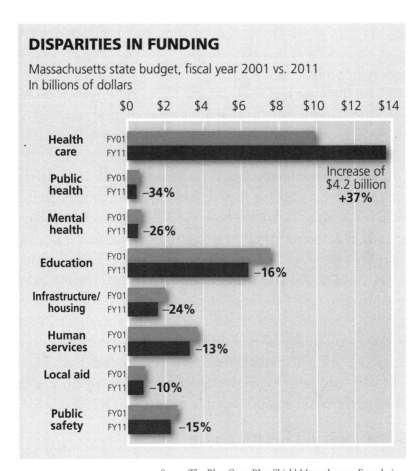

DISPARITIES IN FUNDING
Massachusetts state budget, fiscal year 2001 vs. 2011
In billions of dollars

Source: The Blue Cross Blue Shield Massachusetts Foundation.

The Massachusetts 2011 state budget illustrates how health-care costs squeeze other programs that may have important effects on population health. According to research, education attainment may be the most important social determinant of health. Bay State schools have suffered the largest cuts in absolute dollars in the past decade.

One exception is what is known as the "Hispanic paradox," which reflects the fact that Latino immigrants generally are healthier than non-Latinos of similar income and education. One explanation is that moving to a new country requires resilience and stamina. Other factors may be strong social and family support networks and that they are more likely to hold physically demanding jobs.

The "fight or flight" response to physical threats allowed prehistoric ancestors to summon bursts of physical and mental effort to confront immediate danger. Today's everyday threats are likely to be less dramatic and more persistent.

Low SES is strongly linked to this kind of chronic stress, which is likely to lead to diminished health. It can damage internal organs and impair the body's ability to turn off a constant state of alert. Scientists call this "allostatic load," or the price a body pays for adapting to challenges over long periods of time. Researchers in the MacArthur Study of Successful Aging have attempted to create an index of biological markers to measure allostatic load and assess its effect. They drew body fluids to assess the condition of an individual's nervous, cardiovascular, metabolic and inflammatory systems. They found that a high allostatic load is strongly associated with poor cognitive and physical functioning, cardiovascular disease and risk of death.

Social policy is health policy

If education and income are primary determinants of health, then social policies to improve both should improve health. This is reflected in Great Britain's 1998 Acheson report, an authoritative government-commissioned report that linked health disparities and social class. It noted that death rates had fallen between 1970 and 1990, but at a much steeper rate for higher social classes, creating a larger disparity between the haves and have-nots. The report recommended 39 policy steps in areas such as taxes, education, employment, housing, nutrition and agriculture to improve the health of lower-income citizens, although the entire population could benefit. The goal was to attack the social inequalities that reliably produce health inequalities.

The problem is that funding for social policies is much less stable than for medical care. Programs that address the needs of those who some believe are not deserving struggle to maintain support. Government is more likely to assist those who are considered not at fault for their vulnerability, such as children, the disabled and the elderly. Unwed mothers, substance abusers and ex-convicts attract far fewer sympathizers.

Social programs that boost education, food security, employment and neighborhood stability can be considered investment in disease prevention. However, government is far more inclined to intervene with expensive health-care services when medical conditions present themselves.

University of Oxford researchers analyzed the health effects of deep social-welfare budget cuts in Europe. They looked at funding for programs that support families and children, help the unemployed find jobs and assist the disabled, from 1980 to 2005.

The analysis showed a strong association between social spending and risk of death, especially from heart attacks and binge drinking. They found that when social-welfare spending was high, mortality rates fell. When spending fell, death rates rose substantially. They found no such effect from cuts in spending for the military or prisons.

Low SES is associated with poorer health behaviors. It accounts for higher rates of smoking, binge drinking, obesity and, ultimately, death. Many argue that risky behavior is only an indirect cause of poor health and is itself a consequence of low income and education and powerlessness. A 1998 study examined the degree to which four risk factors—cigarette smoking, alcohol consumption, inactivity and being overweight—contributed to the death rate at various income levels. Researchers found that poor health behavior explained only a small portion of the higher death rate for those with low SES. They concluded the death-rate disparity would persist even if the disadvantaged improved their health behavior to the level of those with more education and income. In other words, there was a wide array of factors involved beyond health behavior.

Many assume prompt, affordable health care improves the health of the socially disadvantaged. This medicalization of social reform encourages the view that health disparities can be solved by improving health-care access, use and quality. The result is that health-care access is overvalued and overemphasized, perhaps because medical interventions are easier to provide than fundamental social and economic reforms.

Canadian researchers wanted to find out whether lack of access to health care explained poor health for those with low SES. They tracked about 15,000 patients in the nation's universal health-care system for more than 10 years. They found that low-income Canadians used the health-care system more. The increased use had little impact on their poorer health outcomes, especially the death rate. Likewise, SES health disparities actually widened after Great Britain established the National Health Service, its publicly funded universal health-care system.

Although medical innovations are intended to improve population health, they actually worsen health disparities. The rich and well-educated have the resources to use them more readily and reap the benefits more swiftly. On the other hand, cost-effective public-health measures aimed at broad populations have the ability to decrease health disparities. Examples include water fluoridation, fortified food and environmental efforts against toxic substances.

Preschool pays big dividends

A group of 89 retired generals in 2009 released a report called *Ready, Willing and Unable to Serve*. According to the report, about 75 percent of young adults age 17 to 24 were ineligible for the military because they had failed to graduate from high school, were physically unfit or had a disqualifying criminal record.

The military leaders said early childhood education was critical to reversing this alarming trend. They urged Congress to pass the Obama administration-proposed Early Learning Challenge Fund, which would give states $1 billion annually for 10 years to pay for early childhood education. By 2011, the Obama administration scaled back the request to $350 million in its proposed 2012 budget.

The generals' report cited a famous study, begun in the 1960s, that followed a group of high-risk, low-income black children in Michigan. Half were randomly enrolled in preschool at ages 3 and 4, while the others were not. Participants were tracked until age 40. The preschoolers had significantly higher scores on IQ tests at age 5, and outperformed the others on basic school achievement, high school graduation and income.

A 2011 study reached similar conclusions. It followed about 1,500 Chicago children from preschool to age 28. The children, most of whom were black, lived in neighborhoods where nearly 40 percent of the residents lived below the poverty line. Those who attended preschool were less likely to have eventual substance-abuse problems or be imprisoned. They also had higher incomes and were more likely to attend a four-year college than those who had not attended preschool.

Education's role in health

The impact of education on health and health disparities is a thoroughly researched topic. Many researchers have found its effect is greater than that of income. There is some debate whether income, in itself, protects health beyond the effect of education. In the U.S., however, it appears they are separately protective.

According to one analysis, giving everyone the death rate of those who attended college would save seven times as many lives as those saved by biomedical innovations. People with bachelor's degrees are four times less likely than those without a high school education to report being in fair or poor health.

A *Review of Economic Studies* journal article examined state-mandated extensions of compulsory education in the first half of the 20th century. According to the study, every extra year of required education translated into an average of up to 18 months of additional life after age 35.

In developed nations, each additional year of educational attainment reduces the death rate by 8 percentage points. Each additional year of education also increases income by an average of 8 percentage points, which also appears to lower an individual's death rate independently from education. Therefore, education reduces mortality twice—directly, and through higher earnings.

If adults who did not complete high school died at the same rate as college graduates, 190,000 fewer Americans would have died in 2006. On average, these 190,000 would have lived an extra 20 years.

The life-course model of health suggests that the ability to protect children from health risks is linked directly to reducing chronic conditions, disability and even premature death. In essence, children who fall behind because of disadvantage never catch up.

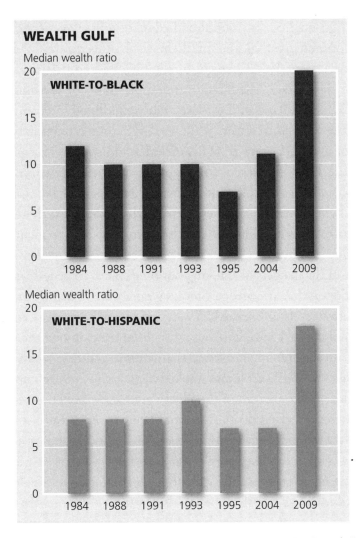

Source: Pew Research Center.

Racial and ethnic wealth disparities have grown significantly during the recent recession. Median net worth of white households is 20 times greater than that of black households and 18 times greater than that of Hispanic households. In dollars, the average white household was worth $113,149, compared with $6,325 for Hispanics and $5,677 for blacks. These wealth inequalities are the worst since the federal government began tracking the data about 25 years ago.

High-quality early childhood education improves cognitive development, verbal and mathematical skills and behavioral function. Less than 3 percent of eligible children participate in Early Head Start, a federally funded program for low-income families with infants and toddlers. Early childhood interventions have been found to return $8 to $14 in lifetime economic benefits for every $1 invested. This includes additional government revenue from increased employment, less incarceration and crime, and lower enrollment in government-assistance programs.

There are several theories on why education has such a large impact on health. Education may be a proxy for being patient and delaying gratification. For example, less-educated people are fully aware of the dangers of smoking but they appear to be less willing to act upon that knowledge. Smoking rates were similar among all education levels before the U.S. surgeon general's landmark report on smoking in 1964. Smoking rates plummeted among the educated after the report, and that disparity remains today. Nearly half of those with GED diplomas smoked cigarettes in 2009, compared with less than 6 percent of those with graduate-school degrees.

Better-educated people are more likely to wear seat belts, eat more nutritional food, have lower body mass indexes and use more preventive medical services. Each additional year of education incrementally reduces the incidence of high blood pressure.

Education's health benefits also span generations. Better-educated parents have healthier children, and they grow up to be healthier adults.

Of all social programs, education enjoys the broadest political support and is the most easily modified component of SES. Unfortunately, low educational attainment is a national problem. About 30 percent of high school freshmen fail to graduate in four years. In the 50 largest U.S. cities, that rate is nearly 50 percent. The U.S. is the only industrialized nation where those in the current generation are less likely to be high school graduates than those in their parents' generation.

The effects of income

Income affects health in two positive ways: a direct effect on material conditions that sustain survival, and the ability to control one's life circumstances and maintain a sense of optimism. Higher income allows people to live in neighborhoods that are safe, have pleasant surroundings for physical activity and an ample supply of nutritious food.

A 25-year-old man living in a family earning more than $84,000 can expect to live nearly eight years longer than a 25-year-old in a family earning less than $21,000. That is approximately the same effect that having heart disease has on life expectancy.

The U.S. poverty rate was above 13 percent in 2008, the highest since 1997. That translates to about 40 million people. The 2008 poverty threshold was an annual income of $22,025 for a family of four. The U.S. has higher rates of poverty and worse health indicators than other affluent nations, which may explain the comparatively low U.S. ranking on life expectancy and infant mortality.

A task force of the Center for American Progress, a progressive public-policy think tank, has proposed a set of policies that it says would cut U.S. poverty in half. The task force estimated that its proposals would cost $90 billion annually, which is about 10 percent of federal health-care spending. The policies include cash transfers similar to those enacted in Great Britain. The proposals include subsidized housing, raising the minimum wage, guaranteeing child care and early childhood education for low-income families.

Such proposals would be difficult to implement in the U.S. Survey data show most Americans are much more willing to

spend tax dollars to redress health disparities in access and outcomes than on unequal conditions in housing, education and
income. However, Social Security set a historic precedent on
reducing poverty. The U.S. elderly poverty rate in 1997 was
about 12 percent. Without Social Security, the rate would have
been more than 47 percent.

Other determinants of health:
Class, race and inequality

Besides education and income, researchers cite other social forces
at work that contribute to health disparities. Income inequality
in a community, rather than an individual's income, appears to
be harmful to health to those at the bottom of the ladder. There
is also a substantial body of research, especially in Great Britain,
indicating that social-class rank has a powerful impact on health.

People who unfavorably compare themselves with others who
have more status and possessions and better life circumstances
create biological changes that negatively affect their health. They
feel shame, worthlessness and envy, which can impair metabolism, immunity and the nervous system. Some attempt to cope
with these feelings by overspending, or overextending themselves
by taking a second job. Others self-medicate with overeating,
smoking or substance abuse.

The notion of social class is a somewhat unfamiliar construct
in U.S. policymaking. Beyond education and income, class distinctions include occupations that boost self-esteem and freedom
to dictate personal working conditions. Perhaps because of the
nation's history, Americans are more attuned to race than class.
There is broad acceptance of the injustice of racial disparities
in health.

Class distinctions draw less attention, perhaps because many
consider them the inevitable results of market forces. The de-

cline of organized labor since World War II has diminished class awareness. Both race and class have distinctive effects on health. However, many U.S. researchers believe class has a more powerful effect. One comprehensive review of evidence that compared race and class concluded: "Socioeconomic differences between racial groups are largely responsible for the patterns of racial disparities in health status."

The U.S. government is one of the few developed Western nations that do not report health statistics by class. For example, the U.S. Census Bureau annually reports life expectancy by age, sex and race. Class-based statistics would include income, education and occupation.

Great Britain tracks markers of social class. Researchers have produced three major studies of the effect of class distinctions on health. The British began including one of five occupational categories, ranging from unskilled to professional, on death certificates starting in 1911. A 1980 study, called the Black report, concluded that there were health inequalities among English social classes. The 1984 Whitehall study of British civil servants found the death rates of those in each job rank were higher than of those in the class above, displaying a classic gradient effect. The 1998 Acheson report showed that death rates between 1970 and 1990 had fallen for all social classes. However, the rate had fallen more sharply in higher social classes, creating an even greater disparity.

The outcomes in the Whitehall study largely were accounted for by the differences in control in the workplace. People in high-status jobs typically have staff support and a high degree of control over their work and working conditions. Many people in lower-status jobs experience chronic stress because of a lack of control over their work and physical demands that inflict wear and tear on the body.

Social status itself, aside from income and control, has health benefits—often a result of self-esteem. One intriguing study found that actors and actresses who win Academy Awards live nearly four years longer than those who were merely nominated. The study, which seems a bit whimsical, had a robust sample of more than 1,600 performers and successfully accounted for a number of confounding factors.

Racial health disparities often are a proxy for class. Blacks are overrepresented in disadvantaged socioeconomic groups. Racial differences also tend to disappear once statistics are adjusted for class-based indicators. In addition, the majority of those below the poverty line in the U.S. are white.

The alleged role of racial genetic differences in health has been debated and discredited by authoritative research. The controversy over supposed racial differences in biology dates back to the Civil War. In fact, both sides of the slavery debate looked to medical science to determine the answer to a critical question: Are blacks innately inferior to whites and therefore fit only to be slaves?

Social circumstances and class differences trump genetics. For example, the rate of hypertension of blacks in the Caribbean was up to five times lower than that of blacks in the U.S. and Great Britain. More starkly, a man is more likely to live past the age of 40 in Bangladesh than in New York City's Harlem.

U.S. income inequality is greater than that of other industrialized nations, and is widening. From 1997 to 2007, those in the top 10 percent of households generated nearly two-thirds of overall income growth. The income growth for the bottom 20 percent: 0.4 percent.

The combined net worth of the 400 wealthiest Americans in 2007 was $1.5 trillion. The combined net worth of the poorest 50 percent of U.S. households was $1.6 trillion. The average hourly wage in 1972, adjusted for inflation, was $20.06. In 2008, it was $18.52.

Between 1978 and 2005, the average compensation of corporate chief executive officers increased from 35 times the average worker's pay to 262 times. The typical CEO earned more in an hour than a minimum-wage worker earned in a month.

The racial and ethnic wealth gap widened significantly during the recent recession. The median wealth of white U.S. households was $113,119 in 2009, compared with $6,325 for Hispanics and $5,677 for blacks. The white-to-black household wealth ratio was 20 to 1 and the white-Hispanic ratio was 17. The ratio for both groups was 7 to 1 in 1995.

The American Dream increasingly seems unattainable. Only 8 percent of U.S. men make the "rags to riches" climb from the lowest to the highest fifth in income in one generation, compared with 11 to 14 percent in other industrialized nations.

The widening income gap seems to be eroding American confidence. Less than one-third of U.S. voters in 2006 election exit polls said they believed the next generation would enjoy a better life than they did. In fact, this appears to be happening to the current generation. Men in their 30s in 2004 had a median income of about $35,000. Men in their fathers' generation who are now in their 60s had a median income of $40,000, adjusted for inflation, when they were in their 30s. In a separate poll, more than half of U.S. adults said they believed the American Dream was no longer attainable for most Americans.

Environmental justice

Environmental risk factors are underappreciated as causes of disease and death. A World Health Organization (WHO) report attributed about one-quarter of the world's disease to environmental risk factors. It also estimated that those risk factors contributed to nearly 85 percent of the diseases it reviewed.

Pollution and chemical exposures affect everyone. More than 80,000 synthetic chemicals have been introduced in the U.S. in the last 50 years and are used in millions of consumer products. The Environmental Protection Agency has identified about 3,000 high-volume chemicals produced in the U.S. in quantities of more than a million pounds annually. In surveys by the Centers for Disease Control and Prevention, traces of 200 of these high-volume chemicals have been found in the blood and urine of nearly every American, including pregnant women. The health effects of these chemicals largely are unknown.

However, numerous studies have documented how poor people are more likely to be exposed to environmental hazards in their homes and neighborhoods and on the job. They live closer to hazardous waste and industrial facilities. They are also more likely to have greater exposure to air pollution, pesticides and lead—all of which can impair health.

The concept of "environmental justice" emerged in the 1980s. Its proponents have fought the increased exposure to environmental hazards that is suffered by disadvantaged groups.

Nearly one-fifth of the U.S. population lives in neighborhoods where at least 20 percent of residents are poor. Poor neighborhoods represent the intersection of heightened environmental risks and a population already vulnerable to disease and death because of low socioeconomic status.

Substandard housing also increases exposure to lead paint, mold, dust and pest infestation. About 2.6 million blacks and 5.9 million whites live in housing that violates residential building codes. However, the National Center for Healthy Housing estimates as many as 1 out of 3 homes in U.S. metropolitan areas have at least one problem that can harm health, such as water leaks, peeling paint or rodent infestations.

In addition to residential environmental hazards, the poor and minority groups disproportionately encounter hazardous occupational exposures. They are also more likely to bring chemicals home on their clothing, further contaminating their residences. Toxins from cigarette smoke also are more likely to be present. Smoking is two to four times more prevalent among those with less than a high school education.

Disparities also exist in rural areas close to agricultural facilities. Livestock and produce bring pesticide exposure, soil contamination and water pollution. Agriculture also is among the most hazardous occupations because of frequent accidents, lung disease and cancer from chemical and sun exposure.

The WHO blamed one-third of childhood disease on environmental factors, primarily in developing countries. Children have greater exposure to toxic chemicals because they weigh less than adults. A 6-month-old drinks seven times more water and has twice as much air intake per pound of body weight as an adult. A child eats three to four times more calories per pound of body weight than an adult. These differences heighten the risk of toxins in air, water and food.

A study of Michigan public schools found that those located in areas with the highest air-pollution levels had the lowest attendance rates and highest proportions of students who failed to meet the state educational-testing standards.

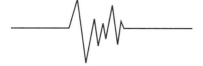

Chapter 11

Prevention
What's too much and what's too little?

When 2008 Democratic presidential candidate Hillary Clinton unveiled her $110 billion health-care plan, one of her strategies for paying that bill was savings resulting from disease prevention and "wellness."

Not to be outdone, her Democratic rival Barack Obama said improved disease prevention and chronic-disease management would save $81 billion toward his plan for reform.

As with most presidential-campaign proposals, there were few details, such as how prevention was being defined and how savings would result. But these claims were reminiscent of presidential candidate Ronald Reagan's pledge to balance the federal budget by eliminating government mismanagement, fraud and abuse. Relying on people to change their health habits, thus ultimately creating the funds to help cover the cost of health reform, was and is a fairy tale.

The Congressional Budget Office (CBO) estimated the 2010 health-reform law would reduce the federal deficit. However, it refused to attribute any savings to the law's requirement that insurance plans cover preventive services for free. The CBO cited a lack of clinical evidence of the effectiveness of many prevention measures, and said that widespread use of preventive services might cost more than is later saved on treating preventable disease.

No one opposes preventive health measures. As a political stance, none is safer. Bad habits do not have many advocates. All of us grew up hearing the aphorism: "An ounce of prevention is worth a pound of cure." Hardly anyone challenged that.

Prevention is one of the most popular components of the new health-reform law. Nearly 3 out of 4 Americans favor increased investment in disease prevention. And nearly the same number believes prevention will save money.

Advocates correctly point out that the U.S. spends billions on medical services of questionable value while pennies on the dollar are spent on preventive services.

What is it—and does it pay off?

There are three kinds of prevention.

Primary prevention focuses on community-wide efforts to reduce disease in everyone. This is usually called public health. Some examples are mass immunizations, air-pollution controls and public-service campaigns to reduce smoking and other risky behavior. So-called "sin taxes" on cigarettes and alcohol are a form of primary prevention.

Secondary prevention is primarily screening to detect diseases such as cancer and heart disease in their early stages, in an effort to reduce severity. But screening does not prevent them.

Tertiary prevention attempts to keep disease under control after it has developed. This is also known as chronic-disease management, and is the most expensive form of prevention. There is an entire chapter devoted to this subject later in this book.

The bottom line is that most preventive services do not save money immediately. But that might not be the point. Prevention advocates correctly argue that most medical treatment does not

- Eliminates cost-sharing for preventive services that are recommended by the United States Preventive Services Task Force (USPSTF) in Medicare and Medicaid. Effective in 2011.
- Offers Medicare beneficiaries free access to a comprehensive health-risk assessment and creation of a personalized prevention plan. Effective in 2011.

HEALTH CARE REFORM

Prevention

- Requires health plans to provide government-recommended preventive services and immunizations recommended by the USPSTF without deductibles or copayments. Effective in 2010.
- Creates the Prevention and Public Health Fund to expand research, outreach campaigns and access to preventive services. Effective in 2010.
- Creates the National Prevention, Health Promotion and Public Health Council and authorizes $2 billion in initial funding to coordinate federal prevention, wellness and public-health activities. Effective in 2010.
- Initiates a five-year grant program aimed at strengthening prevention services, reducing rates of chronic disease and addressing health disparities. Effective in 2010.

save money, and that holding prevention to the different standard is unfair. The larger issue, they say, is to determine the best way to allocate health-care dollars to improve Americans' health.

Steven Woolf, a physician and Virginia Commonwealth University professor, argues that health is a commodity, just like a new car or a loaf of bread. Those are bought for their non-monetary value—in this case, transportation or nourishment. They are not meant to save money. But they are expected to provide good value.

How much should an additional healthy year of life cost? The rule of thumb seems to be $100,000 or less for what health-policy experts call a "quality-adjusted life year." It is easy to spend far more than that when disease-prevention efforts include a mostly healthy, low-risk population.

Placing an economic value on life is a tricky business. The Environmental Protection Agency valued an individual American's life at $9.1 million when it proposed more stringent air-pollution controls in 2010. That is up from $6.8 million, the figure the agency used during when George W. Bush was president. The Food and Drug Administration's number is $7.9 million, up from $5 million in 2008.

It is likewise difficult to tote up prevention cost-effectiveness. For example, adult cigarette smoking causes multiple chronic conditions and sickens children in the household. Secondhand smoke affects the public in places where smoking is not banned. How do you account for the value of tobacco-cessation programs for the damage *not* caused by smoking?

Timing can also be an issue. Obese children almost inevitably become obese adults. If the condition could somehow be altered early in life, the personal and societal payoff would be enormous and compounded annually.

How much prevention costs depends on how it is delivered. An out-of-shape, overweight man can transform his health by deciding to change his diet and frequenting a local hiking trail. That cost is no more than an adjustment of the weekly grocery bill and a pair of sneakers, and it stays within the household. He profits by having a longer and healthier life. His insurance company pays less for his medical bills. His employer has a more energetic and engaged employee. Everyone wins, and the cost is peanuts.

If the man is not self-motivated, the costs start to mount and effectiveness becomes less certain. Perhaps his doctor has to spend time counseling him about potential health risks. Or his company has to offer him a cash incentive to work out.

Woolf contends that people often conflate the value of programs with the effectiveness of the behavior. The programs encouraging exercise cost money. But the resulting behavior likely saves money. This confusion can obscure positive public-health messages.

A final, and perhaps more cynical, point is that preventive services account for a tiny percentage of health-care costs. The big money is in treating disease. It is not that the health-care system wishes people ill. But most health-care marketing is about the wonders of medical technology and dealing with expensive conditions.

Public health

Of the 30-year increase in U.S. average life expectancy in the last century, only five years can be credited to advances in medical care. The 25 other years are credited to public health, yet less than 1 percent of Americans can define the mission of public health.

Public-health measures virtually eliminated the scourge of infectious disease through efforts to provide clean and fluoridated drinking water, better sanitation, widespread immunization, motor-vehicle and occupational safety, family planning, smoke-free public places and chronic-disease management.

Public health differs from medical care in two distinctive ways. First, public health is aimed at prevention rather than the curative aspects of health. Second, it deals with collective, population-level health, while medical care generally is individual.

Public health more broadly promotes healthier lifestyles and addresses environmental factors to prevent widespread illness on a community level. Medicine focuses on diagnosis and treatment of specific diseases with drugs, surgery and medical technology.

Because public health addresses large populations, it has more potential to lessen health disparities cost-effectively. Research has repeatedly shown that effective public-health programs and disease-prevention initiatives can reduce cancer, heart disease and diabetes, as well as continue to suppress infectious diseases.

Despite widespread support for disease prevention, less than 5 percent of U.S. health-care spending goes toward public health. Public-health activities primarily are carried out by state and local governments. Departments vie for scarce resources from government entities that by law usually must balance their budgets. As a result, public health is destined to be underfunded, especially in a difficult economy.

By contrast, the economics of medicine are immune from these constraints, as evidenced by the fact that health-care costs rise at a significantly higher rate annually than the overall Consumer Price Index.

Trust for America's Health (TFAH), a nonpartisan advocacy group, estimates that an annual $10-per-person investment in proven disease-prevention programs based in communities could save more than $16 billion annually in medical costs within five years—a return on investment of more than 5 to 1.

Local public-health funding varies dramatically. The top 20 percent of communities in public-health funding spend more than 13 times the amount of the lowest 20 percent. More spending translates into better health surveillance and research, and lower mortality rates. A 2011 *Health Affairs* journal study found that death rates fell between 1 and 7 percent for each 10 percent increase in local public health spending.

More than half of local health department budgets are funded by federal and state governments. Federal funding in recent years has remained relatively flat, while state and local support has waned because of the recession. The average state budget's projected deficit was 24 percent in 2010, and 29 states projected deficits for 2011.

About 15,000 local public-health jobs were eliminated in 18 months from 2008 to mid-2009, according to a survey by the National Association of County and City Health Officials. In 2009, 51 percent of existing jobs were affected by reduced hours and salaries. About 55 percent of local health departments and 76 percent of state health departments were affected by cuts.

The $35 billion spent on U.S. public health each year is about $20 billion short of optimum funding for critical programs, according to a 2008 analysis by TFAH and the New York Academy of Medicine.

Clinical services

Only about half of Americans use clinical preventive services—counseling, screening, immunizations—every year. That is the case even when insurance pays the entire bill.

Preventive measures have uneven value, and some of the most effective are not promoted nearly enough. Only 28 percent of smokers are advised to quit by their physicians. Only about one-third of adults get an annual flu shot. Fewer than half take aspirin daily to prevent heart disease. Partnership for Prevention calculates that 100,000 lives a year would be saved if Americans took advantage of the five most effective preventive services.

A New York City Health Department simulation estimated that 50,000 to 100,000 lives per year would be saved by a 10 percent increase in use of nine preventive services, including cardiovascular screening and treatment, cancer screening, smoking cessation and daily aspirin use.

If 90 percent of Americans used the 20 most effective preventive services, 2 million years of life and $3.7 billion would have been saved in 2006, according to a 2011 *Health Affairs* journal study. The dollar savings only represent 0.2 percent of U.S. health-care costs.

The best source for advice on preventive services is the U.S. Preventive Services Task Force (USPSTF), an independent panel of non-government experts sponsored by the U.S. Agency for Healthcare Research and Quality. The USPSTF rigorously assessed the latest scientific evidence regarding effectiveness of about 200 clinical preventive services, including screening, counseling and medications.

The 16-member panel calculates the benefits and risks of individual services, and recommends which ones should be included routinely in primary care for specific populations. The group assigns grades from A to D, based on effectiveness. Because of the health-reform law, nearly 90 million Americans with employer or individual insurance—as well as Medicare—will not have to pay a deductible or co-payment for services the USPSTF has graded A or B.

The USPSTF does not weigh cost-effectiveness, only scientific effectiveness. However, many others do.

For example, the National Commission on Prevention Priorities reviewed 21 services recommended by the USPSTF as of December 2004. It found that five reduced costs while the 16 others increased medical expenses.

TFAH argues that prevention programs would save $16 billion over five years, a return of $5.60 per $1 invested.

A 5 percent reduction in the number of people diagnosed with diabetes and high-blood pressure through preventive efforts would save $9 billion a year immediately, and savings would rise eventually to nearly $25 billion.

That is an enticing number. But many such calculations do not take into account the cost of prevention services applied to a broad population.

A 2008 study estimated the cost of treating heart disease and diabetes would be $9.5 trillion. A comprehensive cardiovascular disease prevention program of up to 11 services would cut treatment costs by 10 percent, but at the hefty price tag of $8.5 trillion. Therefore, total treatment and prevention costs would be an extra $7.6 trillion.

One of the reasons for the sticker-shock price tag: The study calculated that more than 3 out of 4 adults ages 20 to 80 were candidates for at least one heart-disease prevention intervention.

A 2007 study illustrated how expensive it is to combat heart disease, especially in those with a low risk. Prevention expert Louise Russell calculated that broad use of statins to lower cholesterol would cost $85,000 to $924,000 for every healthy year gained, depending upon the risk profile of the patient.

How broadly are statins used? One out of 4 Americans 45 or older take them, compared with about 2 percent 20 years ago.

Cardiovascular prevention can be expensive even without procedures or statins. Researchers had Australian doctors watch a video and read a booklet on how to help their patients prevent heart attacks. The patients also received a series of videos and a booklet. For low-risk women, this seemingly harmless intervention cost $9.8 million for every year saved from a premature heart attack.

Even high-risk patients can be expensive. Russell determined that an intensive program of personalized exercise and diet plans and ongoing counseling could cut diabetes cases in half, but the cost would be $192,000 for every healthy year gained.

Researchers reviewed hundreds of preventive-care studies for a *New England Journal of Medicine* article and concluded that less than 20 percent of the methods studied saved money.

Prevention becomes more cost-effective when it is targeted to narrower, at-risk populations, and at the proper frequency.

For example, screening 35-year-olds for diabetes costs $130,000 for every healthy year gained. Screening 75-year-olds for high blood pressure costs $32,000 per healthy year gained. Russell illustrated the effect of frequency. Pap smears to screen for cervical cancer every three years would cost $41,000 per healthy year gained. The cost rises to $1.3 million if the screening is done every two years, and $3.3 million if done annually.

Consumer Reports, better known for rating cars and kitchen appliances, surveyed its subscribers about nine medical screenings for cardiovascular risk. The organization concluded that 44 percent of health adults were getting unnecessary heart disease screenings that may even be harmful for people without symptoms.

The pros and cons of screening

Many consider routine screening almost a duty, not unlike voting. But there are disadvantages as well as advantages.

Screening can detect medical conditions before symptoms present themselves. The best-case scenario is that treatment is more effective in a disease's early stages and perhaps lives are saved.

But there are several downsides:

- Screening people with low disease risk is expensive and needlessly clogs the medical system.
- Screening can produce anxiety, discomfort, and exposure to radiation and chemicals.
- A false positive can be stressful and lead to additional expensive tests and possibly unnecessary treatment.

- A false negative, on the other hand, creates a misleading sense of security that could delay a definitive diagnosis.

False-positive screening results can be unsettlingly high. One in 5 falsely tested positive for syphilis, according to a recent CDC study of five U.S. laboratories. This no doubt led to unnecessary treatment and untold anguish.

In a national survey, nearly 9 out of 10 adults said they believed that cancer screening is almost always a good thing, and 3 out of 4 said it saves lives. But more than 1 out of 3 had received a false-positive screening test, and more than 40 percent of those called it "very scary" or the "scariest time of my life." Remarkably, 3 out of 4 said they would choose to get a full-body CT screening instead of $1,000 in cash—despite no scientific evidence of the screening's benefit or safety.

Many credit widespread cancer screening for an increase in the five-year survival rate of cancer patients. But a comprehensive review of the 20 most common tumors from 1950 to 1995 showed that screening simply identified the cancer earlier and patients were aware of it longer. There was little effect on the death rate.

The sad truth is that the deadliest cancer sprouts and kills so quickly that routine screening rarely catches it. Cancer screening finds lots of what Dr. Gilbert Welch of Dartmouth Medical School calls pseudo-disease. That is an abnormality that meets the criteria of being cancerous but will never grow to become harmful. High-resolution MRIs and CT scans are especially good at discovering these. However, the doctor and patient often feel compelled to do something. This often leads to unnecessary treatment that can create harmful side effects.

Dr. Laura Esserman is director of the breast cancer center at the University of California, San Francisco. She was co-author of an essay in the *Journal of the American Medical Association* reflecting on her experience. She wrote: "After (25 years) of screening for breast and prostate cancer, conclusions are troubling: Overall cancer rates are higher, many more patients are being treated, and the absolute incidence of aggressive or later-stage disease has not been significantly decreased. Screening has had some effect, but it comes at a significant cost, including over-diagnosis, overtreatment, and complications of therapy."

Oddly, people with advanced cancer continue to be screened long after there is any useful purpose. Up to 1 in 5 Medicare patients with poor-prognosis cancer were screened for cholesterol, prostate cancer and breast cancer. Researchers speculated that screening is such an ingrained habit that the terminal patients believed they should continue to do what they have always done regardless of their circumstances. Why health-care providers indulged them is another issue.

The number needed to treat (NNT) is a useful health statistic that measures the effectiveness of a preventive service to avoid one additional bad outcome, such as death or a heart attack. The idea is that one person would benefit by a screening or medication while everyone else would incur the expense, anxiety and potential harm of the intervention.

Welch calculated NNT for mammography to save the life of a 50-year-old woman. Five women out of 1,000 would die of breast cancer without mammography. To lower that rate to four women, 1,000 women would be screened annually for 10 years. What happens to the other 999 screened women?

- 2 to 10 women will be overdiagnosed and treated needlessly.
- 10 to 15 will learn they have breast cancer earlier than they would have otherwise, but their prognosis will not change.

- 100 to 500 women will have at least one "false alarm," and about half of these will have a biopsy.

In another example, 53,000 men ages 55 to 74 with a history of heavy smoking received CT scans to detect early lung cancer. News reports hailed the results, saying the risk of lung cancer was reduced by 20 percent. But according to the NNT in this study, 300 would need to be screened to extend the life of one person. What about the other 299? One out of 4 had a false positive, resulting in a cascade of more tests, radiation, anxiety and biopsies. The cost of each CT scan is about $300.

An earlier study showed a false-positive rate of 33 percent for those who had two lung CT scans. Among those, 7 percent had either a biopsy or surgery, or both.

Patients don't do it anyway

Many patients do not pursue preventive care even when someone else is paying for it. Americans use preventive services at about half the recommended rate. A survey by the Midwest Business Group on Health found that 88 percent of workers do not value preventive services, and 56 percent said they have no motivation to stay healthy.

That might not be a completely bad thing.

If everyone received the services recommended by the USP-STF, every U.S. physician would have to spend 7.4 hours a day on prevention.

Unlike screening, immunization has a stellar track record. The CDC named vaccination as one of the 10 greatest public-health achievements of the 20th century. Infectious diseases such as diarrhea and tuberculosis that were among the leading causes of death around 1900 have been virtually wiped out as fatal diseases.

The health-care system correctly is a strong advocate of infant and child immunization. Pediatric offices have well-established protocols to administer vaccines. School systems mandate that children be immunized to enroll.

Adult immunization is a different story. Patients and health-care providers tend to undervalue it. As a result, adults represent 95 percent of the more than 50,000 annual deaths that could be avoided with immunization.

Patients have a hard time grasping the value of prevention, unlike disease treatment. A National Foundation for Infectious Diseases poll showed less than half of respondents knew influenza was a vaccine-preventable disease. Less than 1 in 5 could name a second example, such as pneumonia. About half were either not very concerned or not "at all" concerned about a family member or themselves getting a vaccine-preventable disease.

People question the safety of the vaccines themselves. For example, nearly half of Americans still believe there is a link between autism and vaccines. The original research by a British physician asserting such a connection was retracted, and the doctor has been barred from practicing medicine.

Health-care providers are nearly as unenthusiastic as their patients about adult immunization. They often lose money administering adult vaccines, and the supply pipeline has been unreliable. But nearly 9 out of 10 patients said they likely would be immunized if their doctor recommended it.

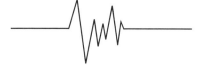

Workplace Wellness

Health as a tangible asset

Enlightened businesses correctly treat employee health as a precious asset. To be competitive in the marketplace, a company needs healthy and productive workers.

Many companies offer incentives to change destructive behavior. They provide tools and guidance for employees to manage their health. In return, these companies have healthier, happier and more productive employees who take fewer sick days. The best-run "wellness programs," as they are customarily called, have a return on investment (ROI) far in excess of program costs. Those programs essentially have no health-related expense increases from year to year.

Businesses have an enormous incentive to control costs. Nearly 60 percent of an average company's after-tax profits are spent on corporate health benefits. Starbucks, for example, spends more on health benefits for its workers than it does for wholesale coffee beans.

If government insurance programs and all health insurance plans could do the same for all Americans, there would be a similar ROI. Unfortunately, this is not politically feasible. Public policy maintains a laser focus on accessibility and affordability for those who are sick. That does not lower health-care costs or improve the quality of constituents' lives.

Forward-thinking businesses believe that employee health is too important to rely on the broader health-care system. They create healthy environments that reward individual effort and build self-esteem. They help pay for the treatment of illness, but they place equal emphasis on keeping employees' health from deteriorating. In short, they play offense (offering compelling programs) rather than defense (waiting for employees to get sick).

Dee Edington, a University of Michigan professor, has been studying workplace health for decades. His research shows that the correlation between disease and health-care costs is highly predictable. High-risk employees produce high costs 70 to 83 percent of the time and low-risk employees are low-cost 90 percent of the time. A company's health-care costs follow the same direction as its employees' aggregate health risks. As risks rise, so do costs. As they fall, so do costs.

The goal, according to Edington, is to achieve what he calls "zero trend." That means health-care costs do not rise faster than the Consumer Price Index. When employees "don't get worse," a company is rewarded with a zero cost trend.

Employee wellness is an imprecise term with several meanings. It customarily refers to programs offered by businesses to enhance the health and happiness of employees and thus improve productivity and lower health-care costs. They typically identify employee health risks and poor behaviors, and attempt to address them systematically before they become expensive chronic conditions. They most frequently address tobacco use, poor nutrition, excess weight, chronic stress and substance abuse. Some programs broaden wellness efforts to include financial planning, career guidance and community involvement.

- Allows employers to offer rewards of up to a 30 percent discount of the cost of insurance coverage for participating in wellness activities and meeting health standards beginning in 2014. The law authorizes that reward to be increased to 50 percent by the executive branch of the federal government.

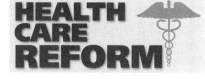

- Provides grants for up to five years to small employers that create wellness programs beginning in 2011.

According to a 2010 international survey of 1,200 organizations, two-thirds had a formal wellness strategy, compared with less than half three years earlier. Three out of 4 North American employers offered wellness programs. About 12 percent without them plan to offer them within two years.

In most of the world, employee stress is the major driver of wellness strategies. In the U.S., where two-thirds of employees are obese or overweight, the primary goal is physical activity, followed by nutrition. The top U.S. strategic objective is to reduce health-care and insurance costs. Elsewhere, the main objective is employee productivity.

Large employers consider wellness programs nearly as important as processing insurance claims. More than three-quarters of large employers believe wellness programs are important, compared with about half of small businesses.

These programs enjoy broad political support because they have little government funding or oversight, and they help reduce health-care costs without rationing care. Many businesses take on wellness as a responsibility because employees spend almost half of their waking hours in the workplace. Safe working conditions and a corporate culture of healthfulness can have a big impact on individual health. Workplaces suffered 5,000 fatalities and 4 million work-related injuries and illnesses in 2007, costing businesses nearly $90 billion in treatment expenses and lost productivity.

The 21st-century U.S. economy is increasingly reliant on knowledge and service workers and less so on manufacturing. Workforce health issues have slowly shifted from workplace accidents to sedentary- and stress-related ailments such as anxiety, lower back pain and obesity.

The corporate responsibility for wellness has been heightened by the spread of consumer-directed health plans (CDHP) that feature higher deductibles. If a CDHP is not complemented by a wellness program, it is tantamount to shifting the costs of health care to the employee. CDHP is about giving the employee more responsibility. Wellness programs provide the tools.

Wellness programs typically include employee health-risk assessments (HRA), followed by interventions targeted at the risks that have been revealed. Management of chronic conditions, such as diabetes, heart disease and high blood pressure, receives the greatest attention because it is responsible for about 75 percent of health-care costs.

Employers are certainly grumpy about having to play such an active role in their employees' health. About 2 out of 3 employers blame their workers' poor habits for rising health-care costs. The majority believe some of their employees simply are not engaged enough in their health to change their destructive habits.

Health reform will provide added incentives for businesses to augment wellness programs. The law will allow employers to offer deeper premium discounts to reward healthy behavior, such as not smoking or maintaining a healthy weight. Reform also expands coverage to include preventive services without a deductible. According to a survey by Chicago-based Midwest Business Group on Health, 60 percent of businesses said they were more likely to create or expand wellness programs because of reform.

Some argue the health law should have gone even further to encourage the programs. However, there is not enough evidence of broad-based success to justify taxpayer-supported subsidies. Many businesses have ineffective programs because they are poorly designed or managed.

Anything less than a robust wellness program is likely to fail. Efforts such as online tools and health-risk assessments without personalized follow-up are largely ineffective. Programs can take several years before they begin to pay off, and ROI is difficult to measure. The best programs do ongoing, effective communication. Part of that message should be senior management's linking the wellness program to company goals.

Most programs pay employees to participate in wellness activities rather than achieve certain performance targets, such as weight-loss goals or low blood-pressure metrics.

Programs spreading quickly

A Kaiser Family Foundation survey reflects the rapid increase in wellness programs. Nearly 3 out of 4 businesses offered at least one of the following programs in 2010: fitness newsletter or website information, weight-loss program, personal-health coaching, or classes in nutrition or healthy living. That compares with 58 percent of businesses in 2009.

An Integrated Benefits Institute survey of 500 companies listed 26 health and productivity initiatives that included management of health, disease and disability. Nearly every company provided at least one. The average small company had adopted about 10 of the 26 practices, compared with an average of about 18 for businesses with more than 5,000 employees.

The tip of the spear for most company wellness programs is the health-risk assessment (HRA). According to a review of three dozen wellness studies, 81 percent of companies offered them. These questionnaires ask employees about their health status and risk factors. Employers use the information to persuade their employees to participate in activities that address warning signals. They also hope the information will motivate the employee to act without being prodded.

There is little evidence that HRAs alone change behavior. They rely on self-reported information, and those who volunteer to participate tend to be the healthiest employees. They are more likely to be women, have high-deductible insurance plans and have fewer chronic conditions.

Participation in wellness programs is increasing. About 57 percent of employees were involved in 2009, compared with 46 percent in 2008. Those who did so tended to be successful on a number of fronts. More than 8 out of 10 lost weight, exercised more, improved eating habits, managed stress better, and reduced cholesterol and blood pressure.

Despite the recession, several large businesses have established on-site clinics as a way to control health-care costs. Clinics were common at large manufacturing and industrial companies until the 1980s to handle work-related injuries. As these jobs migrated overseas, the clinics began to fade from the industrial landscape. They are being reborn as patient-centered medical homes for many employees. They offer convenient, inexpensive care tailored to the company's workforce. They coordinate care with specialists and avoid expensive procedures and tests of marginal value. They lower absenteeism and help retain employees.

Many companies that have taken the plunge have seen a positive return on investment. Pitney Bowes, for example, reports that for every $1 spent on clinics, it saves $1 in health-care costs and gains an additional $1 in worker productivity.

The clinics provide traditional occupational-health and typical doctor-visit care, as well as preventive care, wellness services and management of chronic diseases. These clinics help businesses control prescription costs and specialist referrals, and they proactively treat patients to avoid emergency department visits, hospitalizations and more expensive care later on for untreated complicated conditions.

Return on investment

One of the most comprehensive studies found that medical costs fall $3.27 for every $1 spent and absenteeism costs fall $2.73 for every $1 spent. A *Harvard Business Review* study also concluded that properly run wellness programs could save up to $6 for every $1 spent.

Wellness programs are relatively inexpensive to fund. The average business spends about 2 percent of its total health-care claim dollars on them. Yet most program administrators have no clue how well they are performing. Two out of 3 have no measurable program goals, and 60 percent do not know their return on investment.

Some of the bigger payoffs are less obvious. Two types of ROI are typically calculated. "Hard ROI" consists only of direct medical costs. "Soft ROI" also includes productivity gains. The indirect costs of poor health can be double or triple those of direct medical costs. They include productivity losses from absenteeism or attempting to work with a brief illness or chronic condition, also known as presenteeism. The payback rises to as much as $15 for every $1 invested when indirect costs are included.

It typically takes a few years to have adequate information to determine the return on investment. Start-up costs can be substantial, and improving employee health behavior takes time. The long payback period is enough to deter some organizations, especially small businesses with limited resources. Such programs also make less sense in industries with high employee turnover and younger employees, such as hospitality, restaurant and retail.

Businesses prefer to measure the impact of their programs by overall health-cost increases. The most consistent performers have kept cost increases to about 2 percent over the last four years, compared with nearly 7 percent for all companies.

Participation is key

Employers increasingly are becoming irritated at the damage that skyrocketing health costs are doing to their bottom lines. They spend about $10,000 a year on health care for every active employee. They resent employees' engagement in their health. They blame medical vendors' ineffectiveness for not producing healthier employees and lower costs. They especially are angry at government for below-cost Medicare and Medicaid reimbursement, because the health-care system shifts the additional cost to private employers, resulting in escalating insurance premiums.

There is an inverse relationship between wellness-program participation and a business's health-care costs. For example, Dallas-based Baylor Health Care System has an award-winning wellness program called "Thrive." Health-care costs for participants have risen 1.1 percent annually, compared with 9.9 percent for nonparticipants. The participation rate is 75 percent, which is high for a voluntary program.

According to Edington, a business with 85 to 100 percent participation will control health-care costs if 75 to 85 percent of its workforce has two or fewer health risks. To get 90 percent participation, businesses need to provide per-employee incentives of about $1,000.

Unfortunately, employees in poor condition are the least likely to manage their health. In this group, only 1 in 5 uses programs to manage chronic conditions. These people represent the biggest health-care expense. About 80 percent of a business's health-care costs is created by 10 to 20 percent of the employees.

A Midwest Business Group on Health survey of employees revealed a stunning disregard for personal health. Nearly 9 out of 10 lacked an understanding of the value of preventive services and more than half said they have "no motivation to stay healthy."

The presence of insurance does not mean employees will take advantage of preventive services, even when they are free. In a federal government survey of 160,000 working adults, 3 out of 4 did not get an influenza vaccination. About half had not been screened for colon cancer.

According to a survey, about 7 percent of employees used nurse help lines, and less than 5 percent of those eligible for smoking-cessation and weight-management programs used them.

In focus groups, employees say they lack the confidence to make health changes, and need support and tools to get started. They are increasingly reliant on their companies to provide information about quality of health plans and how to improve their health.

Many, however, do not trust their employers to have their best interests at heart. For example, health "coaches" are often seen as an extension of the employer rather than as a health-care provider. Some also admit they lie on health-risk assessments to qualify for participation bonuses.

Presenteeism is a menace to workplace health. The U.S. does not require employers to provide paid sick days—despite the fact that 86 percent of Americans favor legislation that would guarantee seven sick days a year. Connecticut became the first state in July 2011 to require companies to provide paid sick leave.

More than 8 out of 10 low-income workers are not paid for sick days. That includes businesses with frequent human contact, such as food service, hotels, nursing homes and day-care centers.

More than half of workers without paid sick days have gone to work ill. They are twice as likely to go to the hospital emergency department after work hours for care because they could not get time off work for medical care. That results in higher cost of care for the employer and the employee. One out of 4 workers say they either have lost a job or were told they would lose their job if they took time off for a personal or family illness.

Getting paid to do what is right

The idea of earning money for breaking bad habits—or forming good ones—rubs many the wrong way. People should be responsible enough to do the right thing in the first place. However, changing behavior is hard work, and people often will act only if they are nudged.

According to a University of Pennsylvania survey, people were evenly split on whether they thought it was a good idea to pay smokers to quit, lose weight, control their diabetes or lower their blood pressure.

Businesses are willing to pay for this because research shows that every employee health risk increases costs. It is cheaper and easier to snuff out such risks if they can. In many large companies, employees who address bad habits or health risks become eligible for bonuses.

An Integrated Benefits Institute survey found that nearly 3 out of 4 employers have at least one such incentive program. However, fewer than 20 percent of employers use disincentives, or penalties, to change behavior. Companies generally are not strategic in how they employ these carrots and sticks. For example, the most prevalent incentives are discounts on services or nonmonetary gifts, although companies consider these among the least effective. Conversely, premium reductions and reduced co-payments are considered among the most effective but are used far less often.

Incentives also tend to reward mere participation in programs, when what employers really want is evidence of employee behavior change. However, according to a Towers Watson survey, two-thirds of companies say they are going to pay only for results by 2012.

Employers are investing substantial amounts of money in incentives, and they are increasing the stakes rapidly. The average per-employee incentive was worth $430 in 2010, up from $260 in 2009. Two-thirds of employers expect to increase them again in 2011. Half of the companies that provide incentives also do so for dependents.

How much incentives actually change behavior is questionable. There have been several studies on this. Most indicate that incentives produce initially higher rates of tobacco cessation and moderate weight loss, but few follow up to see if progress is sustained over a longer period of time. For effective wellness programs, the proof is the positive ROI. For businesses, that is the whole point.

Healthy employees can earn a 20 percent discount on insurance. Health reform will increase that percentage to 30 percent in 2014, and allows federal regulators to raise that to 50 percent.

Harvard researchers calculated that a 30 percent discount would amount to about $1,500 for an average individual policy and more than $4,000 for a family policy. A 50 percent discount would be worth nearly $2,500 on an individual policy and exceed $6,688 for a family policy.

A 2005 *Wall Street Journal* and Harris Interactive poll reflected strong public opposition to charging more for those with health problems. However, the healthy often are silently disgusted by fellow employees puffing on cigarettes in designated smoking areas or obese co-workers with overflowing lunch trays in the company cafeteria. A company's health-insurance premiums reflect the collective health of its workforce. The healthy do subsidize the unhealthy.

Companies that reward employees with premium discounts for certain health outcomes are required to offer an alternative way for those who cannot reach those goals for medical reasons. High blood pressure, high cholesterol and excess weight can be caused by factors other than behavior: genetics; physical or mental disability; lack of access to healthy food and exercise facilities, or other priorities such as working multiple jobs or being a caregiver.

Ironically, increased insurance discounts allowed by health reform could undermine another important goal of the law: that insurance companies not discriminate against those with substandard health. Businesses will have to be careful that incentives reward behavior rather than health-status factors.

Businesses that pursue deep discounts will have to tread carefully. Some business executives seem to be telling employees: Your right to an unhealthy lifestyle ends at my balance sheet. People who blame lack of personal responsibility for bad health really are asking for a different model of health insurance, one based on actual risk. The sick, they suggest, should pay more regardless of how they got that way.

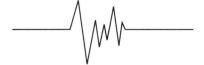

Chapter 13

Patient Engagement
Paying attention pays off

Better health outcomes and more years of healthy life require patient engagement. An engaged patient actively and consistently does what needs to be done to gain the greatest benefit from available health resources.

How many do this? Americans can be divided into thirds. One-third is engaged. Another third is tentative and inconsistent. The final third is disengaged. People with more education, income and self-confidence are more likely to be in the first group.

People who do not take charge of their health will fare poorly under health reform, and will be a drag on the performance of their health-care providers.

Hospitals will be penalized if they do not provide a high level of patient-centered care. That means they must provide a comfortable, emotionally supportive environment. However, it also means patients will be encouraged to be involved in their own care. They will be asked to participate in decisions about their care and follow treatment plans so they are not readmitted needlessly.

Organized systems of care emerging from health reform, such as accountable care organizations (ACOs) and patient-centered medical homes (PCMHs), will be paid based on the health of their patients. That is a shared responsibility. Physicians can only improve their patients' health if the patients are willing to do their part. Access to physicians increasingly will become difficult as the number of insured patients increases. Providers may end up "firing" patients if they are not compliant.

High-deductible health-insurance plans will increase rapidly under health reform. They will be a central feature of the health-insurance exchanges established by the new law. An increasing number of companies will offer them—in some cases exclusively—as a means of controlling costs. These plans assume that consumers will make wiser personal-health choices to minimize their out-of-pocket costs.

What do engaged patients do? They are not deterred by the complexity and fragmentation of the health-care system. They practice good health habits. They manage over-the-counter medications, minor wounds and injuries on their own. They collaborate with their providers and participate in making treatment decisions. They successfully navigate the health-care system, paying attention to provider quality and performance. They seek out reliable information on their own.

Ultimately, personal health requires self-care. Consider that physicians spend about two hours annually with their diabetic patients. Otherwise, those patients log an average of 8,758 hours a year managing their condition on their own.

Research consistently shows that engaged consumers have better health, make better choices and avoid medical errors. Engagement leads to better compliance with treatment, lower health-care costs and better-quality care. Patients do not have the power to change the health-care system. However, they do have the power to change their own care.

The disengaged are overwhelmed. They are less likely to have a usual source of care. They forget 40 to 80 percent of what

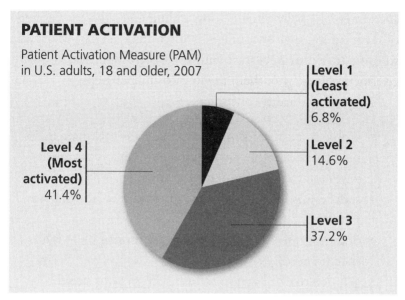

PATIENT ACTIVATION

Patient Activation Measure (PAM)
in U.S. adults, 18 and older, 2007

**Level 1
(Least
activated)**
6.8%

Level 2
14.6%

Level 3
37.2%

**Level 4
(Most
activated)**
41.4%

Source: HSC 2007 Health Tracking Household Survey.

The Patient Activation Measure identifies four levels. Level 1 (least activated): Passive and unwilling to manage his or her health. Level 2: Lacks basic knowledge and confidence. Level 3: Takes some action toward positive behavior. Level 4: Adopts many of the ideal healthy behaviors.

the physician tells them in the exam room. Six out of 10 with employer-based insurance blame their disengagement on not knowing where to go for information. One in 4 Medicare beneficiaries is disengaged, and would "rather have someone else tell me what I need to do." One in 3 of those who are uninsured is simply "not interested."

Many of the patient behaviors needed in the evolving healthcare system are being done only by the one-third most active consumers. Researcher Judith Hibbard has developed a way to measure this, called the Patient Activation Measure. The model includes four stages to becoming a fully competent health-care consumer. She believes activation is fluid and subject to a range of flash points that encourage or discourage engagement. She suggests that providers start with the easiest behaviors to instill confidence and break them down into smaller steps.

The typical health consumer:

- is able to perform simpler tasks such as making a list of medications, rather than more complex tasks such as participating in treatment decisions.
- seeks out information about a provider or health plan but tends not to use it.
- does not research health information until there is a specific need.
- is quick to cite barriers to care such as poor health, insufficient knowledge or lack of external support.
- uses the Internet to learn about a condition or symptoms, but it is less clear whether the newly gained knowledge changes behavior.

Patients are too passive

All of this puts the patient in the back seat. Physician opinion, rather than patient preference, drives treatment decisions. In his book *Tracking Medicine*, John Wennberg asserts that a commonly overlooked medical error is what he calls operating on the wrong patients—meaning those who would not have wanted the operation if they were fully informed of the risks and benefits.

This is an inherent problem in health-care transactions. Patients do not know what they need. Physicians understand medical problems and select what they believe are the right treatments, often without patient input. Physicians, as sellers, can create demand. Economists call this asymmetry of information.

Improved communication between providers and patients can improve health outcomes, health-care quality and patient satisfaction. These are among the federal government's goals for satisfactory communication skills by the year 2020.

Increase the proportion of patients who say their provider always listens to them carefully

Starting point: 59 percent of people reported in 2007 that their health-care provider always listened carefully to them

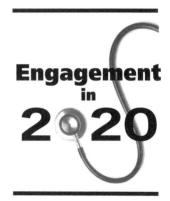

Goal: 65 percent (10 percent improvement)

Increase the proportion of patients who say their provider always explains things so they can understand them

Starting point: 60 percent of people reported in 2007 that their health-care provider always explained things so they could understand them

Goal: 66 percent (10 percent improvement)

Increase the proportion of patients who say their provider always shows respect for what they have to say

Starting point: 62 percent of people reported in 2007 that their health-care provider always showed respect for what they had to say

Goal: 68.2 percent (10 percent improvement)

continued

Increase the proportion of patients who say their provider always spends enough time with them

Starting point: 49 percent of people reported in 2007 that their health-care provider always spent enough time with them

Goal: 54 percent (10 percent improvement)

This is not unlike the auto mechanic who tells the customer what needs to be done. In both cases, the buyer is afraid to ignore the seller's advice.

Physicians are not particularly skilled at figuring out patient treatment preferences. Few medical schools train physicians on how to do this. Effective communication takes time, which is often not paid for by insurers. Health plans pay physicians primarily for the volume of service, rather than quality. Many doctors have developed "efficient" styles that keep them from listening to patients.

The average physician visit lasts 18 minutes. The average patient is able to speak for 23 seconds before the physician interrupts. Trying to have a meaningful discussion under these circumstances is difficult. Physicians often select treatments based on what they believe their patients would want, absent an actual conversation.

However, patients and physicians may have different priorities. In a University of Michigan study, about one-third of physicians and patients with diabetes differed on treatment priorities. About 38 percent of physicians ranked high blood pressure as the most important priorities, compared with 18 percent of diabetes patients. Patients were more likely to place a higher priority on treating pain and depression.

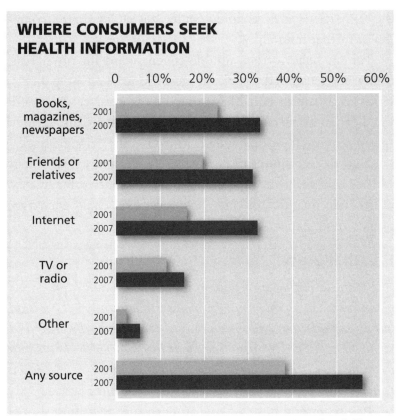

WHERE CONSUMERS SEEK HEALTH INFORMATION

Source: HSC 2001 and 2007 household surveys.

According to a 2007 survey, more than half of American adults sought information about a personal health issue. Every medium showed an increase in use of health information from 2001 to 2007. More than half who sought information said the results changed their approach to health, and 4 out of 5 said the information helped them better understand an illness or condition.

Nonetheless, most patients are fine with physicians making the decisions. Many are uncomfortable making decisions they are not sure of, and that potentially have enormous personal implications. Seven out of 10 are confident in the accuracy of their physician's advice, and do not feel a need for a second opinion or further research.

Patient behavior is a double-edged sword for physicians. Many are frustrated by disengaged, noncompliant patients. However, many are equally frustrated by aggressive, highly activated patients who enter the exam room wanting to discuss their Internet research—disparagingly known as the "Google stack."

New delivery innovations such as ACOs and PCMHs may address this problem. Providers will be reimbursed for quality, rather than quantity, of care. New incentives could encourage deeper, more patient-centered discussion.

Health literacy

A 2-year-old is diagnosed with an ear infection and is prescribed an antibiotic in liquid form. Her mother understands that her child has an ear infection and knows the girl should take the prescribed medicine twice a day. After looking at the label on the bottle and deciding that it does not tell how to take the medicine, she fills a teaspoon and pours the antibiotic into her daughter's ear.

As preposterous as this true story seems, one-third to one-half of U.S. adults do not have the literacy skills to navigate the health-care system. Studies have shown that poor health literacy is associated with higher rates of hospital readmissions, treatment complications and death.

Health literacy is the capacity to obtain, process and understand basic health information and services to make appropriate health decisions. Reading comprehension and understanding numbers are the key components.

One hospital study found proportions of patients could not understand simple instructions on prescription bottles, comprehend the statement of rights and responsibilities on a Medicaid application, or understand an informed-consent form.

Americans have a difficult time with simple math. Almost half of the U.S. population has difficulty calculating the difference between a regular and sale price or estimating the cost per ounce of a grocery item. One out of 4 patients cannot understand information about when an appointment is scheduled.

Educational attainment certainly is important for health literacy. Yet 17 percent of high-school graduates and 10 percent of those with higher education have inadequate health literacy. For example, 16 percent of highly educated people could not correctly answer questions about risk magnitudes (i.e., which is the greater risk: 1, 5 or 10 percent?).

A classic example: Former New York City Mayor Rudolph Giuliani believed he was cancer-free when his doctor told him that his prostate biopsy was "positive." A positive biopsy indicates cancer is present.

Unfortunately, patients often either hide their lack of knowledge or do not acknowledge it. Of those scoring at the lowest level on a 1992 National Adult Literacy Survey, only 29 percent said they did not read well and only 34 percent admitted they did not write well. In a study at a women's clinic, physicians could identify only 20 percent of those with low literacy.

Literacy skills predict health status more accurately than age, income, employment status, education level, or race and ethnicity do. Adults with measurably limited reading and math skills have less knowledge of disease management and proper health behaviors, report poorer health status and seek fewer preventive services.

A review of 96 studies found that low health literacy was associated with poor health outcomes. They include more hospitalizations, greater emergency-room use, fewer flu vaccinations, fewer mammogram screenings and poor medication compliance.

This problem is not entirely the patient's fault. Anyone can have difficulty navigating densely written medication-inserted instructions or medical-consent forms loaded with jargon and technical language. More than 300 studies have found that such health-related reading materials are written beyond the average reading comprehension of U.S. adults.

Medicaid recipients include some of the poorest and least educated Americans. An analysis of Medicaid application forms revealed that nearly all of the directions were at or above a fifth-grade reading level despite the fact that 40 million Americans read below that level. This suggests that inability to understand the forms may be a barrier to enrollment. Forty-six states have established reading-level guidelines for their forms, but nearly half of those fail to meet their own standards.

Health-literacy skills are used in many settings. Examples include taking a child's temperature, assessing nutrition labels on grocery products, applying for health insurance, reading safety instructions on a new tool or trying to follow the rules of a weight-loss diet.

The majority of the estimated 90 million with limited literacy skills are native-born white Americans. Although poor English skills contribute to the problem, others most likely to have low health literacy are those 65 and older, those who have fewer years of formal schooling or those in a racial or ethnic minority group.

Low health literacy is especially problematic for the elderly. Chronic-disease management requires a high level of self-care. They must follow complex treatment instructions with uncertain risks and benefits, monitor their conditions, enact lifestyle changes and decide when and where to seek professional help.

Yet an emergency-room study found that 4 out of 5 patients over 60 could not read or understand basic medical instructions.

While many call for greater patient education, the health-care system also will need to adapt. Magically eliminating health illiteracy is simply not going to happen. The National Work

Group on Literacy and Health recommends that physicians rely less on written communication and that health-care material be written at a fifth-grade reading level or lower.

Shared decision-making

The research on whether or how consumers want to be involved in treatment is mixed, and there is no consensus on a systematic approach. Many are advocating a more formal approach to what is called shared decision-making. The American Medical Association, the American College of Critical Care Medicine and the American Academy of Pediatrics all endorse that model.

Shared decision-making means informing patients of the risks and benefits of various treatments or services when there is more than one option. Ideally, the patient carefully considers the alternatives in light of personal preferences and agrees on a course of action with the physician.

Medicine will have to change its traditionally paternalistic culture of care if it is to become more participatory. The patient-doctor encounter is not an ideal venue for joint decision-making. The physician and patient have unequal positions, and the patient is in a compromised physical and mental state. The physician, under pressure to generate revenue, is in a hurry.

Patients make a large number of medical decisions annually. More than 80 percent of adults over age 40 have made a decision about a surgery, new medication or screening test in the last two years. More than half had to make two or more of these decisions. About one-third of these decisions, in turn, have two or more treatment options. When faced with options, about 70 percent of uninformed patients say that doing what the doctor recommends is important.

When the patients become involved, things change. One study found a 20 to 30 percent reduction in aggressive treatment. This suggests that informed patients are more conservative than their health-care providers are. There are other benefits: better quality of care, increased satisfaction for the patient and provider, and improved self-esteem.

Wennberg and several colleagues interviewed patients who had undergone hysterectomies. It was clear that patients considered depression and decreased sexual drive to be important surgical outcomes—neither of which their physicians seemed to acknowledge.

In another study of treatment for benign prostate enlargement, symptoms were the driving force in patients' decisions. Only 11 percent with moderate symptoms and 22 percent with severe symptoms chose surgery. Most were more concerned about potential impotence because of surgery than whether they would have to live with their condition. For most physicians, by contrast, symptom relief is a major priority.

The paternalistic approach to health care often violates a basic ethical principle of patient autonomy. Patients should be given enough information about their conditions and treatment options to make informed decisions.

A study of nine common medical decisions, such as whether to have cancer screenings and whether to prescribe medication to alleviate a condition, found that U.S. patients were not well-informed. The research also showed that physicians tend to stress the advantages of the treatments they recommend rather than the disadvantages or risks. They also were unlikely to ask patients which treatment they would prefer.

Patient decision aids

There are tools that facilitate shared decision-making. These decision aids, as they are called, offer evidence-based information on treatment options, and probabilities on risks and benefits.

They also attempt to draw out a patient's personal values. They enhance a patient's knowledge and participation without increasing anxiety. Videos and written brochures are the most common formats.

Decision aids can save money and have tremendous potential for curbing excessive medical services. Many physicians have a bias toward overtreatment. They have been taught to use every possible means of curative treatment. The threat of medical-liability lawsuits encourages more testing and services than would be used under normal circumstances. Also, physicians are paid more when they perform procedures or tests.

Use of decision aids has reduced rates of major elective surgery by one-quarter without affecting patient outcomes or satisfaction.

In one study, less than 50 percent of men knew that prostate cancer grew so slowly that they would likely die of something else. After viewing a video, nearly all understood the risk. Routine screening requests subsequently decreased from 97 to 50 percent afterward. Similarly, patient choice of an invasive treatment for stable angina decreased from 75 to 58 percent after watching a video about risks and benefits.

Washington State enacted a law in 2007 supporting the use of shared decision-making. According to the law, patients acknowledge in writing they have participated in shared decision-making.

Senator Ron Wyden, D-Oregon, introduced the Empowering Medicare Patient Choices Act of 2009. The legislation would withhold 20 percent of a Medicare payment for some medical procedures if there is not documented use of a patient decision aid. The bill never emerged from the Senate Committee on Finance.

In theory, physicians are in favor of decision aids. A 2009 study showed that 93 percent believed the principle was positive. However, they also cited lack of time during a typical office visit as a significant barrier. Although decision aids represent an ideal direction in patient-centered care, they are unlikely to be used without financial incentives for health-care providers.

Paging Dr. Google

One out of 2 patients worldwide looks first to the Internet for health advice. It is a stunning development that half of the world consults a digital device initially when making health decisions. Nearly 1 in 5 say they find useful information for making decisions on social-media websites such as Facebook and disease support groups. Only 1 out of 4 rely on traditional media—newspapers, magazines and television—for health advice.

In fact, seeking health information is the third most frequent use of the Internet, behind exchanging email and using search engines. Nearly 8 out of 10 Internet users do this at least occasionally. Unlike your physician, the information is there 24/7. Women are voracious consumers of online health information, especially if they have children or are conducting research for family members or friends.

These avid users have a nickname: cyberchondriacs. They troll the Web for information six times a month. One out of 3 Americans did that in 2010, up from 1 in 5 in 2009. Most of the top 20 health websites in the world are U.S.-based.

The most frequent reasons for looking online: medicine information; taking a stab at self-diagnosis; reading about other patients' experiences, and researching hospitals or clinics.

The Internet does have a significant impact on health behavior. More than half who sought information said it changed their approach to personal health, and 4 out of 5 said they gained a deeper understanding of a condition or illness.

How trustworthy is the information? It depends. Researchers reviewed 343 website pages on breast cancer and found inaccuracies on only 18 of the sites—an impressive error rate of about 5 percent. By comparison, websites promoting alternative medicine were 15 times as likely to have false or misleading information as conventional-medicine websites.

Many have gone from simply reading health information to participating in discussion groups and sharing information. This deeper engagement has been called Health 2.0, which is the use of social media that encourages collaboration among patients, caregivers, medical professionals and other stakeholders. Social media, with its worldwide reach, often have been called "word-of-mouth on steroids."

The simple act of reaching out has a medicinal effect. A large 1979 California study found that people with the least social contact had a death rate 2 to 4.5 times higher than those with strong social connections.

People trust information from "a person like me" more than from other authority figures such as government or the media. Social-network participants are also more likely to be engaged in their health.

There also are practical reasons for this online involvement. Consumers facing high deductibles are motivated to take a more active role in their care. A 2009 poll found nearly half of health consumers changed their behavior because of cost: skimping on medication, postponing care and relying more on home remedies. Even when they want to see a doctor, patients are also finding it more difficult to secure physician appointments promptly.

While the Internet can be useful for research, it can become counterproductive. Dr. Michael Fisch, chairman of the oncology department at the University of Texas M.D. Anderson Cancer Center in Houston, cautions patients about information over-load. He told The New York Times: "Just like with medicine, you have to ask yourself what dose you can take. For some people, more information makes them wackier, while others get more relaxed and feel more empowered."

Most U.S. adults still trust offline sources more for health information. Most consult health professionals, friends or family members for advice, with the Internet playing a supplemental role.

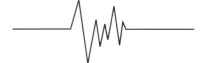

Chapter 14

Chronic Disease
Health care's big-ticket item

Chronic disease is the greatest single source of health-care spending in the United States. Of every Medicare dollar, 96 cents is spent on patients who have one or more chronic conditions. In Medicaid, it is 83 cents. Chronic conditions account for about three-quarters of total U.S. health costs, causes of death, hospital admissions and physician visits, and nearly 9 out of 10 drug prescriptions.

Viewed optimistically, the prevalence of chronic disease is a testament to medical and public-health advances in the 20th century. In 1900, life expectancy was 47 years. Most died of infectious disease, accidents and childbirth, well before today's chronic conditions could develop.

Now more than 1 in 4 adult Americans copes with two or more chronic conditions. Many struggle with fundamental activities of daily life—bathing, dressing, eating and basic mobility. Chronic illness is usually incurable and requires ongoing medical attention. It shortens lives, erodes quality of life and burdens caregivers. Lingering conditions such as cardiovascular disease, stroke, diabetes, cancer and chronic obstructive pulmonary diseases (COPD) require, but often do not receive, ongoing treatment. Asthma, arthritis, obesity and depression are also highly prevalent chronic illnesses. Mental illness and chronic disease are interrelated: One aggravates the other.

Chronic disease is increasing. It is closely tied to the aging of the U.S. population and to the rising obesity rate, which contributes to diabetes, high blood pressure and heart disease. Four out of 5 Americans 50 or older have at least one chronic condition. The percentage of those 65 and older who have five or more conditions increased from 30 percent in 1987 to 50 percent from 2002.

Other factors have contributed to this increase. The thresholds of disease definitions have been lowered, creating millions of new patients overnight. For example, new guidelines for diagnosing high blood pressure resulted in more people with less severe cases receiving treatment. This also occurred for high cholesterol. For both conditions, new medications have allowed patients to receive treatment with fewer side effects. Because of these developments, about 60 percent of Medicare patients with five or more conditions rated their health as good or excellent in 2002—about twice the rate in 1987.

The course of the illness, also known as its "trajectory," varies widely depending on the number of conditions, severity, life expectancy, treatment cost and quality of life.

Despite their expense and prevalence, chronic diseases represent the medical system's stepchild. Physicians and hospitals focus primarily on short-term illnesses, accidents and recovery from surgery.

Patients and providers seem to spring to life only when there is a temporary flare-up or potentially life-threatening episode. Long-term control, also known as tertiary prevention, does not fit the quick-fix ethos of a society bent on instant gratification.

Chronic-disease sufferers also bear the stigma of supposedly having caused their circumstances by gluttony and sloth. People

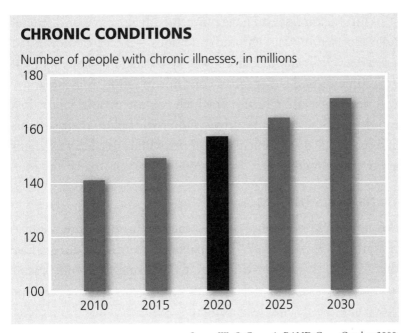

CHRONIC CONDITIONS

Number of people with chronic illnesses, in millions

Source: Wu S, Green A. RAND Corp. October 2000.

The number of people with chronic conditions is expected to grow by 16 million in each of the next two decades. That is more than 1 percentage point of growth each year.

with infectious diseases are more likely to be considered genuine victims. Unquestionably, the four major modifiable health behaviors—smoking, excessive alcohol intake, poor nutrition and inactivity—cause most chronic disease and premature death. A person who turns 65 years old with one chronic condition can expect to live another 22 years—or about six years more than a 65-year-old does with three or more chronic conditions.

Regardless, more than two-thirds of adults say the health-care system should invest more in chronic-disease prevention, and more than 4 in 5 say government should step up its financial commitment.

Chronic diseases do have powerful advocates. World federations representing four chronic conditions—cancer, cardiovascular disease, COPD and diabetes—jointly warned in a statement, "If governments and aid agencies continue to ignore this threat, we will sleepwalk into a future in which healthy people will be in a minority, obese and unhealthy children die before their parents, and economic development and already vulnerable health systems are overwhelmed."

Transitions of care

People with chronic disease bear the full brunt of the medical system's fragmented care. This balkanization is encouraged by the way health-care providers are paid. Usually, no one is paid to manage a patient's overall condition. Providers are paid for procedures, visits and dispensing prescriptions. There is no direct relationship between how much physicians earn and whether the patient improves. Chronic-disease patients see health-care providers in a number of unrelated venues, many of which do not communicate with each other.

Transitional care, which patients receive after discharge from a hospital or other health-care facility, occurs during an especially vulnerable period. Patients often do not understand the purpose of their medications or receive a detailed care plan. These oversights are especially critical in chronic-disease care because the conditions are managed largely by patients and their caregivers. As a result, nearly 1 in 6 is readmitted to the hospital within 30 days of having left a health-care facility. Hospitals are paid when again the patient is readmitted.

About 1 in 7 does not make a follow-up doctor appointment within four weeks of discharge. Patients' physicians often are not informed about the details of the care provided in the hospital.

Chronic disease is the major battleground in 21st-century health care. Baby boomers will add 15 million to the 65-or-older population between 2010 and 2020. The biggest predictor of chronic disease is age. About 81 million people are expected to have multiple chronic conditions by 2020, compared with 51 million in 2000.

Here is what is expected for three of the most expensive conditions by 2020.

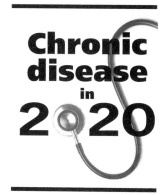

Cancer: The National Cancer Institute (NCI) expects spending on cancer treatment to rise 27 percent, to $158 billion, in 2020. NCI officials expect increases in the numbers of prostate- and breast-cancer patients. If new treatments and diagnostic tools add 2 percent to the annual cost, the 2020 price tag will be $173 billion, or a 39 percent increase.

Heart disease: The cost of treating cardiovascular disease is expected to rise by 75 percent, to $470.3 billion, in 2020. The cost estimate also assumes no major changes in treatment. About 37 percent of U.S. adults have some form of heart disease.

Diabetes: More than 50 percent of Americans may have diabetes or prediabetes by 2020, according to UnitedHealth Group's Center for Health Reform & Modernization. Treatment is expected to account for 10 percent of health-care spending and cost about $500 billion annually. Pre-diabetes refers to elevated blood-glucose levels that are not high enough for a diabetes diagnosis.

About 1 in 5 chronic-disease patients say their physicians did not do a good job of communicating about their care.

Nearly 1 out of 4 was a victim of a medical error, and nearly two-thirds of those errors created a major problem.

Chronic-disease management

Care for chronic disease does not fit neatly into the standard 15-minute physician appointment. Fee-for-service payment discourages services that are not paid for under insurance plans, including prevention and care coordination. The typical clinical focus is a particular problem, rather than dealing with a nonurgent general condition.

More than half of people with chronic disease say their physicians have not asked whether they need help to manage their disease. Nearly half say they rarely or never receive referrals to resources such as coaching or health education.

Good chronic-disease management requires considerable engagement by the patient and provider.

The patient must exercise, practice good dietary habits, faithfully take prescriptions and closely monitor symptoms.

Providers must practice good health-coaching skills and co-ordinate care with community services and specialists. This is time-consuming—and poorly reimbursed by insurers. According to one estimate, a physician would need to practice 18 hours a day simply to provide all of the recommended preventive and chronic-disease control for a typical client base. That, of course, would not include treatment of the short-term illness that usually fills a doctor's daily appointment schedule.

Unfortunately, most U.S. physicians lack the staff and electronic health-record systems to manage chronic disease and coordinate care effectively. Physicians, actually, are not the best-equipped to do the

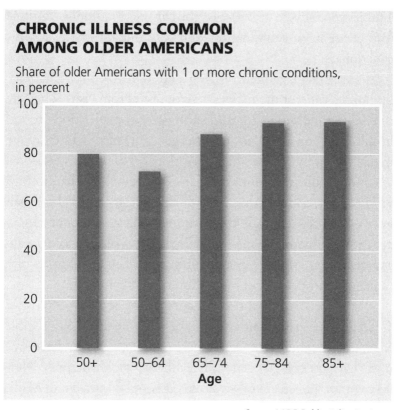

CHRONIC ILLNESS COMMON AMONG OLDER AMERICANS

Share of older Americans with 1 or more chronic conditions, in percent

Source: AARP Public Policy Institute.

As infectious diseases receded as a public-health threat during the 20th century, chronic illnesses replaced them as the most pervasive medical problem in the U.S. About 8 out of 10 Americans age 50 or older have at least one chronic condition.

job. A 2005 review of studies found that nonclinical staff does the most effective job of managing patients with diabetes.

In a 2001 survey, most physicians agreed that the current health-care system is poorly organized to deal with chronic conditions. They also said that it was difficult to coordinate care and that they were poorly trained to handle those kinds of patients.

This is especially disturbing because chronic conditions continue to increase in an aging nation, and consume most U.S. health-care dollars.

Disease-management programs attempt to educate patients on how to care for themselves between physician visits. They are disease-specific and focus on ensuring proper medication use and health behavior. High-risk patients generally receive intense care management by nurses while low-risk patients receive occasional telephone calls from nonphysician educators. Less than a third of U.S. physician practices have nurse managers, and about half have educators. They are concentrated in large group or HMO practices, while most one- or two-physician offices lack the resources to have them. The predominant method of chronic-care management: the brochure or photocopied handout.

Effective chronic-disease management is labor-intensive. Chronic disease hits hardest those people who are dually eligible for Medicare and Medicaid. These 7 million people have two of the greatest risk factors for ill health: being old and poor. They account for 42 percent of Medicaid costs and 25 percent of Medicare costs. Of the most expensive 1 percent of Medicaid enrollees, 83 percent have three or more chronic conditions, and about 60 percent have five or more. However, government reimbursement rates are inadequate to support disease management. The continually strapped Medicaid programs generally do not invest in these kinds of services unless they can provide immediate cost savings.

Thirteen out of 15 Medicare pilot programs for management of chronic illness failed to reduce hospitalizations, which is a key aim of any such effort. The few successful programs had substantial in-person contact, which is expensive for the health-care provider and is generally not reimbursed well. Politicians become discouraged by so little success. Providers are equally discouraged by the effort's expense.

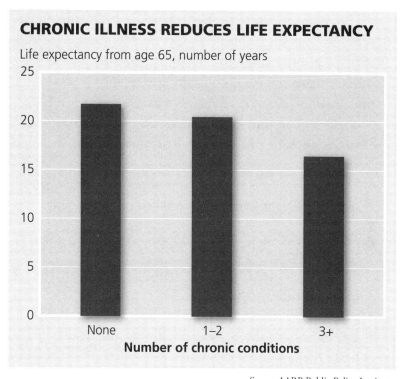

CHRONIC ILLNESS REDUCES LIFE EXPECTANCY

Life expectancy from age 65, number of years

Source: AARP Public Policy Institute.

Each chronic disease a person acquires, on average, lowers life expectancy. A 65-year-old with no chronic conditions is expected to live more than five years longer than a 65-year-old with three or more conditions.

A 2008 *Health Affairs* survey compared the care of chronic conditions in eight industrialized nations, including the United States. The results underscored the weak U.S. primary-care infrastructure and comparatively high cost of care. According to the study:

- More than half of U.S. patients skipped filling prescriptions, or seeking a doctor when ill, because of cost. Other nations ranged from 7 to 35 percent.

- U.S. patients experienced the most medical errors, such as incorrect prescriptions or incorrect test results, as well as the greatest amount of disorganized care, such as unavailable test results or duplicate testing.
- Only one-quarter of ill Americans could get a same-day doctor appointment, compared with one-half or more in the Netherlands, New Zealand and the United Kingdom.
- U.S. patients paid the most out of pocket, with more than 40 percent spending $1,000 or more annually.

According to research, effective disease-management programs share common characteristics. They include:

- Individual case management.
- Face-to-face contact between patients and providers.
- Use of hospital discharges as opportunities to alter health behavior and outcomes.
- Minimizing patient expense to maximize effectiveness and adherence.

Other factors that contribute to success: a large enough patient base to support additional staff; simple design and execution; patient-centered focus; data that can be gathered and analyzed easily, and financial incentives for all stakeholders.

The gold standard in disease management is the Chronic Care Model, developed by Dr. Ed Wagner of the Group Health Cooperative of Puget Sound. The model's components include: patient support to instill confidence; interdisciplinary teams that include nonclinicians; decision support tools and clinical information systems for providers to track care; community resources for ongoing education and support, and strong commitment to the concept.

Chronic-disease management nationally increased 23 percent between 2000 and 2006. The greatest progress was at physician practices that were rewarded financially for quality care and were committed to quality initiatives. Adequate financial compensation is key to supporting necessary staffing.

'Polypharmacy'

People with chronic conditions consume a prodigious amount of prescription drugs. They account for $3 of every $4 spent on pharmaceuticals. Those with five or more conditions filled an average more than 57 prescription medications a year.

Taking so many drugs, also known as "polypharmacy," can create problems. A patient may not react to one drug on its own. When drugs are used together, the risk of adverse consequences increases exponentially. Unfortunately, health-care providers often react to these events by adding still more drugs to the mix—called "prescribing cascading"—which can increase the chance of additional adverse reactions.

On the other hand, about half of people who have three or more conditions do not take medicines as directed—often because of cost. Therefore, the risk of taking too many or too few medications is high for those with chronic illness.

The costs

Chronic disease is an unquestionable financial drain on the health-care system. It accounted for 85 percent of all U.S. health-care spending in 2004.

The average cost of medical care for an adult 50 and over in 2005 was about $6,400. For those without a chronic condition, it was $1,425. The cost for those with five or more conditions was nearly $16,000. The expense per person rises with each additional condition. Several conditions tend to cluster together, such as obesity, high blood pressure, high cholesterol and diabetes. How much a person with chronic disease spends over a lifetime depends on the cost of treatment and life expectancy. For example, diabetes is more costly than cancer per year—$15,052 vs. $13,503. Likewise, high blood pressure is far more expensive than stroke—$11,143 vs. $4,397. High blood pressure treatment requires life-long expensive medication. Stroke generally occurs late in life.

Chronic-disease sufferers often pay more for health insurance, in addition to their treatment costs. Either insurance companies charge them more because they require more costly care, or they choose more expensive policies with more extensive services because of their chronic conditions. About half spend more than 10 percent of their income on their condition—the expense threshold at which health-care costs are considered a financial burden.

Therefore it is not surprising that 1 in 4 people with chronic conditions delay care because of cost, including 22 percent of those with household incomes over $50,000. More than 1 out of 3 women ages 50 to 65 and nearly half of Latinos in that age group forgo care.

The uninsured often simply suffer in silence. About 1 in 3 uninsured working-age adults never receive care to manage their conditions. If they make it to age 65, they enter Medicare in poor condition and use more health services than those who were insured prior to program eligibility.

The Milken Institute calculated current and future treatment costs and lost productivity for seven common chronic diseases that afflicted 1 in 3 Americans in 2007: cancer, diabetes, hypertension, stroke, heart disease, pulmonary conditions and mental disorders. Total annual economic impact was $1.4 trillion, of which $1.1 trillion represented lost productivity and $277 billion was needed for treatment. If current trends continue, the cost for treatment and lost economic output is expected to rise to $4.2 trillion in 2023.

Two decades ago, Medicare spending growth was driven by inpatient hospital services, especially for heart disease. Recent cost increases largely are attributed to chronic diseases, chiefly arthritis, high blood pressure, kidney disease and diabetes.

Patient engagement is the key

A patient's engagement in his or her health can be measured using a survey called Patient Activation Measure (PAM). According to an AARP survey, those with high PAM scores described themselves as highly activated, more confident and proactive about their health, compared with those at lower PAM levels. The least activated chronic-disease patients were more likely to report health problems, appear sicker, use the health system more, and yet were less likely to follow the doctor's advice.

Chronic-care patients are themselves the principal caregivers. Most care behavior—medication adherence, diet, exercise and vital-sign monitoring—is up to the patient. Self-management is essential to good chronic-disease control. Correct medication and diet and exercise advice are useless if they are not carried out. Some people intentionally do not follow orders because they rebel against difficult lifestyle restrictions. Indifferent chronic-disease patients often fail to reach out for help.

Reasons for not following health advice differed for the engaged and disengaged. Proactive patients who ignored medical advice did so because they did not agree with it. They generally are better-informed and more likely to question instructions from a provider. The less-interested chronic-disease patients did not follow advice because they believed it was poorly communicated.

Use of technology

There is a great deal of enthusiasm about the remote monitoring of chronic conditions. Research has confirmed that remote monitoring devices and telephone contact can lower the cost of chronic care while maintaining quality. The side benefit is that using the device makes people more interested in their health. The Department of Veterans Affairs has successfully used such care for years.

Cost, and discomfort with technology, can be barriers for older patients. Insurance companies have been slow to reimburse patients for equipment and personnel to do the monitoring. An AARP survey indicated that patients and caregivers were willing to spend up to $50 a month for a monitoring device. The most patients 50 years or older would pay for software such as iPhone applications was $35.

People over 50 with chronic conditions are less likely to use a computer regularly. However, once they go online, they become avid health consumers. Nearly 3 out of 4 look for websites specific to their condition, and 2 out of 3 research specific medical treatments or procedures. They are also more likely to look for alternative treatments, medications and procedures, and study information on Medicare and Medicaid payment.

Those with chronic diseases also want to find others like themselves and communicate online. They tend to blog and participate in online health discussions.

Policymakers looking for big health-care savings need to look no further than preventing and controlling chronic disease. Health reform's creation of payment models for keeping people healthy is a start. However, the fragmented U.S. health-delivery system and the failure to reimburse for educating and monitoring chronically ill patients represent almost insurmountable barriers.

Part 3

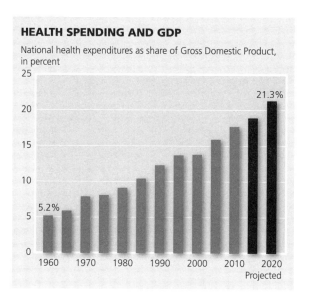

HEALTH SPENDING AND GDP

National health expenditures as share of Gross Domestic Product, in percent

Health-Care Finances

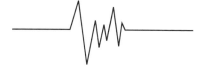

Chapter 15

National Health Costs
Technology, market power dominant

Health-care costs grew about 4 percent in 2009, which was the slowest rate in half a century. Job losses mounted that year, with concurrent loss of employer-sponsored insurance and, as a result, more people delaying care.

Health costs reached another historic benchmark in July 2010: They actually fell 0.1 percent, which was the first monthly decline in 35 years.

This good news would appear to be short-lived. Employer health costs were expected to rise 8.5 percent in 2012. Businesses were forecast to counter that by shifting more costs to employees and providing leaner benefits—tactics that are becoming an annual rite at many companies.

Health spending is rising faster than the rates of incomes and other consumer prices in most developed nations, raising worldwide concern about how future medical costs will be met. Annual per-person spending, adjusted for inflation, has exceeded income growth by an average of about 2 percentage points for the past 50 years. The U.S. spends more per capita than any other nation, and its absolute costs are increasing the most.

The U.S. is expected to spend 17.6 percent of its gross domestic product (GDP), or $8,650 per person, on health care in 2011. In contrast, food and housing costs each represent 10 percent of GDP. European nations spent about $3,000 per person and an average of 9 percent of GDP on health care. The Centers for Medicare and Medicaid Services predicts the U.S. will be spending $13,710 per person and nearly 20 percent of GDP by 2020.

Peter Orszag, then-director of the Congressional Budget Office, said in Congressional testimony, "The nation's long-term fiscal balance will be determined primarily by the future of health-care cost growth."

The current trend is sobering. Health-care spending is on track to consume 119 to 142 percent of current U.S. per-capita spending over the next 75 years. That means health care would crowd out other valuable areas of the budget, such as national defense and education.

This would happen despite the fact that the U.S. population is smoking less, suffering fewer heart attacks and living longer, healthier lives.

Federal Reserve Chairman Ben Bernanke has warned that Americans will have to either allow higher taxes or change Medicare and Social Security, or else budget deficits will suffocate economic growth. The two programs account for about one-third of U.S. government spending.

Americans clearly do not like budget deficits, but they do not want to alter these revered entitlements either. More than three-quarters of U.S. adults say it is unacceptable to cut either Social Security or Medicare. About half believe neither program needs to be cut to balance the budget. Even 70 percent of Tea Party members oppose cutting Medicare.

Meanwhile, the health-care sector continues to be robust, despite a lagging economy. From late 2007 to February 2011,

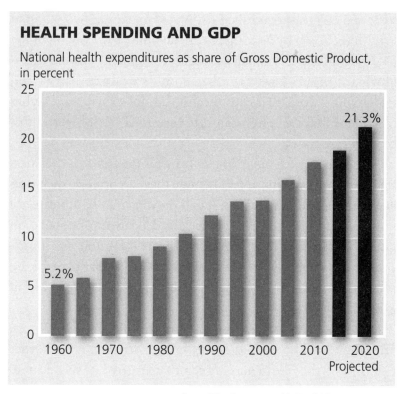

HEALTH SPENDING AND GDP

National health expenditures as share of Gross Domestic Product, in percent

Source: The Commonwealth Fund; The Lewin Group.

This 2020 projection of health-care spending as a percentage of the gross domestic product illustrates the steady ascent of the sector's percentage of the U.S. economy. This estimate is slightly higher than that of Medicare's Office of the Actuary.

heath-care employment grew 6.3 percent. In all other sectors, employment contracted 6.8 percent. One out of 10 U.S. workers is now employed in health care.

Why costs are rising

Wealthier nations all spend more on health. However, the U.S. spends well above what would be expected, compared with its peers. McKinsey Global Institute used data from 13 industrialized nations to develop a measure it called Estimated Spending According to Wealth (ESAW). By McKinsey's calculations, $477 billion of the $1.7 trillion the U.S. spent on health care in 2003 was in excess of what it should have spent based on its wealth. Analysts said the condition of Americans' health did not explain the higher costs. Hospital and physician care accounted for 85 percent of the excess spending.

McKinsey said a huge driver of costs is the fact that providers are expanding capacity, in part because they can produce their own demand. This echoes ample research showing that health-care use rises when facilities expand or open, independent of population health. McKinsey also cited technological innovation that invariably delivers more expensive care, and the fact that patients are insensitive to high prices because their out-of-pocket costs are, in general, so low.

In a classic *Health Affairs* journal study called "It's The Prices, Stupid: Why The United States Is So Different From Other Countries," the researchers argued that Americans spend more on health care even though they use fewer health services than other developed nations. The difference, they said, was that the U.S. health-care providers charged higher prices.

For example, the U.S. consumes 10 percent fewer drugs per capita than other industrialized nations. However, the U.S. spends 70 percent more for drugs. The U.S. also has comparatively lower disease prevalence because it has a younger population and lower smoking rates. It also has the lowest hospital usage compared with 10 peer nations and ranks eighth out of 10 in the number of physician visits.

The reason for higher U.S. prices is that purchasers lack negotiating power—or choose not to exercise it. Other nations consolidate their bargaining power either in their governments or as cooperatives. They negotiate one standard—and invariably

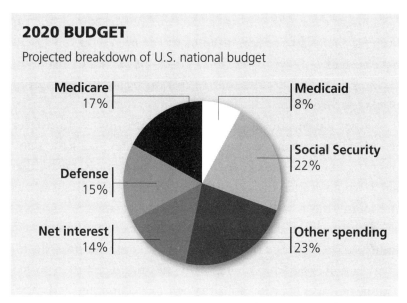

2020 BUDGET

Projected breakdown of U.S. national budget

- Medicare 17%
- Medicaid 8%
- Social Security 22%
- Defense 15%
- Net interest 14%
- Other spending 23%

Source: Congressional Budget Office.

By 2020, Medicare and Medicaid are expected to account for about 25 percent of the federal budget, exceeding both Social Security and defense. The Children's Health Insurance Program and other health-related spending under "other spending" would account for an additional 2 percent. The combined health programs comprised about 21 percent of the 2010 budget, compared with the 27 percent projected for 2020.

lower—price for health services and pharmaceutical drugs. In the U.S., there is no government purchaser willing to bargain on behalf of constituents. The continuing consolidation of hospitals and physicians leaves health plans in weaker negotiating positions.

The government shies away from using its buying power. Mike Leavitt, Health and Human Services secretary under President George W. Bush, said he opposed negotiating Medicare drug prices because "it really isn't about government negotiating drug prices. It's a surrogate for a much larger issue, which is really government-run health care."

During the health-reform debate, the Obama administration dropped the "public option" insurance plan, even though it would have been one of several available options on the health insurance exchanges. It also decided not to seek to negotiate lower drug prices for Medicare.

Other nations do not have a choice on whether to drive a hard bargain with health-care providers. If they spent the same portion of GDP as the United States did, the required tax burden likely would cripple their economies. The United States is not at that point, but is well on its way.

The International Federation of Health Plans surveyed 12 industrialized nations on the costs of 14 common procedures. Every nation except the U.S. reported one price. The U.S. reported a range of prices because of its fragmented negotiating landscape. The price differences were significant. The cost of delivering a baby was $2,667 in Canada, $2,147 in Germany and an average of $8,435 in the U.S. A comparable length of hospital stay cost $1,679 in Spain, $7,707 in Canada and ranged from $14,427 to $45,902 in the U.S.

Even though U.S. physicians deliver less care than doctors in other industrialized nations do, their average income is about three times greater. The ratio of physician income to that of the average U.S. employee is 5.5, compared with 1.5 in Great Britain and Sweden.

Health reform attempts to reduce the amount of care consumed, rather than attempt to control prices. It will encourage doctors and hospitals to form accountable care organizations (ACOs) and pays them a fixed sum to discourage unnecessary care. The law also funds comparative-effectiveness research in an effort to reduce less effective treatments. However, many health-policy analysts consider these measures too weak to counteract

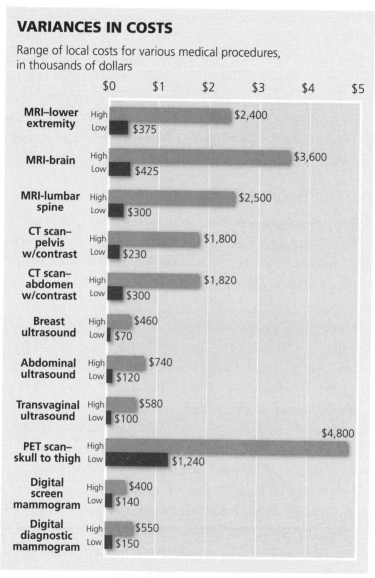

VARIANCES IN COSTS

Range of local costs for various medical procedures, in thousands of dollars

MRI–lower extremity	High	$2,400
	Low	$375
MRI-brain	High	$3,600
	Low	$425
MRI-lumbar spine	High	$2,500
	Low	$300
CT scan–pelvis w/contrast	High	$1,800
	Low	$230
CT scan–abdomen w/contrast	High	$1,820
	Low	$300
Breast ultrasound	High	$460
	Low	$70
Abdominal ultrasound	High	$740
	Low	$120
Transvaginal ultrasound	High	$580
	Low	$100
PET scan–skull to thigh	High	$4,800
	Low	$1,240
Digital screen mammogram	High	$400
	Low	$140
Digital diagnostic mammogram	High	$550
	Low	$150

Source: Change: healthcare. Q2 2011 healthcare transparency index.

Patients can pay as much as 683 percent more for the same medical procedure at two locations within a 20-mile radius. The price disparity is a reflection of the power of dominant health-care organizations to determine prices.

the proliferation of expensive procedures and emerging, costly technologies.

The fragmented health-care sector is also larded with excessive administrative costs. The McKinsey Global Institute estimated that administration accounted for 21 percent of ESAW. Most of that is because of the incredibly complex U.S. private insurance system. The U.S. spends about six times more on insurance administration than other industrialized nations.

Why health care is different

The health-care market does not operate like other economic sectors. The players—insurance companies, hospitals, doctors and pharmaceutical companies—rarely compete for consumers on the basis of price, because consumers do not pay much of the cost.

There also is an asymmetry of information: The sellers know more than the buyers about what needs to be done. Doctors and hospitals decide which of their services best suit the patients.

Consumers clearly are in the back seat and have little room— or inclination—to negotiate on price or shop around. Televisions and cellphones are commodities, and price comparison is easy. Patients do not know what mix of health services they need for a given condition, so they do not know what to shop for.

Inefficiency is tolerated, even encouraged. Providers are able to do pretty much whatever they want to address medical conditions, with little or no accountability for results. In other markets, efficient companies drive out inefficient competitors by offering lower prices and superior quality. That rarely happens with health-care providers. There is a lack of transparency on pricing, and consumers do not know how to determine quality. Because someone else is negotiating prices with providers and paying the bills, most patients do not really care about price or quality.

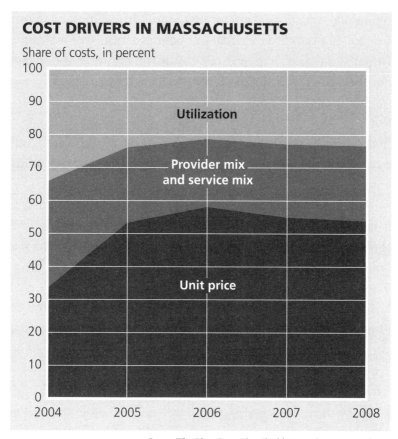

COST DRIVERS IN MASSACHUSETTS

Share of costs, in percent

Source: The Blue Cross Blue Shield Massachusetts Foundation.

An investigation of rising health-care costs by the Massachusetts attorney general's office found that rising prices—not volume or change in provider or service mix—were the main culprit. Market power has allowed prestigious health-care organizations to command premium prices for their services.

The comparative lack of productivity gains stems from virtually nonexistent price competition and payment policies that encourage volume rather than efficiency. Increased productivity requires that prices decrease for the same services, or more care is provided at the same cost. That rarely happens in health care.

Paying one price for treatment of an episode of illness or injury, often called a bundled or global payment, is a means for increasing efficiency and discouraging excess treatment. However, the savings must be shared with the payer for productivity to increase.

Cost driver No. 1: Technology

Medical technology is the engine that drives health-care costs. It accounts for an estimated one-half to two-thirds of spending growth.

Technology can come in the form of new procedures, drugs, medical devices or support systems such as telemedicine or electronic health records. The National Center for Health Statistics took a snapshot of technology changes from 1996 to 2007. Use of advanced imaging technology in outpatient facilities tripled during that time. Knee and hip replacements increased 60 to 70 percent. Angioplasty surgeries open blocked or narrowed coronary arteries. Nearly two-thirds of angioplasties involved no stents in 1996. By 2006, more than 90 percent included stents— and more than three-quarters of those were coated with drugs.

All of these procedures are expensive. Technology expansion contributed mightily to the fact that Medicare Part B reimbursement, which covers doctor and outpatient services, more than doubled, to $14.1 billion, from 2000 to 2006.

Outpatient care does not require an overnight stay in a hospital. It can take place in a doctor's office, hospital or outpatient surgery center. Health-care providers have aggressively expanded outpatient care for a number of reasons. The centers are highly profitable, sometimes exceeding a 25 percent margin. Outpatient procedures often result in quicker patient recovery and can be performed less expensively than during hospitalization. However, lucrative fee-for-service reimbursement and customer convenience encourage excessive use of services. In other words, it is doubtful that the *need* for advanced imaging tripled in a decade. Moreover, health outcomes were not twice as good for a Medicare patient in 2006 as they were in 2000.

Technology serves a useful purpose for providers, beyond the possibility of improved treatment. Health-care innovation leads to higher prices for services. There is scant resistance to this from patients, because they pay so little of the bill. Government programs and health plans also offer little resistance, because they do not want to be accused of denying patients access to the latest medical tools.

Hospitals also like to market their cutting-edge technology to attract physicians and their patients, because it serves as a proxy for quality. The consequence in many markets is a medical arms race as hospitals try to match their competitors, creating an oversupply of facilities and a temptation to overuse the equipment to justify the expense. Even the most efficient health-care organizations must grapple with acquiring technology and charging high prices for procedures. This can offset—even overwhelm—their best efforts at supplying more cost-efficient care in other services.

At best, the evidence is spotty that all of this technology is bettering health outcomes—or even is an improvement over the services they replace. Health care arguably is not an important determinant of health. Other factors—health behavior, genes, education and income—play much greater roles in health outcomes. Health care rarely cures disease. It mostly helps patients cope with what they have.

Cost driver No. 2: Market power

Market power is an underappreciated contributor to medical inflation. Four major players compete on the health-care economic stage: buyers, providers, insurers and suppliers. Buyers include employers, governments and individuals. They pay insurers, who in turn pay the providers. More specifically, governments are both purchasers and insurers. They collect money from taxpayers and ensure that qualified constituents receive care by paying providers. Providers include doctors, hospitals and pharmacies. Suppliers include medical-device manufacturers and pharmaceutical companies.

Money flows from payers to providers and suppliers. Providers and suppliers seek to exercise their pricing power whenever possible.

Hospitals and physicians have been consolidating at a rapid rate. An average of 2,200 U.S. physicians have been involved in mergers and acquisitions each year since 2007. This is expected to increase, because health reform is encouraging hospitals and physicians to form ACOs to test new health-care delivery models and payments based on quality and patient outcomes. Some analysts fear that ACOs will encourage greater market power for providers.

A major reason for hospital-physician consolidation is to increase market power. A health-care organization with a dominant market share and sturdy brand can raise prices well above what it needs to meet rising expenses. Insurers consider these organizations "must haves" in their networks and are willing to pay a premium price to include them, especially if there are several health plans competing for local employers. The opposite happens in markets with dominant insurers and several hospitals. Providers accept lower price increases because they must compete and have fewer options.

The Center for Studying Health System Change monitors 12 nationally representative metropolitan areas for health-care trends. It found that health plans were no match for consolidated hospital and physician groups in Miami and the prestigious academic medical centers in Boston. Those providers won large rate increases in 2010, which were passed on to employers, and ultimately to individual employees, as premium increases. Conversely, the highly dominant Blue Cross Blue Shield plans in Lansing, Mich. and Syracuse, N.Y. were able to win comparatively modest rate increases.

This negotiating battle occurs all across America annually. In short, health-plan market power keeps price increases low. Hospital market concentration results in higher prices. Hospitals appear to have the edge in most markets.

There is no hard evidence on the contribution of market power to medical inflation because these price agreements remain secret. However, Massachusetts Inspector General Gregory Sullivan wants the legislature to give the state the ability to review the hospital-insurance company agreements and reject them, if necessary.

After a wave of hospital mergers from 1990 to 2003, about 90 percent of metropolitan area hospitals acquired what the Federal Trade Commission considered excessive market power. Health economists estimate the mergers lifted prices by as much as 40 percent over what they would have otherwise been.

According to an investigation by the Massachusetts attorney general, the state's insurance companies paid some physicians and hospitals twice as much as others in the same market for the same services, with no better quality. The report attributed the higher prices to provider market power.

Market power also allows hospitals to shift costs. For many hospitals, Medicare and Medicaid reimbursement often is less than the cost of care. They typically compensate by charging commercial insurance companies more. In 2009, Medicare and Medicaid paid hospitals about 90 percent of the cost of care. Private plans paid 134 percent of the cost of care.

On average, the commercial-insurance rate is nearly 30 percent more than what Medicare pays. Hospitals with market power can exceed that rate. For example, some California "must have" hospitals and physician groups are able to charge health plans twice the rates they receive from Medicare for the same procedures. Annual increases of 10 percent or more are now commonplace.

Consumers weigh in

Few health consumers blame technology and market power for rising health-care costs. Instead, they point to favored demons, real and imagined. In a HealthDay/Harris Interactive poll, 6 out of 10 put the same blame on insurance companies and pharmaceutical firms. About felt that hospitals were culpable.

Health economists say insurance and drug-company profits account for about 2 percent of total health-care spending. A 2009 analysis of hospital finances found that the median profit margin for U.S. hospitals was zero.

More than 1 in 3 poll respondents blamed obese and overweight people. The least-cited reason: Their own excessive use of health services.

Should costs be controlled?

Perhaps controlling medical costs violates basic American values. Medical ethics and government policy dictate that human life be extended as long as possible. Individual choice—for the patient and the physician—seemingly is non-negotiable. Equal rights is interpreted to mean all Americans should have access to the best possible care.

Exercising these principles in health care translates into a blank check. There are no financial limits, as long as payers are willing to shell out whatever is necessary. Any talk of limiting or rationing care is politically toxic. Health care is considered a necessity, even life-saving, so insurers and government ultimately pick up the tab regardless of whether someone has insurance. People see little reason to deny themselves care, especially when they do not benefit from the savings that would result. Cost constraints are immaterial to patients when they can commit someone else's money to whatever treatment they or their physicians choose. Economists call this "moral hazard," or behaving differently than if patients bore the full cost of care.

However, this cannot continue without high taxes. Historically, federal taxes have accounted for about 20 percent of the economy. According to a 2007 Congressional Budget Office analysis, financing a 1 percent gap between health-care costs and income growth would require a tax increase of 70 percent by 2050. The analysis assumed no cuts in other government programs. The highest federal tax rate would be a currently unfathomable 60 percent.

No easy solutions

There are no easy answers on how to harness medical costs. After five decades of excessive inflation, rising medical costs have taken on a life of their own. Many on the left of the political spectrum favor a single-payer, Medicare-for-all system. The government could exercise its monopsony, or single-buyer, power to negotiate the most favorable prices. Some employers favor this because they would escape the tyranny of providing health benefits to employees. Most conservatives and moderates hate this idea, saying that it gives government too much power and eliminates market forces.

Many conservatives believe government should subsidize low-income people through tax credits and have them shop for insurance policies that best fit their needs. Pulling back the government's obligation to supply insurance to the elderly, the poor and disabled would shrink the size of government and expose people to the true cost of health care, thereby reducing utilization. It would also force market players to compete for business. Unfortunately, consumers are poor judges of quality in the health-care arena and do not know what health care they need. Current consumer tools are of little value.

Government's favorite cost-control method is to pay providers less for the same services. Recession-plagued state governments have been cutting Medicaid rates to help balance their budgets. The health-reform law lowers Medicare reimbursement to hospitals immediately and lowers payment to all providers over time. This strategy increasingly is ineffective. As reimbursement rates decline, more physicians withdraw from the programs, making access more difficult for government-insurance enrollees. Doctors who continue to see these patients often try to make up for the reimbursement cuts by seeing more patients for shorter periods of time—arguably providing lower quality of care for all patients.

For the past 50 years, there has been a steady redistribution of resources from employers, households and government coffers to the health-care system. There are few signs that trend will abate.

Steven Schroeder, distinguished professor of medicine and health policy at the University of California, San Francisco, concluded in a 2011 *Archives of Internal Medicine* essay, "In the long run, reining in costs will require mobilizing political forces that can withstand the inevitable claims of rationing sure to come from industries currently benefiting from the 17 percent of the economy spent on health care, and from consumers who have come to expect unlimited access to what they feel they need."

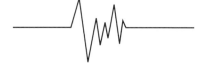

Chapter 16

Consumer Health Costs
Struggling with bills and deductibles

As state and federal lawmakers grapple with skyrocketing health-care costs, households across America are doing the same.

Expecting health reform to provide relief is wishful thinking.

In less than a decade, the annual health-care costs for a typical family have more than doubled, to $19,400. That is the price of a 2011 Hyundai Sonata. The average family bears about 40 percent of that cost, with employers paying the rest. However, a more realistic view is that employees pay for all of it because most wage-and-benefit increases go toward health-insurance costs.

Most people have only a vague notion of how valuable health insurance can be. The median household income for a four-person U.S. family in 2009 was about $70,300. However, the Congressional Budget Office (CBO) estimates the true figure to be $94,900. A footnote on page 65 of a CBO budget forecast said this: "All income is assumed to be from compensation, which includes employment-based health insurance and the employer's share of payroll taxes."

That additional value does not mean much to those living paycheck to paycheck. Each family has a different financial pressure point. The media often focus on catastrophic costs inflicted on people with no insurance. The broader story of health-care costs is about financial strain spread across a wide swath of American households. The pain affects much of the middle class and some of the upper middle class as well, including those with employer-sponsored insurance.

Americans actually pay a far lower share of health expenses than they used to. The main purpose of health insurance originally was to cover catastrophic episodes. Before the introduction of Medicare and Medicaid in 1965, patients paid more than half the cost of care out of pocket. That shrank to 15 percent in 2008. Meanwhile, private health plans' share of the bill rose from 21 to 35 percent and government's portion doubled, to 50 percent. The perception that medical bills are the responsibility of someone other than the patient has been a prime contributor to health-care demand over the past four decades.

A Deloitte study estimates that consumers pay an additional 15 percent out of pocket on personal health not captured by government statistics. These costs include unpaid caregiving, over-the-counter medications, and complementary and alternative medical care not covered by insurance.

The inability to pay medical bills and buy prescription drugs is the most persistent household finance problem, according to a recent Consumer Reports poll. About 40 percent of Americans had trouble paying medical bills in 2010, up from 34 percent in 2005. More than one-quarter of insured households reported problems with medical debt.

Even more disturbing is widespread self-rationing. Nearly 6 out of 10 adults said they delayed care because of cost. About 40 percent of those in fair or poor health did not fill at least one prescription in the past year. People with chronic conditions who fail to take medication are flirting with disastrous consequences.

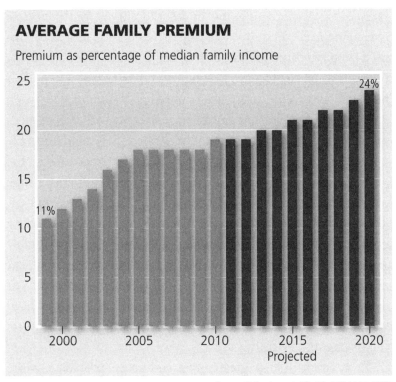

AVERAGE FAMILY PREMIUM

Premium as percentage of median family income

Source: Sisko A, et al. Health Aff. 2009;28(2)

The projected average family health-insurance premium in 2020 excludes out-of-pocket costs. The 2020 premium cost as a proportion of family income is expected to double between 2000 and 2020, from 12 percent to 24 percent.

Americans generally cite lack of access as the greatest obstacle to health care, followed by costs. Lack of access can mean several things. In some instances, people cannot see a physician or specialist promptly. Nearly 60 percent say they cannot find care after physician office hours, 40 percent cannot get service by phone and 30 percent cannot get a timely office appointment.

Increasingly, though, lack of health-care access means not being able to afford it.

According to an ongoing household survey, the incidence of delaying needed care rose sharply between 2003 and 2007. Insured people are among those facing cost pressures. They are paying more out-of-pocket for care, finding fewer doctors who accept their insurance and facing more limits on what insurance will cover. During those four years, the percentage of those with unmet medical needs increased more among the insured than the uninsured.

It is difficult to pinpoint when health-care costs become burdensome. The Center for Studying Health System Change found that financial pressures increase significantly after out-of-pocket spending exceeds 2.5 percent of family income. Unlike a mortgage, groceries and utilities, medical costs are less predictable and often unexpected. High medical expenses generally are urgent and associated with serious conditions. Significant injury or disease may also result in loss of income. Even two-thirds of Americans earning more than $75,000 a year worry about getting or paying for future care.

Women experience greater cost and access problems. More than half of women have trouble getting care, and more than 60 percent under age 65 have difficulty paying medical bills. Women use the health-care system more than men do. They often must make choices between getting care or paying credit-card bills, the mortgage or for basic necessities.

Recession's impact on health-care use

For the 40 percent who struggled to pay medical bills in 2010, the worst recession since the Great Depression was an albatross. Layoffs added 9 million to the ranks of the uninsured. One out of 4 U.S. adults said they or their spouse lost a job in the past two years.

A recession is a worldwide phenomenon, yet Americans reduced routine care far more than their European counterparts

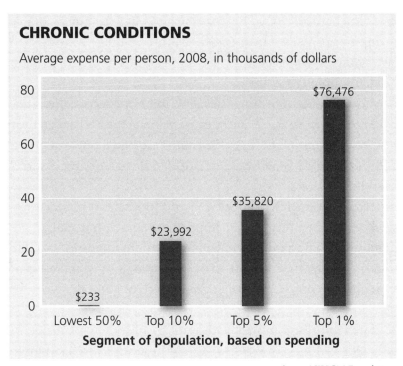

CHRONIC CONDITIONS

Average expense per person, 2008, in thousands of dollars

Source: NIHCM Foundation.

Per-capita health-care costs are heavily skewed. The lowest-cost, or healthiest, 50 percent of the population spends an average of $233 a year, compared with more than $76,000 for the sickest 1 percent. The average for the top 50 percent is well above the deductible for most high-deductible health plans.

did. More than 25 percent of Americans have cut back on regular medical care since the global economic crisis began in 2007. Comparable figures elsewhere were about 5 percent in Canada, less than 8 percent in Great Britain and 12 percent in France.

The ripple effects have also hit hospitals hard. About 70 percent of U.S. hospitals reported fewer patient visits and elective procedures. Nearly all say they are treating more patients who cannot pay at all. The inevitable result is staff reductions and curtailment of services. The recession also put a dent in charitable giving to hospitals. Historically, health-care usage continues to lag as long as five years after a recession ends. The latest recession officially ended in 2009.

Insurers are confirming the falloff in health-service use. They have profited from this, because employers and insurers design their health plans far in advance. Premiums are based on anticipated volume of care. When that care does not materialize, insurers keep the balance.

Health plans have reported record profits and rich cash reserves. However, this has not stopped insurers from seeking state approval for infuriatingly enormous premium increases. In some states, employers with more than 20 employees saw increases of 20 percent in one year. Smaller groups received bills that were 40 percent higher than the previous year, or even more.

Such hubris prompted Kathleen Sebelius, the U.S. secretary of health and human services, to require insurers to justify rate increases of more than 10 percent beginning in September 2011. However, the federal government does not have the power to stop rate increases it believes are unjustified.

A February 2010 Moody's Investors Service report asserted that the reduction in consumer health care may be the new normal. Its analysts said the likely trend is a more permanent shift in consumer behavior. They cited a number of factors, including an increase in high-deductible health-insurance plans and greater demands by insurers for treatments whose effectiveness can be proved.

However, according to a forecast of 2012 medical costs by PricewaterhouseCoopers, employers and health plans are reporting a rising frequency of employee claims. They credit the rise to workers who deferred care during the recession, creating more complicated conditions and pent-up demand.

- Prohibits the purchase of over-the-counter drugs with money from health reimbursement accounts, flexible spending accounts (FSA), health savings accounts (HSA) or Archer medical savings accounts (MSA). Effective in 2011.
- Increases the tax on distributions from HSA or MSA that are not used for medical expenses to 20 percent (currently 10 percent for HSAs and 15 percent for MSAs). Effective in 2011.

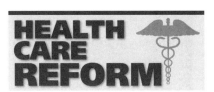

Cost sharing

- Limits contributions to an FSA to $2,500 annually, which will be adjusted yearly based on cost of living. Effective in 2013.
- Increases the threshold for itemized deduction for unreimbursed medical expenses from 7.5 percent to 10 percent. Effective in 2013.

Difficult economic times definitely take a toll on mental health. About 40 percent of employees report increased stress and anxiety. The Occupational Safety and Health Administration has declared stress a workplace hazard. An American Psychological Association survey showed that the top three causes of stress from 2007 to 2010 were money, work and the economy. Yet demand for psychiatric services slackens during recessions.

The economy's impact on physical health is more complex. Many studies point to a profound impact from layoffs on health outcomes, but other research has found that health actually worsens during good economic times.

The risk of heart attack and stroke doubled when older workers lost their jobs. A 2006 study found the risk of developing stress-related chronic conditions nearly doubled. The death rate of high-seniority male employees rose as much as 100 percent within the first year of a layoff, and an increased risk persists for as long as 20 years.

On the other hand, people tend to work and play harder during economic expansion—often to the detriment of their health.

A University of North Carolina economics professor found that the death rate fell during recessions in the 1970s and 1980s and rose when the economy recovered. He also discovered that smoking and weight decline in hard times because idled workers are more physically active with their increased leisure time.

Increased economic activity creates more vehicle traffic and its associated dangers, and more industrial accidents. Other health behaviors associated with a robust economy include greater consumption of tobacco and alcohol, weight gain, lack of exercise, sleep deprivation and less time with family and friends—all of which compromise immunity to disease. Low-income workers are especially vulnerable because they juggle multiple part-time jobs and, in some cases, literally work themselves to death.

Difficult economic times can also cut both ways in the workplace. Employees who ordinarily miss work often for health-related reasons attend work more frequently. People who abuse alcohol or drugs may curb their behavior to be more productive and perhaps become healthier.

In 2010, employers and health plans said they were beginning to see an uptick in claims related to stress caused by the recession, as well as an increase because of deferred medical care because of tight household budgets.

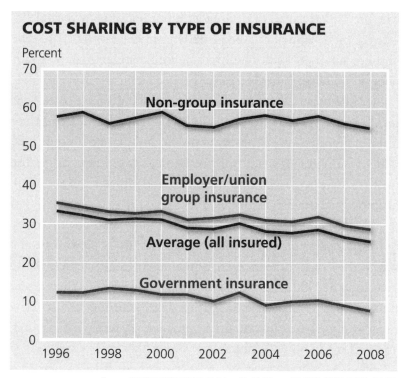

COST SHARING BY TYPE OF INSURANCE

Source: MEPS 1996-2006; Baicker K, Goldman D. JEP. 2001;25(2):47-68; Barro J. Manhattan Institute, March 2011.

Cost-sharing differs significantly based on the source of health insurance. People who buy individual policies pay for more than half of their expenses out of pocket. Public-sector employees pay the lowest percentage out of pocket. The average government worker earns $4.65 per hour in health benefits, compared with $2.10 for nongovernment employees.

A recession even affects family planning. According to a 2009 survey of women ages 18 to 34, nearly half said they planned to reduce or delay childbearing until the economy improved.

Bankruptcy: The household nuclear option

Access to care is normally measured nationally by the percentage of Americans who are uninsured. This deflects attention from people who are underinsured or dealing with burdensome medical debt. The typical benchmark for being underinsured is paying 10 percent or more out of pocket for health care. People under financial strain often forgo needed medical care.

Unlike other expenses, medical costs are difficult to budget for. The uninsured are especially disadvantaged because they receive bills up to 2.5 times what public and private insurers pay. Unlike individuals, health plans can negotiate lower prices for treatment costs. Only 1 out of 8 uninsured families can pay their hospital bills in full.

Nearly half of the uninsured did not fill at least one prescription in the past year and more than half had medical problems for which they did not seek care. One out of 5 had medical debts exceeding $8,000. They lose one-third to one-half of their assets to medical expenses when tragedy strikes. According to a government study, most uninsured people have "virtually no" savings and had median financial assets of just $20.

Medical bills are playing more prominent roles in personal bankruptcies. Medical expenses contributed to nearly two-thirds of bankruptcies filed in 2007, according to a Harvard research study. The share of bankruptcies associated with medical bills increased 50 percent between 2001 and 2007.

The authors were blunt: "The U.S. health-care financing system is broken, and not only for the poor and uninsured. Middle-class families frequently collapse under the strain of a health-care system that treats physical wounds, but often inflicts fiscal ones."

Lead researcher David Himmelstein, who advocates a single-payer system, said in a statement: "Unless you're Warren Buffett, your family is just one serious illness away from bankruptcy. For middle-class Americans, health insurance offers little protection."

Three-quarters of those filing for bankruptcy had medical insurance when they became ill or injured. Many found that they were underinsured and had large out-of-pocket expenses. One-quarter of employers cancel coverage immediately when an employee suffers a disabling illness, and another quarter do so within a year. Medical bankruptcy is rare in developed nations other than the United States. Besides having better medical safety nets, Europeans pay about half as much as Americans do for out-of-pocket expenses.

Some conditions are financially devastating. According to the study, people with multiple sclerosis paid an average of more than $34,000 out of pocket in 2007. Those with diabetes paid nearly $27,000 and those with serious injuries paid about $25,000.

Himmelstein also examined the impact of the 2006 Massachusetts health-reform law. The percentage of bankruptcies tied to medical bills changed little after reform, indicating that federal reform will not have much effect.

Himmlestein said, "Massachusetts' health reform, like the national law modeled after it, takes many of the uninsured and makes them underinsured—typically giving them a skimpy, defective private policy that's like an umbrella that melts in the rain. The protection's not there when you need it."

Other researchers say such bankruptcy figures are overblown. They estimate that medical bills contribute to less than 20 percent of bankruptcies and primarily affect those with incomes closer to poverty level.

A study of medical financial burden and mortgage foreclosures found a strong link. Seven of 10 homeowners had a significant medical episode in the two years prior to foreclosure proceedings. More than one-third had outstanding medical bills greater than $2,000 and 1 out of 8 used home equity to pay for care.

Retirement health-care costs

People on Medicare are often viewed as being shielded from bankruptcy. Medicare coverage is extensive, but it does not cover everything. A study focusing on the elderly found that medical-related bankruptcy for those ages 65 to 74 rose 178 percent between 1991 and 2007—just prior to the beginning of the current recession.

Seniors spend about 10 percent more of their incomes on health care than working-age adults, even excluding prescription-medication costs. The elderly have greater medical needs, and their fixed incomes are less capable of absorbing rising medical costs.

Health care is a major retirement expense, and rising at a significantly higher rate than consumer inflation. According to Fidelity Investments, health-care expenses for those 65 or older rose more than 4 percent in 2010, compared with 1.1 percent for consumer prices overall. Retirees are paying 56 percent more for medical expenses than in 2002. Health-care expenses average $535 a month, second only to food costs.

The Center for Retirement Research at Boston College estimates that a married couple age 65 will spend $197,000 out of pocket for their remaining life expectancy. The figure rises to $260,000 when nursing care is included.

The good news is that health reform will close the "doughnut hole" in the Medicare Part D prescription drug benefit. Medicare beneficiaries pay out-of-pocket for medication after the initial coverage limit is met and before catastrophic coverage begins. In 2009, Medicare did not cover the first $295 of prescription expenses or those incurred between $2,700 and $6,154 annually. The latter gap gradually will close by the end of the decade.

The bad news is that Medicare inevitably will shift more costs to retirees in future years. Retirees spend about 10 percent of their income on health-care expenses. That is expected to rise to 19 percent by 2040.

Three out of 4 baby boomers say health care is their No. 1 or No. 2 retirement concern. Almost all consider health care a basic need rather than a discretionary expense.

Reform boosts high-deductible plans

Conservative politicians advocate health policies that ensure consumers have "more skin in the game." For them, a favorite solution has been high-deductible health plans (HDHPs). Consumers pay the first $1,000 or more of medical expenses before insurance takes over. Traditional health insurance plans insulate the patient from the true cost, conservatives say.

Health reform will take HDHPs to an entirely new level. For those participating in the health-insurance exchanges in 2014, the most popular health plans will be HDHPs. According to one estimate, the annual deductible on the least expensive plan could be $6,530.

The conservatives who sneer at "Obamacare" fail to acknowledge that health reform could help establish HDHPs as the most prevalent form of private-sector health insurance coverage when exchanges begin operating in 2014.

Employers increasingly will rely on HDHPs because they want to avoid the law's 40 percent excise tax beginning in 2017 on high-cost plans. This was already the case before health reform became law. The number of workers enrolled in employer plans with a $1,000 or higher deductible tripled between 2006 and 2010. That includes nearly half of all workers in small companies. The average deductible for employees enrolled in a preferred provider organization (PPO)—the most popular and comprehensive plan offered by most employers—reached $1,200 in 2010. This certainly blurs the distinction between conventional PPOs and HDHPs.

HDHPs have been growing for individuals and businesses squeezed by enormous annual increases in health insurance costs. Each year, the tendency is to gravitate toward skimpier coverage and higher deductibles to maintain affordability. Companies with at least 50 percent of their employees in HDHPs pay about $1,000 less per employee for health benefits. Nearly two-thirds of large companies offered HDHPs in 2011, and the percentage that offered only HDHPs doubled to 20 percent from 2010.

Nearly 25 percent of working-age adults and about half of individually insured adults have an HDHP.

Types of plans

HDHPs, often called account-based plans, come in several flavors. Standard HDHPs are simply high-deductible plans. Consumers pay lower premiums in exchange for paying more of the initial cost, a higher portion of each medical bill, or both. In 2008, the IRS tax-free threshold was $1,100 for individual coverage and $2,200 for family coverage.

A consumer-directed health plan (CDHP) is an HDHP with a special tax-favored savings account to pay for medical expenses. With CDHPs, consumers make tax-free deposits into health savings accounts (HSAs) that accompany HDHPs. Balances accumulate year to year, earning tax-free interest. Health reimbursement arrangements (HRAs) are often used by employers to help shape their benefit packages and to provide incentives for prevention and wellness. With HSAs, people make their deposits and own the balances. With HRAs, companies make the deposits, roll over from year to year and usually keep the balances when the employee leaves the company.

The typical CDHP member is more likely to be young, single, higher-income, healthier and better-educated than those on traditional plans are. The plans are also popular with healthy employees over 55 who consider HSAs a tax-free retirement investment account. The average household income for people with HSAs was $139,000 in 2008, compared with $57,000 for all other taxpayers. They are less likely to smoke or be obese, and more likely to exercise and be involved in a workplace health-promotion program than traditional-plan enrollees.

People who are sick or have an ill family member are less likely to choose account-based insurance. Some fear that, if many healthier people switch to CDHPs, traditional plans may become more expensive because they include a higher percentage of people with chronic conditions.

Regardless of the arrangement, HDHPs are more like true insurance by covering unforeseen, high-cost events while the consumer pays for low-cost health expenses that are more predictable and amenable to a household budget.

Effects on health-care use

People with HDHPs almost invariably use less health care. They usually use self-diagnosis, followed by self-rationing. They generally cut back equally on unnecessary and necessary care. Patients tend to give less weight to the future state of their health than to present costs.

RAND Corp. conducted groundbreaking research in the 1970s that illustrates what happens with high consumer cost-sharing. The so-called Health Insurance Experiment randomly assigned 5,800 working-age adults to different levels of cost sharing, ranging from free to 95 percent. The results showed:

- As the percentage paid by the patient rose, physician visits decreased.

- The total amount of treatment received was unaffected once they began medical care, meaning consumers tended to lose control of costs.
- Health outcomes were unaffected regardless of cost-sharing and medical usage.

Another, more recent RAND study showed that HDHP enrollees cut back on care regardless of their income or health.

People on Medicare are especially sensitive to higher cost-sharing, even to increases of just a few dollars. One study of health plans that raised co-payments modestly for drugs and physician care showed a dramatic impact—and ultimately more costly care. For every 100 people who had to pay more, there were 20 fewer doctor visits, two additional hospitalizations and 13 more days in the hospital. Unlike the younger participants in the 1970s RAND study, Medicare beneficiaries have far more chronic conditions that can flare up without consistent care.

Some companies are employing a strategy called value-based insurance design. The format varies the cost-sharing with employees based on the scientific evidence of a drug or procedure's effectiveness. For example, Pitney Bowes reduced the co-payments of several medications for conditions such as diabetes, high blood pressure and asthma. The company's higher pharmacy costs were offset by fewer Emergency Department visits and avoidable hospitalizations.

A 2007 study concluded that the optimal co-payment for cholesterol-lowering medication was $0 or even negative—meaning patients should be paid to take the drugs in order to lower overall costs.

Americans have been using fewer medical services for the past couple of years. Some analysts say the recession makes it more likely that consumers forgo medical care. Others say the increase of HDHPs is having an impact. Health-insurance companies have enjoyed record profits because they are paying for less care than anticipated as premiums have continued to rise. It is hard to know whether this is a temporary lull or the new normal in health-care usage.

What is puzzling is that HDHPs prompt patients to cut back on preventive care, even when it is free. This suggests either they did not understand that their policies paid for the services completely, or they are leery of the health-care system generally. They also may fear that the doctor may find something wrong that will result in a costly expense.

The long-term effects of this are unknown. However, forgone care can lead to greater complications and care that is more expensive in the future. For example, high cost-sharing causes those with newly diagnosed chronic conditions to delay filling their prescriptions.

HDHPs work well for a significant percentage of the population. However, they will do little to hold down national health costs, because a small percentage of consumers account for a large percentage of U.S. health costs. The healthiest 50 percent of Americans spend about $250 a year on health care. The sickest 5 percent spend more than $43,000 a year. Even an HDHP would not make a dent in costs for these patients. Once the deductible has been met, the incentive to minimize health-care costs vanishes.

The harsh reality of HDHPs: Eight out of 10 families earning about $52,000 do not have enough savings to cover the deductible. More than 40 percent of adults with HDHPs spent 10 percent or more of their income on household medical expenses—a threshold many consider a financial burden on the average family.

HSAs are meant to be an incentive to set aside money to pay for future medical expenses. However, many have difficulty saving for retirement or even vacations—both more pleasant prospects and worthy goals. If people cannot do that, it is unlikely they will save for an unpleasant circumstance such as an unforeseen bout with cancer.

A 2008 consumer survey delivered one of the most depressing commentaries on the American health-care system: People were more concerned about the prospect of paying for the treatment of an illness than about the illness itself.

Shopping around

One of the key principles behind HDHPs is to create more discerning health-care consumers. In theory, health-care providers will compete for customers on price and quality, lowering the former and increasing the latter. However, the existing tools to do this are primitive and mostly useless.

For example, California requires hospitals to publish their official prices, known as charge masters. However, these have little value because hospitals charge any of dozens of prices for the same procedure, depending on negotiations with different health plans. UCLA Medical Center included this unexplained entry on its published charge master: GRMS EXT PIECE HOWMED STRYKER. Price $10,290. That, by the way, is a prosthetic bone.

Contrast this with other consumer goods, for which prices are clearly marked and easily compared. Product details are listed and readily available. Expert and consumer reviews usually exist. These tools do not exist in health care.

More than 30 states are considering or attempting to pass legislation to increase price transparency. Three bills were introduced in Congress in 2010 to do the same.

There has been little urgency to help HDHP enrollees up to this point. They remain a small, if growing, segment of the insured population. Most patients are fully insured and pay a small portion of their health-care costs.

Patients shopping based on price are at a disadvantage because they do not know what they need. Every disease or condition needs a different mix of care. Attempting to figure that out without a physician's guidance can be a foolhardy exercise. Consumers have a much easier time with simple procedures such as those offered in retail health clinics, or for prescription prices.

And, of course, few feel like shopping when they are ill.

Patients also have a difficult time trying to determine quality of care. This is an example of how efforts to provide the consumer with more detailed information may backfire. Many erroneously believe higher cost of care means higher quality. That line of thinking might encourage providers to raise their prices simply to enhance the perceived value of their services.

Consumers do not even shop around for health services not customarily covered by insurance, such as LASIK surgery and dental crowns. These services are ideal for comparison shopping: they are not urgent; there is no need for further diagnosis; there is usually one price per provider, and the out-of-pocket cost can be steep.

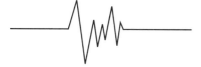

Chapter 17

Waste and Overtreatment
No incentive for efficiency

American health care is bloated with waste. A 2005 report by the Institute of Medicine (IOM) estimated that 30 to 40 percent of health-care spending represented "overuse, underuse, misuse, duplication, system failures, unnecessary repetition, poor communication, and inefficiency."

Gross inefficiencies exist largely because there are no incentives to economize. Consumers generally use more health care than they would otherwise because generous insurance shields them from the true costs. Providers are paid for services they supply, rather than on efficiency, outcomes or quality. The inexact nature of medical diagnosis and fear of malpractice litigation encourage even more services. Insurance companies offer little resistance to stiff annual price increases, preferring instead to pass along the costs to private payers through higher premiums.

Rooting waste out of the health-care system is difficult. What is waste to one person is another's revenue stream. Any medical service can be justified in some way. The key is figuring out which spending can be eliminated without compromising quality and care.

It is difficult to fathom that a health-care system that consumes 17 percent of a nation's economy only delivers 55 percent of recommended care. However, delivering all of the recommended preventive care and chronic-disease management would require physicians to work 17 hours a day on only those.

Many organizations have attempted to calculate the amount of waste in the U.S. health-care system. Most agree roughly with the 2005 IOM report. All say the figure is staggering in size.

The Congressional Budget Office estimated that one-third of the money spent on health care in 2006 did nothing to improve health outcomes. That amounted to about $700 billion, or 5 percent of gross domestic product.

Dr. Jack Wennberg, founding editor of the Dartmouth Atlas of Health Care, which tracks patterns of health-care use, has said, "Up to one-third of the over $2 trillion that we now spend annually on health care is squandered on unnecessary hospitalizations; unneeded and often redundant tests; unproven treatments; over-priced, cutting-edge drugs; devices no better than the less-expensive products they replaced, and end-of-life care that brings neither comfort, care nor cure."

PricewaterhouseCoopers' (PwC) Health Research Institute came up with the largest waste estimate, claiming that more than half of health spending is squandered. That figure is $1.2 trillion, out of $2.2 trillion spent. PwC included in its calculations the cost of care provided because of Americans' poor health habits.

A Thomson Reuters analysis asserted that $3.6 trillion in wasted spending could be eliminated over 10 years by encouraging efficiency and better health behavior while attacking fraud and medical errors.

A 2008 RAND Corporation study built a framework for considering wasted resources in health care. It distinguished among administrative, operational and clinical waste. *Adminis-*

Fake surgeries work

Pharmaceutical drug trials traditionally test new medicines against fake pills, or placebos. In essence, the goal is to determine whether the new drug is better than nothing.

Why not fake surgeries?

Medical ethicists have debated the propriety of this. Nonetheless, scientists have "sham" procedures to test the validity of surgical techniques—with startling results.

In 2002, 180 patients with osteoarthritis were randomly assigned to undergo either arthroscopic knee surgery or fake surgery, although neither group was aware of the parameters. The results indicated that knee surgery provided no more pain relief or added mobility than the fake surgery. Predictably, the results were attacked by those who do knee surgeries. A second set of researchers did a similar study in 2008. The results were the same. Regardless, more than 500,000 patients spent $3 billion on arthroscopic surgery for arthritic knees in 2009.

Two recent randomized trials involving procedures for repairing vertebral fractures—kyphoplasty and vertebroplasty—found that they provided no more relief than sham surgeries. Medicare pays annually for about 100,000 of these procedures, which have significant risks, at a cost of about $1 billion.

trative waste is the excess administrative overhead associated with the complexity of the U.S. insurance and provider payment systems. *Operational waste* includes needless duplication and excessive price of services, system inefficiency and medical errors. *Clinical waste* is services that add little or no value, and may even be harmful.

Brookings Institution economist Henry Aaron described the U.S. health-care system as "an administrative monstrosity, a truly bizarre mélange of thousands of payers with payment systems that differ for no socially beneficial reason, as well as staggeringly complex public systems with mind-boggling administered prices and other rules expressing distinctions that can only be regarded as weird."

For example, Johns Hopkins Health System in Baltimore deals with about 700 different health plans, employers and other payers. Each payer has an annually negotiated rate for each service. Each also has different payment cycles and eligibility rules that must be tracked. The sheer complexity creates its own redundancies in several Hopkins departments, which the organization calculated to be more than $40 million annually.

Simply moving money from the payer to the provider based on negotiated rates is extremely expensive. Billing and insurance-related functions can account for more than half of administrative expense at a hospital or large physician practice. For an insurance company, the share can exceed 80 percent. Health-care clerical workers outnumber physicians 9 to 1, and registered nurses 3 to 1.

The U.S. spends about three times as much on health administration and insurance per capita as Canada. Brookings economist Aaron estimated in 2003 that the U.S. would save more than $213 billion annually if it had a single-payer system similar to that nation's.

Operational waste has myriad examples. Brand-name drugs are prescribed when generic medications will do. Expensive services are substituted for less expensive and equally effective ones. Physicians supply care that can easily be provided by a nurse practitioner or physician assistant. Duplicate tests or procedures are performed because of poor record-keeping or lack of communication between providers.

- Attempts to reduce waste, fraud and abuse in government insurance programs by allowing more rigorous provider screening, and longer oversight periods for new providers and suppliers.

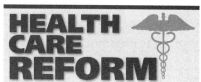

- Develops a database to share information across federal and state programs, and increases penalties for submitting false claims.

Waste

Effective dates vary.

One barrier to eliminating operational waste is a lack of incentives for providers. Efficiency benefits the payers. Forgoing services that are more expensive hurts provider profitability.

A service that delivers less value than its cost is considered clinical waste. This is often difficult to avoid when a physician is legitimately attempting to solve a medical riddle. However, it can also result in what is called "treatment creep," which means delivering a medical service to a larger population than was originally intended.

In an essay in *The New England Journal of Medicine*, Howard Brody, a family physician at the University of Texas Medical Branch at Galveston, challenged every medical specialty to identify five diagnostic or therapeutic procedures that are performed frequently, have a high price tag and offer no benefit to most patients.

Brody told *Newsweek* magazine: "We doctors are extremely good at rationalizing. Somehow we manage to figure out how the very best care just happens to be the care that brings us the most money."

Using medical guidelines is one way to avoid clinical waste. However, there is shockingly little scientific basis for much of today's medical treatment. Evidence on which treatments work often is incomplete or unavailable. When it is available, it is frequently ignored.

Only 40 percent of osteoporosis patients receive appropriate therapy, as well as two-thirds of stroke patients. Statins are underprescribed for stroke patients. Antibiotics are overprescribed for children with upper respiratory infections, despite evidence that they do not work.

There are several barriers to adopting medical evidence as the standard for treatment, including the difficulty of changing physician practice patterns and the sheer volume of research. Translating science into medical practice takes an average of 17 years, and monitoring the more than 10,000 randomized, controlled trials published annually is impossible for a busy clinician.

Some of this research makes its way into guidelines created by government agencies and medical associations. The U.S. Department of Health and Human Services lists more than 7,000 guidelines on one of its websites. However, some of these guidelines are no more than opinion.

For example, a 2011 study in *Archives of Internal Medicine* found that only 1 of every 7 treatment recommendations from the Infectious Diseases Society of America were based on high-quality clinical data. More than half of the more than 4,200 recommendations were based on opinion or anecdotal evidence.

Another 2011 study in the same journal found that more than half of the experts who wrote treatment guidelines for the American Heart Association and the American College of Cardiology had private financial conflicts of interest.

Zapping prostrate cancer with protons

Proton beam therapy was an extremely expensive medical solution in search of a cost justification.

It found one in prostate cancer. Billions of dollars later, there still is no evidence that it works better than conventional therapy.

The exotic treatment requires a nuclear particle accelerator to shoot protons at the speed of light into tumors. They are considered more precise than conventional X-rays used in radiation therapy. Theoretically, that means fewer side effects from stray radiation, and perhaps a higher cure rate.

The accelerator weighs more than 220 tons and is housed in a facility the size of a football field. Construction can cost as much as $200 million. There are nine centers in the U.S., with seven more being built.

The therapy is ideal for tumors in parts of the body vulnerable to collateral damage, such as eyes, the brain, the neck and the spine. Children are especially sensitive to radiation's side effects. However, these cancers are relatively rare and cannot support the cost of construction and operation of proton facilities.

Hello, prostate cancer.

The National Cancer Institute estimates that about 220,000 American men discovered in 2010 that they had prostate cancer. About 2.2 million have been diagnosed at some point.

Proton radiation therapy (PRT) needs that market. Of the 150 patients treated at an Oklahoma City facility in its first year, 109 had prostate cancer.

Medicare will pay for PRT despite a lack of scientific evidence of its superiority over conventional radiation

continued

treatment. A course of PRT can cost as much as $90,000, which is twice the cost of traditional radiation therapy.

Anthony Zietman is a radiation oncologist at Harvard and Massachusetts General Hospital, which owns a proton center. He told *The New York Times* that PRT was not much better than X-ray technology for fighting prostate cancer.

"You can scarcely tell the difference between them, except in price," he said. Of the rapid expansion of PRT facilities, Zietman said, "This is the dark side of American medicine."

Prostate cancer is an ideal candidate for speculative high-tech solutions, because there is little clinical-trial research comparing therapies. The latest U.S. research was a federally funded study of surgery versus what is called "watchful waiting," or closely monitoring the patient and withholding treatment until symptoms appear or change. The study found there was no survival benefit for those who had their prostates removed, up to a dozen years after diagnosis.

In an academic journal article, Zietman and colleagues explained why PRT would continue to rely on prostate cancer: "When a hospital invests in (PRT) ... it takes on a very substantial amount of financial risk... It needs to amortize its costs rapidly, and it needs ultimately to generate a profit. Thus, the use of protons becomes as much a business decision as a clinical one."

Sometimes less is more—and sometimes more is less

Many patients believe more health care is better health care. However, in most cases, it is simply more. Less-expensive interventions are often more effective. For example:

- One study found that a greater percentage of strokes have been prevented in the last decade by making sure patients took aspirin than by developing more potent anti-platelet medication.
- Older men diagnosed with low-risk prostate cancer can choose active surveillance rather than invasive treatment without losing quality of life.
- Recovery from small heart attacks was as successful on drug therapy as with invasive vessel-clearing procedures.
- Similarly, 22 percent of elderly Americans had coronary bypass surgery or balloon angioplasty in 1990, compared with 2 percent of Canadians. However, the 30-day death rate after a heart attack was the same for each nation.

There are other examples of expensive care that does not do much good:

- One out of 5 heart defibrillators is implanted without solid evidence that the devices will be helpful. They are implanted to shock an irregularly beating heart back to a normal rhythm. They work well in patients with advanced heart failure, but they have been ineffective in other patients. The procedure costs $35,000 and may cause unnecessary harm.
- Americans spent nearly $86 billion in 2005 on imaging, physician visits and medication for back and neck pain—most of which did not improve the patients' conditions.
- Medical imaging—which includes CT, PET and MRI scans—has become a $100 billion business. However, studies show 20 to 50 percent of the procedures should not have been done because they

neither helped diagnose patients nor helped determine their treatment.

The apparent heart-defibrillator overuse is an example of what is often called "technology creep." After a device is approved for use in a high-risk population, its use expands to a larger, lower-risk population, for whom risks outweigh the benefits. This, in a nutshell, is a major contributor to runaway medical costs and clinical waste. It is not the technology itself. It is technology utilized beyond its original intent—often to recoup its original cost and to bolster profits.

Imaging costs have grown at about twice the rate of other health-care technologies, including laboratory procedures and pharmaceuticals. A contributing factor is the financial incentives of self-referral. Federal regulations bar physicians from referring Medicare or Medicaid patients to services in which they have a financial interest. However, an exception is allowed if physicians have equipment in their offices—presumably for patient convenience.

Patients of doctors who own or lease MRI equipment are more likely to be scanned for lower back pain. A 2011 study showed an increase of nearly one-third for primary-care physicians and 13 percent for orthopedists. Orthopedic patients who were scanned were 34 percent more likely to have back surgery—meaning the scans induced more surgery. The study's authors point out there is no definitive evidence that either MRIs or surgery improve outcomes for lower back pain.

In a 2006 essay, two Johns Hopkins physicians blamed the overuse of technology on "gizmo idolatry"—a belief that more technological care is intrinsically better than less, regardless of the evidence. They said sophisticated techniques seem to ward off the risk of malpractice litigation, and technology provides a halo

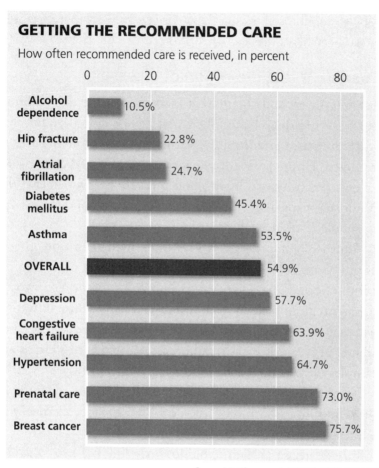

GETTING THE RECOMMENDED CARE

How often recommended care is received, in percent

Condition	Percent
Alcohol dependence	10.5%
Hip fracture	22.8%
Atrial fibrillation	24.7%
Diabetes mellitus	45.4%
Asthma	53.5%
OVERALL	54.9%
Depression	57.7%
Congestive heart failure	63.9%
Hypertension	64.7%
Prenatal care	73.0%
Breast cancer	75.7%

Source: McGlynn, et al. NEJM. 2003;348:2643.

On average, Americans receive evidence-based treatment only 55 percent of the time. The delivery of recommended care varies widely depending on the condition.

of competence for doctors who use it. Nevertheless, the biggest reason is money.

"Business models, having more to do with money than health care, are created around gizmos ... Physicians offered the choice between poorly reimbursed, careful, painstaking, uneventful diligence or a well-reimbursed exploit may... behave in ways that are not in the patients' best interests," they wrote.

Broadening the definition of disease

One way to expand the market is to change the definition of who is not healthy. The thresholds for disease have been lowered for a number of conditions, creating millions of new patients overnight. Doing so increased the number of diabetics by 14 percent; patients with high blood pressure by 35 percent; the number of overweight Americans by 42 percent, and those with high cholesterol by 86 percent.

Another cost pressure is known as medicalization, or re-defining nonmedical problems as conditions that need medical attention. Some marketers call it "condition branding," which transforms an unpleasant aspect of everyday life into a pressing need that requires a clinical solution. Baldness, frequent need to urinate, unpleasant breath and occasional bouts of sadness are examples for which medical products have been created. A 2010 study estimated that about 4 percent of health-care spending in 2005, or about $77 billion, was devoted to such medicalized conditions.

Expanded use of high-resolution scanning has also created a significant amount of "pseudo disease," or the presence of abnor-malities that will not harm a patient if left untreated. However, it is difficult for patients and their physicians to ignore these abnormalities. It can lead to a cascade of further testing and perhaps unnecessary treatment that may cause harm.

Quality: getting value for what we pay for

Cost and quality are not the same in health care. Many health-care providers charge high prices because they can. However, there are physicians and organizations that deliver high-quality care at 20 percent below the average price. If everyone could do the same, the percentage of GDP devoted to health care would decline from 17 to 13 percent—an annual savings of about $640 billion.

Most Americans have two perspectives on health-care quality and costs: the nation's and their own. About 80 percent say they are dissatisfied with the cost of health-care nationally, and more than half are dissatisfied with overall quality. However, nearly 9 out of 10 are satisfied with their own insurance coverage and the quality of care they receive. More than half are satisfied with their own health-care costs.

Those who are dissatisfied with national costs point to several culprits. About half blame what they believe are excessive profits for drug and insurance companies. About a third blames fraud and waste, physician and hospital profits and medical-malpractice lawsuits for rising costs. About 30 percent say unnecessary treatments and Americans' unhealthy lifestyles are boosting costs. Only 28 percent agree with health-policy experts who say expensive technology is the main culprit. One in 8 says higher costs are yielding better care.

The U.S ranks poorly in international comparisons of health systems. A 2000 World Health Organization report ranked the U.S. 37th in the world. The report measured the extent to which investments in public health and medical care improved health, reduced disparities and protected citizens from medical impoverishment.

The Commonwealth Fund ranked seven industrialized nations in 2010 on quality, efficiency, access to care, equity and the ability to live long, healthy and productive lives. The U.S. was last.

In these rankings, the glaring conclusion is that the U.S. does not create value in proportion to what it spends.

Waste, fraud and abuse

A politician's favorite campaign pledge is to cut budgets and taxes by eliminating "waste, fraud and abuse." These so-called savings are usually illusionary, and seldom specified. However, the phrase never fails to add energy to a stump speech.

However, the slogan implies there is a painless solution to often-intractable government-financing problems. Gov. Mitch Daniels, R-Ind., said that going after waste, fraud and abuse is inadequate, especially in addressing the deficit. "(The slogan) trivializes what needs to be done, and misleads our fellow citizens to believe that easy answers are available to us."

The often-used estimate of unnecessary care is 30 percent. Fraud is a separate issue. The FBI estimates 3 to 10 percent of health-care spending is lost to fraud. By comparison, credit-card fraud accounts for only .07 percent, or 7 cents, of every $100 spent. Health-care fraud schemes cost Americans $234 billion annually, or roughly the size of Finland's gross domestic product.

Health reform augmented efforts to combat fraud. The Congressional Budget Office did not include savings from Medicare-fraud crackdown efforts. However, Health and Human Services Department officials say the return on investment on previous efforts to combat fraud is nearly $5 for $1 invested since 1997, and $6.80 for every $1 since 2008.

Unfortunately, government systems for analyzing Medicare and Medicaid are not up to the task. According to the Government Accounting Office, its technology is inadequate and underused. The government has trained less than 10 percent of analysts needed to fight fraud. Medicare processes about 4.5 million claims daily, making it one of the largest payer systems in the world. Its "pay and chase" policy reimburses medical providers quickly but makes it difficult to follow up suspicious claims after-the-fact.

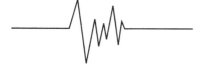

Chapter 18

Private Insurance
Heart and soul of reform

Private health insurance—whether supplied by an employer or bought individually—is the heart and soul of health reform. Many hoped reform would mean fundamental changes to how health care was delivered and paid for. Instead, the new law can best be described as a collection of incremental adjustments and insurance-coverage expansions.

Employers are unimpressed by the legislation. Less than 1 in 4 say health reform will lower costs, improve quality or encourage healthier lifestyles.

The people most affected by the law are only dimly aware of its impact. Less than 1 in 10 with private insurance say they are very knowledgeable about the legislation.

Historians call employer-supplied health insurance an "accident of history." Companies began offering health benefits when wages were frozen during World War II. In 1954, the Internal Revenue Service ruled that health-insurance premiums paid by employers would be tax-exempt. That exemption will cost the U.S. government $660 billion between 2010 and 2014. It represents the most expensive tax giveback in the U.S. tax code.

Despite skyrocketing costs, employers largely have remained loyal to this self-imposed obligation. However, there has been a steady erosion in health-insurance coverage, hastened by two recessions in the past decade. About 52 percent of employees had health insurance in 2009, compared with more than two-thirds in 2000. According to the U.S. Census Bureau, 2009 was the first year the number of people with health insurance declined since it began collecting that data in 1987.

There are a number of reasons for this trend. More employers, especially smaller ones, stop offering health insurance as the price rises. The U.S. economy has been shedding manufacturing jobs that provided steady incomes and ample benefits. And more employees simply are declining health insurance because of the cost of the premiums.

Employers have been gradually shifting premium costs to employees. The percentage paid by employees only increased slightly, to more than 21 percent, in 2010. However, while employee pay has increased 16 percent in the past five years, employee contributions to insurance premiums have risen 49 percent. Health-insurance costs are continuing to consume a greater share of employee compensation.

Employer-sponsored insurance (ESI) is a lifeline to health coverage. Without a job, health insurance can be unaffordable. More than one-third of those who left a job with ESI became uninsured for at least six months afterward.

The current recession illustrates how health insurance is tethered to employment. The unemployment rate was 4.4 percent in May 2007 and rose to 9.4 percent in July 2009. ESI fell by 4 percent during that period while the nation's uninsured rate rose 4 percentage points to more than 16 percent. Those who lost their insurance were younger workers, Hispanics and part-timers.

- Penalizes U.S. citizens either $695 a year up to a maximum of three times that amount ($2,085) per family, or 2.5 percent of household income—whichever is greater—for not having health insurance. That penalty, effective in 2016, will be phased in beginning in 2014. It will increase after 2016 based on a cost-of-living formula. Exemptions will be given for financial hardship, religious objections, prisoners, Native Americans and those whose incomes are below the tax-filing threshold (in 2009, it was $9,350 a year for an individual).

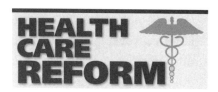

- Requires insurance companies to allow parents to keep children on family insurance policies until age 26. Effective in 2010.

A rule of thumb economists use: A 1 percent rise in unemployment results in a 1 percent decrease in adults with ESI. Another one: A 1 percent rise in unemployment means another 1 million Americans will be uninsured generally.

Health reform's effects on coverage and costs

The new law will help put small businesses and individual health-insurance buyers on a more equal footing with large employers. Health-insurance exchanges, scheduled to begin in 2014, will lower administrative costs and provide a more orderly insurance market. Insurance coverage will be more comprehensive, and plans will be more transparent in their offerings.

Large companies negotiate directly with health plans. Individuals and small businesses buy health insurance through insurance agents or brokers. The sales commissions and marketing costs inflate insurance costs compared with those borne by larger businesses. In fact, small businesses pay up to 18 percent more for identical coverage. Three-quarters of small businesses that do not offer health insurance cite high premiums as the reason for not doing so. More than a quarter of self-employed entrepreneurs are uninsured.

Small-business owners were ready for change well before the current health-reform law. Nearly half called for "radical change" in the health-care system in a poll before the 2008 election because it did not meet their business or personal needs.

Workers not offered health insurance are unlikely to be able to get it as individuals. Nearly 70 percent of small-business employees not offered insurance had difficulty finding quality, affordable insurance. One-third was turned away because of pre-existing conditions, and about half remain uninsured. In 2007, more than half of working adults in small companies were either uninsured or underinsured.

People with high medical needs are motivated to buy insurance, while younger and healthier people are not. This leads to what is called adverse selection. The less-healthy group of buyers raises the rates for everyone buying insurance.

As insurance costs rise, healthier buyers drop out and leave sicker customers with even higher rates. This is often called an insurance "death spiral." Health reform counters adverse selection with the individual mandate, prohibiting exclusion because of pre-existing conditions and ensuring continuous enrollment regardless of health status, age or gender.

Small businesses (no more than 25 employees)

- Exempts them from any penalty for not offering health insurance.
- Offers tax credit temporarily of up to 35 percent of the employer's contribution to the premium if that contribution covers at least 50 percent of the total premium through 2013. Businesses of under 10 employees and average annual wages of less than $10,000 are eligible for full tax credit in 2014

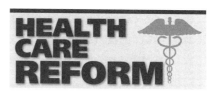

Employer insurance

- Offers tax credit of up to 25 percent of the employer's contribution to the premium to tax-exempt organizations through 2013.

Larger businesses

- Exempts them from any penalty if they have fewer than 50 employees.
- Assesses a fee of $2,000 per full-time employee (in excess of 30 employees) if firms with 50 or more employees do not offer coverage and at least one employee receives a premium credit on the insurance exchange. Effective in 2014.
- Assesses a fee if $3,000 per employee if a company offers health insurance but has employees who receive a premium credit on the exchange. Effective in 2014.
- Imposes an excise tax on insurers of employer-sponsored health plans with values that exceed $10,200 for individual coverage and $27,500 for family coverage. Effective in 2018.

These measures essentially eliminate insurance underwriting, which companies use to evaluate whether to accept or reject customers and to determine the price of their premiums. They use claims history and health status to make their decisions. The goal for insurance companies is to insure as few sick people as possible.

The exchange also will group individual buyers into larger risk pools that imitate those of large companies. Doing so will result in more affordable coverage for people with pre-existing conditions.

The Congressional Budget Office (CBO) predicts that, once health reform is fully implemented by 2016, large companies will not be paying more for premiums than they would have without the law. Smaller businesses will be paying slightly less, or up to 1 percent more. Individuals will pay 10 to 13 percent more, because insurance policies will be more comprehensive. However, more than half of the individual policies bought on the health-insurance exchanges will be eligible for government subsidies, lowering the cost significantly.

Of course, all of these projections are minor compared with the impact of underlying health-care cost increases. Ultimately, health reform itself will have little impact on the price tag.

Reform's effects on employer insurance enrollment

Health reform spared smaller companies from mandates. Employers with fewer than 50 workers will not have to offer health insurance to their employees.

Companies with 50 or more workers may face financial penalties if they do not offer affordable insurance. Their employees will receive subsidies to buy insurance on the exchanges instead. Most large companies already offer affordable insurance and are

- Creates state-based American Health Benefit Exchanges for individuals and Small Business Health Options Program (SHOP) Exchanges beginning in 2014. States may set up their own exchanges, participate in regional exchanges with neighboring states or allow the federal government to run their exchanges.

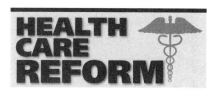

- Allows businesses with up to 100 employees to participate, and states may allow larger businesses to participate beginning in 2017.
- Limits participation to U.S. citizens and legal immigrants.
- Requires health plans to offer a package of "essential benefits." Those benefits include physician visits, hospital care, emergency services, maternity care, lab work, rehabilitation services, prescription drugs, mental-health services and chronic-disease management.
- Establishes four levels of coverage that vary based on premiums and out-of-pocket costs, as well as a catastrophic-coverage plan.
- Establishes premium subsidies on a sliding scale for families between 133 and 400 percent of the federal poverty level ($29,327 to $88,200 for a family of four in 2009).

least likely to be affected, although more employees probably will participate because of the individual mandate.

Analysts have differed widely concerning the law's effect on workplace enrollment. The Urban Institute predicted a slight increase at companies with more than 1,000 employees, and little change in smaller companies. Consulting firm Market Strategies forecasts a 10 percent decrease in the number of workers offered health insurance by 2014.

Companies are weighing whether to continue offering health insurance or simply to pay the $2,000 penalty for each employee. The decision to discontinue health insurance might be prudent for industries with high turnover, such as hospitality, restaurants and retailers. Larger companies are more likely to conclude that offering insurance is too critical for employee recruitment and retention to abandon.

During the health-reform debate, President Obama repeatedly promised that people would be able to keep their current insurance coverage if they wished to. That is unlikely to be the case.

The law exempted, or "grandfathered," health plans in place on March 23, 2010, when the law was signed. However, that exemption places tight restrictions on changes that companies can make to their existing plans. These restrictions include no increases in cost-sharing or coinsurance, and limits on deductible increases and employer-contribution decreases. These are tactics businesses typically use to blunt the impact of medical inflation.

The Obama administration expects 39 to 69 percent of employers to relinquish their exemptions by 2013.

Employers are also concerned about the tax implications of offering high-cost insurance policies to their employees. The so-called "Cadillac" or "gold-plated" plans have low deductibles and generous premium contributions. High-cost plans are defined as annual premiums costing more than $10,200 for an individual or $27,500 for a family, including worker and employer contributions. Employers would have to pay a 40 percent excise tax on the value above those thresholds beginning in 2018.

The law targets executives with cushy benefits. However, union and public employees also have generous health insurance.

- Prohibits denial of coverage or setting the cost of a premium based on a person's health or claim history. Effective in 2010.
- Bars lifetime limits on coverage or rescinding coverage, except in the case of fraud. Effective in 2010.
- Prohibits charging more than three times the lowest premium based on age for the same insurance. Effective in 2014.

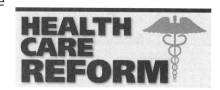

- Requires written justification for annual rate increases of 10 percent or more. Effective in 2011.
- Dictates that insurance companies spend at least 80 percent of premium revenue on medical expenses for individuals and small businesses, and at least 85 percent for large businesses. Those who do not do so must issue rebates to customers. Effective in 2011.
- Allows charging different premiums based on geographical location, age and tobacco use. Smokers may be charged up to 1.5 times more than nonsmokers. Effective 2014.

Reformers believe these expensive policies encourage overuse of the medical system. Businesses and governments likely will respond by offering fewer benefits to lower premiums, and raising deductibles and co-payments for employees.

Expect Congress to revisit the Cadillac plan thresholds. A May 2010 survey by Mercer found that this was the No. 1 employer concern regarding health reform. A Towers Watson analysis predicted that more than 60 percent of large-employer plans will be taxed in 2018.

In contrast, companies with 25 or fewer workers will be eligible for temporary tax credits of up to 35 percent. They will also be able to rely on their own health-insurance exchange, called the Small Business Health Options Program (SHOP), to offer standardized, comprehensive coverage at more affordable prices. This should improve their ability to compete with larger companies for employees.

However, health-reform critics say the tax credits are too complex to attract small businesses and probably will help only those companies already offering coverage. A survey of small California businesses found that more than half were unaware of the tax credits or the SHOP exchange. The CBO estimated that the tax credits would reduce the cost of premiums for small businesses by 8 to 11 percent, which translates into a weak incentive.

The RAND Corporation has a much different outlook. Its analysis showed that the number of workers offered insurance at businesses with 50 or fewer workers will rise from the current 60 percent to more than 85 percent. The researchers say the individual mandate and lower-cost insurance on the exchange will fuel employee demand for insurance.

Reform's effects on individual insurance

People who buy health insurance for themselves are in an awful place. If you can get a policy at all, the deductibles are high and the benefits skimpy. A 2008 survey found that 1 in 4 adults declined another job opportunity, stayed at a job that they would otherwise have quit or decided not to retire in order to retain their employer-sponsored health insurance.

The average out-of-pocket maximums for insurance purchased individually currently average more than $5,200. One out of 8 have no coverage for physician office visits and less than half have maternity benefits in their basic plans.

Viewed from another angle, the average employment-based health plan paid for 80 percent of all health charges in 2007, compared with 64 percent for individual plans.

These are often stopgap policies. About 11 million Americans bought individual policies in 2006, but only 7 million had them for a full year. People used them to plug coverage gaps between jobs or en route to government-insurance eligibility.

Buying individual insurance can be a harsh experience. Nearly one-half of U.S. adults under age 65 have chronic conditions that can result in policies that are more expensive — or outright rejection. One in 7 who applies for individual insurance is denied coverage because of pre-existing conditions. When consumers with pre-existing conditions find insurers who provide coverage, they are more willing to accept high prices and more reluctant to shop around. This is a clear case of market failure.

The reasons for, and the consequences of, being uninsured could fill several chapters of this book. Suffice it to say that more than 20,000 uninsured people die prematurely every year because they lack timely access to care. That is a direct result of the fact that 1 out of 3 uninsured adults have chronic conditions that, if left untreated, have devastating consequences.

Health reform is expected to reduce the percentage of uninsured Americans from about 19 percent to less than 9 percent. The law is expected to insure an additional 32 million, split equally between Medicaid expansion and those buying subsidized coverage from the exchange.

The largest groups remaining uninsured will be young adults eligible for Medicaid who choose not to enroll, undocumented immigrants and adults who will be exempt from the individual mandate because they lack an affordable insurance option.

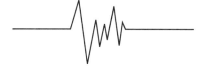

Chapter 19

Government Insurance

Here comes reform—and baby boomers

Medicare and Medicaid, the government health-insurance programs for elderly and low-income Americans, are going to expand significantly by the end of the decade. The number of Medicare recipients is expected to grow from 47 million to 64 million as more baby boomers enter its ranks. Medicaid will nearly double by 2021 to 100 million as health reform expands eligibility. More than half of Americans will be enrolled in at least one of these two programs or the Children's Health Insurance Program (CHIP) by the beginning of the next decade.

According to federal actuaries, these U.S. government programs accounted for more than half of all health-care spending in the United States in 2011. Medicare and Medicaid have been growing faster than the overall economy for decades. They currently make up 5 percent of the gross domestic product (GDP) and are on track to be 10 percent of GDP by 2035. The Congressional Budget Office (CBO) projected that of the three major federal entitlement programs—Medicare, Medicaid and Social Security—the two health programs will represent 80 percent of the spending increases for these three entitlement programs between now and 2035.

Medicare, Medicaid and CHIP accounted for 20 percent of the 2011 federal budget, a higher share than is claimed by either defense spending or Social Security.

Many Americans are confused by the difference between Medicare and Medicaid. Medicare is a federal program for people 65 or older, regardless of income. It also serves younger disabled people and dialysis patients. Patients pay deductibles for hospital and other costs. Medicare beneficiaries also pay small monthly premiums for nonhospital coverage.

Medicaid is jointly funded by federal, state and local governments for people of all ages with low incomes. Enrollees pay no insurance premiums. Deductibles, if they exist, vary by state. Medicaid is administered by state and local governments within federal guidelines. Barely half of Americans can articulate Medicaid's purpose or recognize that it is a jointly funded program.

Commentators had a field day mocking a man who stood up during a town-hall meeting during the reform debate and warned a South Carolina congressman to "keep your government hands off my Medicare."

However, nearly 4 out of 10 Medicare beneficiaries are unaware the program is government-run. The same goes for about 28 percent of Medicaid recipients.

Both programs enjoy broad support in polls, and most people oppose any cuts in either program. Medicare beneficiaries have political power, because they are the age group most likely to vote. About half of Americans either have received Medicaid benefits or had a friend or a family member in the program.

CHIP covers children up to 400 percent of the federal poverty level and varies by state. However, the benefit package is not as comprehensive as Medicaid's.

While Americans specifically support the health-entitlement programs, they have mixed feelings about the federal government's

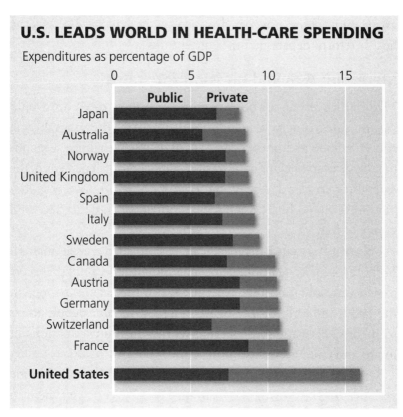

U.S. LEADS WORLD IN HEALTH-CARE SPENDING

Expenditures as percentage of GDP

Source: Kaiser Family Foundation; The Washington Post.

Many criticize other nations for "government-run" or "socialized" medicine. Excluding private-sector spending, the U.S. government spends more as a percentage of GDP on health care than other government-dominated health-care systems such as those in Japan, Norway, Australia, Canada and Switzerland.

role in health care. The Gallup organization has asked the same polling question annually since 2001: "Do you think it is the responsibility of the federal government to make sure all Americans have health-care coverage, or is that not the responsibility of the federal government?" Until 2009, most respondents believed it was the federal government's responsibility—including 7 out of

10 in 2007. That number dropped below half by 2009 as the health-reform debate became contentious.

Medicaid: A mixed blessing for states

Medicaid covers about 60 million people, most of whom would be uninsured otherwise. Under health reform, the program will add 16 million additional people by 2014, when eligibility expands to include everyone under 65 with income up to 133 percent of the federal poverty level. According to current federal poverty guidelines, that would be $14,404 for an individual and $29,326 for a family of four.

Since it began in 1965, Medicaid has provided critical financial support for safety-net public hospitals and health clinics that serve low-income and uninsured patients. When Medicaid expanded in the 1980s and early 1990s, it gave more low-income people access to medical care and was credited with significant reductions in infant and child mortality.

A 2011 study of 10,000 people enrolled in Medicaid for one year in Oregon showed the insurance program allowed them to have better access to and use more health care, be more likely to report good health, and were less likely to suffer depression or have unpaid medical bills.

Medicaid also pays about half of the bill for the nation's long-term care. The elderly and disabled represent about one-third of Medicaid's enrollees but account for about two-thirds of its costs. In 2004, Medicaid spent about half of its budget on the sickest 5 percent of enrollees.

A significant percentage of Medicaid funding goes toward coverage of so-called "dual eligibles," or those entitled to both Medicare and Medicaid. They are among the sickest and poorest people covered by either program. This group of nearly 9 million accounts for about 15 percent of each program's enrollees and

- Phases in full coverage of prescription drugs under Medicare Part D, eliminating the current coverage gap known as the "doughnut hole." It also improves subsidies for drug benefits for people at or below 150 percent of the federal poverty level who also have limited assets. Phased in from 2011 to 2020.

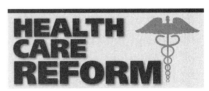

Medicare

- Eliminates co-payments and deductibles for preventive services. Effective in 2011.
- Establishes a 15-member Independent Payment Advisory Board, which will recommend measures to reduce Medicare's per-capita growth rate if it exceeds a target growth rate. First recommendations due in 2014.
- Freezes extra payments to Medicare Advantage plans in 2011 and reduces the extra payments beginning in 2012. The plans also must spend at least 85 percent of premium dollars for medical care.
- Increases taxes for high-income households from 1.45 percent to 2.35 percent on wages earned over $200,000 for a single filer and over $250,000 for married couples filing jointly. Effective in 2013.

about one-third of the two programs' combined spending. Two-thirds have three or more chronic conditions, and more than 60 percent are mentally impaired. Nearly 9 out of 10 live below 150 percent of the federal poverty line.

Medicaid funding ranks behind only elementary and secondary education in most state budgets. On average, about 17 percent of state funds are spent on Medicaid. The program is countercyclical, meaning it grows as the economy contracts. When the economy falters, people lose their jobs and access to employer-sponsored health insurance. According to the Kaiser Family Foundation, every percentage point increase in U.S. unemployment results in an additional 1.1 million uninsured, one million more enrollees in Medicaid and CHIP, and a 3-4 percent decline in state revenues.

Medicaid enrollment rose about 3.8 million between December 2008 and December 2009—the largest annual increase in absolute numbers since the program began in the 1960s. Every state added enrollment during that period, with 11 states growing more than 15 percent. To compensate, virtually every state cut either benefits or payments to health-care providers. The federal government does not allow states to alter eligibility requirements.

Medicaid spending growth primarily has been due to increased enrollment. Spending per enrollee has grown more slowly than aggregate per-capita health-care expenditures. Besides limiting or cutting benefits and rates for Medicaid providers, states aggressively have limited the use and pricing of prescription drugs and expanded community-based long-term care programs at the expense of more expensive nursing-home care.

States also have shifted about half of the nation's Medicaid recipients into private managed-care plans, a trend that is likely to increase as Medicaid grows. Under managed care, states typically pay health plans a set monthly amount per patient. The plans generally limit patient choice of physicians and hospitals. Managed-care arrangements offer states more stable and predictable health-care costs. They also provide a way for states to monitor quality of care.

Attempting to impose greater cost sharing on Medicaid recipients can backfire. Oregon's Medicaid program did so, setting

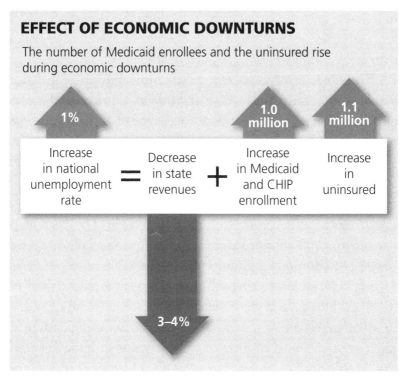

EFFECT OF ECONOMIC DOWNTURNS

The number of Medicaid enrollees and the uninsured rise during economic downturns

1%

1.0 million

1.1 million

Increase in national unemployment rate **=** Decrease in state revenues **+** Increase in Medicaid and CHIP enrollment   Increase in uninsured

3–4%

Source: Kaiser Family Foundation.

Medicaid enrollment grows as the economy contracts, because people lose their jobs and access to employer-sponsored health insurance. Every percentage-point increase in U.S. unemployment results in an additional 1.1 million uninsured, 1 million more enrollees in Medicaid and CHIP, and a decline of 3 to 4 percent in state revenues.

rigid premium-payment deadlines in 2003. In less than three years, enrollment plummeted from 104,000 to 24,000. Those exiting the program were twice as likely as those in the program to have unmet medical needs.

In an attempt to change health behavior and recoup Medicaid costs, Arizona state officials proposed what *The Wall Street Journal* dubbed the "Medicaid Fat Tax." Those who were obese and failed to follow a doctor-ordered weight-loss program would pay a $50 fee. The same levy also would be assessed on smokers and diabetics who failed to follow recommended treatment.

Rising Medicaid costs represent a budgetary thorn to state officials who must balance their budgets. However, the fact that the federal government pays an average of 57 percent of the program's cost is an economic-development boon. For example, every out-of-state dollar spent in Texas on health care generates $3.51 in private-sector spending, according to the state's Comptroller of Public Accounts. The federal government temporarily boosted its Medicaid contribution to an average of 67 percent as part of its 2009 stimulus package to help financially strapped states. The additional funding ended in July 2011.

Republicans have been pushing to convert the federal share of Medicaid into a block grant, which would limit federal spending to a predictable amount without regard to costs and spending at the state level. Stated another way, block grants shift the financial risk directly onto the states. Then-President George W. Bush proposed this in 2004 and the idea was revived by Rep. Paul Ryan, R-Wis. The CBO estimated that a Medicaid block grant begun in 2013 would lower federal Medicaid funding by 35 percent by 2022 and 49 percent by 2030. The grants would give states greater flexibility in running their programs, likely resulting in deep cuts in eligibility, long-term care and provider reimbursement to offset reduced federal support.

Paradoxically, many of the states that oppose Medicaid expansion under health reform have Medicaid-eligible patient populations that have the most to gain. In the 21 states that challenged health reform in court, 39 percent of those who would be Medicaid-eligible residents currently are uninsured, compared with 26 percent elsewhere. The CBO estimated that Medicaid and CHIP expenditures from program expansion

- Expands coverage to non-elderly adults with less than 133 percent of the federal poverty level ($24,352 for a family of three). The Congressional Budget Office estimates that health reform will increase Medicaid enrollment by 16 million. Effective in 2014.
- Requires that states maintain current income-eligibility levels for children in the Children's Health Insurance Program (CHIP) until 2019 and extends funding

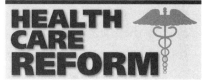

Medicaid

through Sept. 30, 2015. CHIP is designed to cover low-income children whose family incomes are too high to qualify for Medicaid.
- Requires Medicaid to include the essential health benefits available in the exchanges. Effective in 2014.
- Establishes the Community First Choice Option in Medicaid to increase funds for states that supply community-based services for those with incomes up to 150 percent of federal poverty level who require institutional-level care. Effective in 2011.

would rise by the end of the decade by $434 billion, with the states picking up only $20 billion of that increase.

About 40 percent of people who are eligible for Medicaid are not enrolled prior to the expansion. According to a *Health Affairs* study, two-thirds of the 7.3 million American children who were uninsured in 2008 were eligible for Medicaid or CHIP but not enrolled. About 40 percent of those eligible children lived in one of three states—California, Texas or Florida. Some low-income parents either were not aware of the programs or did not believe their children would qualify. Some states also have burdensome enrollment and renewal requirements. Health reform's individual-mandate provision and its requirement that all children have health insurance should cut significantly into the eligible-but-not-enrolled population. States will be responsible for paying their standard share of the Medicaid costs for these enrollees because of their previous eligibility.

Even after children are enrolled in Medicaid or CHIP, they may have difficulty getting care because the programs pay physicians less than private health plans do. For example, Medicaid pays an average of $8 for a flu vaccination—and as little as $2 in Colorado. The average cost of vaccinating a child for a physician's office is $20.

Researchers posed as parents of sick or injured children and called 273 specialty medical practices in the Chicago area. Two-thirds of those who said they had Medicaid or CHIP coverage were turned down for appointments, compared with 11 percent of those who said they had private insurance. Of the clinics that said they accepted both kinds of patients, those who said they had Medicaid or CHIP had to wait 22 days longer for an appointment.

Medicare basics

Medicare and Social Security represent vital social insurance programs for the elderly and younger people with disabilities. Prior to Medicare's enactment in 1965, less than half of those 65 or older had health insurance. Many lacked coverage either because they could not afford the premiums or they were denied coverage because of age or pre-existing conditions.

Nearly half of those on Medicare have incomes below 200 percent of the federal poverty guidelines. That is below $21,660 for individuals and $29,140 for couples in 2010. A Wayne State University Institute of Gerontology study found that more than one-third of Michigan's elderly were unable to meet basic living expenses. About one-quarter of beneficiaries have mental impairments, and about the same percentage describe their health as fair or poor.

Medicare covers basic health services, including hospitalizations, physician services and prescription drugs. Many benefits have deductibles and cost-sharing requirements, and there is no limit on out-of-pocket spending. The program does not cover some services of importance to the elderly, such as long-term care, vision and dental.

Most beneficiaries acquire supplemental insurance to help cover the cost-sharing requirements. The typical sources are employer-sponsored retiree coverage, Medicaid dual eligibility, Medigap policies and the Medicare Advantage program.

Medicare Advantage is composed of private health plans that receive payments from Medicare to administer the program's benefits to its members. About one-quarter of Medicare beneficiaries are enrolled in the Advantage program. The plans differ in their offerings, and many provide additional benefits and reduced cost-sharing, compared with the traditional Medicare plan. However, the Advantage program typically restricts the choice of health-care providers.

Medicare Advantage costs the federal government about 10 percent more than the traditional fee-for-service Medicare program. Health reform intends to close that disparity by changing how it reimburses program providers and lowering the program's cost. The projected savings is $117 billion between 2010 and

2019. Health plans are expected to cut benefits and raise cost-sharing for Advantage program participants to make up for the reduced reimbursement. Because of this, the CBO predicts that the program's enrollment will decline by about one-third, or nearly 5 million members, and return to the traditional Medicare program by 2019.

Medicare financing

The trajectory of Medicare financing is sobering. Annual Medicare expenditures are expected to grow from $519 billion in 2010 to $929 billion in 2020. Spending is highly concentrated on the program's sickest beneficiaries. About 25 percent of recipients account for 85 percent of the program's spending. One study calculated that nearly all of the growth in Medicare expenditures from 1987 to 2002 could be traced back to beneficiaries with five or more chronic conditions.

The number of beneficiaries is expected to rise from 47 million in 2010 to 80 million in 2030. During that same period, the number of workers supporting each Medicare enrollee will decline from 3.5 to 2.3.

Medicare spending historically has grown about 2.5 percentage points faster than the economy, adjusted for inflation. This trend is a greater threat to the program's financial sustainability than the aging of the population, according to the CBO.

The typical couple who turned 65 in 2010 and earned an average household income of $86,200 during their careers paid $109,000 in Medicare taxes over a lifetime. However, that same couple will receive an average of $343,000 in Medicare benefits. The federal government must pay the $234,000 shortfall from other revenue sources or cut spending elsewhere.

Health-care costs are also crimping Medicare beneficiaries' household budgets. Median out-of-pocket spending as a share of income rose from about 12 percent in 1997 to more than 16 percent in 2006.

Yet a majority of Americans are not convinced Medicare is in trouble. A spring 2011 *Wall Street Journal*/NBC News poll showed that only 15 percent believe the program needs a major overhaul and an additional 28 percent say it needs "major changes."

Medicare trustees estimated in May 2011 that the program will run out of money by 2024 because of a sluggish U.S. economy and longer life-expectancy projections for beneficiaries. The Obama administration projected in 2010 that Medicare savings in the health-reform law would extend the solvency of the program from 2017 to 2029.

Congressional resolve continues to evaporate in the face of hard choices on Medicare. The sustainable growth rate (SGR), a formula it created in 1998 to calculate physician fees and control costs, has been overridden numerous times. The SGR attempts to control total Medicare spending on physician services. In theory, the more the volume of care increases, the more prices must be cut the following year. The cuts are supposed to be cumulative and retroactive to 1998.

The overridden fee cut in 2010 was supposed to be 21 percent, with additional 5 percent cuts in subsequent years. Policymakers correctly feared that enacting such cuts would result in a mass exodus of physicians from the Medicare program, and create a potential crisis in access to health-care services for the elderly.

Health reform continues the charade. An SGR fix that would waive the cumulative fee cuts originally was part of the reform bill, but it was abandoned because proponents wanted to keep reform's price tag below $1 billion. The Medicare trustees point out that, if the SGR formula continues, Medicare payment rates would fall to 27 percent of what private insurance pays and less than half of projected Medicaid rates by 2085. It would also render 40 percent of participating health-care providers unprofitable by 2050.

At this point, SGR is little more than an accounting fig leaf that understates the federal government's future financial obligations. It also gives Congress the illusion that it somehow can control escalating Medicare costs, despite its clearly demonstrated impotence.

'Solutions' galore

Several lawmakers and regulators have proposed Medicare reforms. Most of these "solutions" merely shift costs rather than deal directly with the program's larger problems of waste and overuse. Among the proposed solutions:

- Ryan's proposal would convert Medicare from a defined-benefit program to one of defined "premium support" payments and gradually raise Medicare eligibility from 65 to 67 in 2022. The elderly would use the government payments to buy insurance from private insurers. Because the subsidies would be growing at less than the rate of medical inflation, the elderly would pay an increasing share of their medical care. According to the CBO, the average 65-year-old would pay 68 percent of the total cost of his or her coverage by 2030, compared with 25 percent paid under the current law. President Obama's deficit commission, headed by Erskine Bowles, former chief of staff to President Clinton; and former Republican senator Alan Simpson of Wyoming, proposed a similar premium-support program in late 2010.
- In response to Ryan, President Obama proposed strengthening the Independent Payment Advisory Board

(IPAB), created by the reform law to keep Medicare spending growth to the rate of GDP growth plus 1 percent beginning in 2018. Obama suggested lowering the benchmark to 0.5 percent plus GDP growth. The IPAB, appointed by the president and confirmed by Congress, is intended to insulate Medicare payment decisions from political and special-interest influence. The IPAB would propose cuts if cost projections exceeded the guidelines. Unless Congress comes up with alternatives that achieve the same savings, the IPAB decisions would be enacted. Obama also suggested using Medicare's buying power to negotiate drug prices.

- Sens. Joseph Lieberman (I-Conn.) and Tom Coburn (R-Okla.) proposed raising the eligibility age from 65 to 67 immediately and charging higher premiums to wealthier seniors. The senators claimed the plan would save $600 billion over 10 years. According to a Kaiser Family Foundation analysis, raising the eligibility age to 67 in 2014 would save the federal government $7.6 billion for that year. However, it would increase net out-of-pocket costs for 65- and 66-year-olds by $5.6 billion and cost retiree health plans an additional $4.5 billion.

The real problems: Waste, fraud and abuse

In a March 2010 report, the U.S. Government Accountability Office (GAO) designated Medicare and Medicaid as "high-risk programs because they are particularly vulnerable to fraud, waste, abuse and improper payments."

The Office of Management and Budget tracks "high-error" government programs. All of the major health-care government insurance programs are listed: Medicare fee-for-service, Medicare Advantage, Medicaid and CHIP. Medicare Advantage's improper payment rate was more than 14 percent and the fee-for-service improper payments exceeded 10 percent.

According to The Centers for Medicare and Medicaid Services, Medicare improperly paid $48 billion, which amounts to about 9 percent of the program's costs.

As an example, the GAO report pointed out that Medicare erroneously paid $3.1 million for ineligible erectile-dysfunction medications such as Viagra and Levitra in 2007 and 2008.

The Dartmouth Atlas Project has tracked geographical variation in Medicare spending. Dartmouth researchers found that health-care providers in New York City spent more than $12,000 per capita on Medicare patients, compared with about $6,700 in Minneapolis. These differences could not be explained by sicker patients or better health outcomes. The researchers also found that physicians in higher-spending regions were more likely to recommend discretionary services and admit patients directly into intensive-care units, and were less likely to suggest palliative care with patients and their families. The researchers recommend Medicare payment policies that encourage high-cost regions to behave more like low-cost regions by adopting their practices.

In a June 2011 report to Congress, the independent Medicare Payment Advisory Commission said Medicare cannot control costs for two reasons. First, it pays a set rate for services so there is no incentive for a provider to be more efficient. Second, doctors who bill a greater volume of services—regardless of whether they improve outcomes—make more money than doctors who do not.

True Medicare reform will require that the program shift payment incentives away from quantity and toward quality, efficiency and evidence-based medicine. Otherwise, Medicare's march to insolvency will continue without interruption.

Part 4

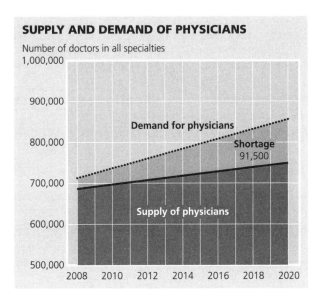

SUPPLY AND DEMAND OF PHYSICIANS

Number of doctors in all specialties

Demand for physicians

Shortage
91,500

Supply of physicians

1,000,000

900,000

800,000

700,000

600,000

500,000

2008 2010 2012 2014 2016 2018 2020

Health-Care Delivery

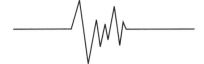

Chapter 20

The Doctor

Overworked and underappreciated

Family doctors are mad. Who can blame them? There are too many forces arrayed against them.

Primary-care physicians are the front line of medicine. They are the first stop for people who need care. They treat the patient as a whole person, not a body part or disease. They determine where to send the patient for more care if necessary.

Their income essentially has stayed the same since the 1990s, while their practice expenses have steadily increased. After accounting for inflation, their average income fell 7 percent from 1995 to 2003. This obviously is an unsustainable business model.

Their workdays are brutal. A Philadelphia practice kept track of what its physicians did in a day's time. The average doctor saw 18 patients, wrote 12 prescriptions, reviewed 14 consultation reports from specialists, studied 11 X-rays or other imaging reports, and wrote or answered 17 email messages.

Many patients do not get the recommended care. If everyone did, it would destabilize the U.S. primary-care system. A physician with a typical 2,000-patient base would have to spend more than 17 hours a day to meet all of the guidelines for preventive care and chronic-disease management.

Physicians have to fight for every dollar. Plumbers and attorneys do not have to call a third party to verify that they will be paid when they fix leaky faucets or draw up wills. Doctors must follow strict health-plan guidelines or they will not be reimbursed. State and federal health-insurance programs continue to squeeze the rates they pay physicians to compensate for rising costs. Many practices lose money when they treat Medicaid and Medicare patients.

Primary-care physicians' share of the U.S. health-care dollar is only 7 cents. If payers cut reimbursement for physician services by 25 percent—not as a body part or disease—the average rate of medical inflation would only decrease from 6.2 percent to 5.7 percent.

However, primary-care doctors control 80 cents of the health-care dollar by sending their patients to hospitals, referring them to specialists and handing out prescriptions. This is a key paradox: Primary-care physicians arguably are the most powerful players in the health-care system but are underappreciated and comparatively undercompensated. In a 2006 survey, nearly 8 out of 10 characterized themselves as "junior partners" or "second-class citizens" in the health-care galaxy.

The threat of malpractice suits weighs heavily on physicians. Medical-liability system costs, including defensive medicine, represent less than 3 percent of total health-care spending. However, physician concerns are the same regardless of whether they live in states that have adopted medical malpractice reforms.

Physicians are deeply suspicious of health reform. Two-thirds said their initial reaction to the law was negative. Almost 90 percent said primary care is on "shaky ground" or "is a dinosaur soon to go extinct."

Lou Goodman, president of the Physicians Foundation and chief executive officer of the Texas Medical Association, predicts

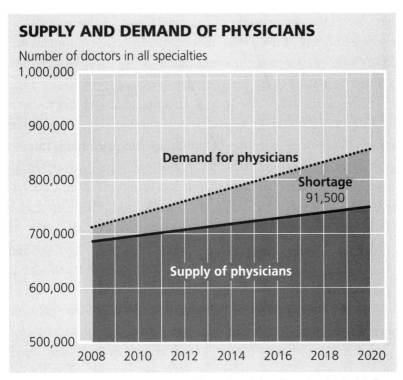

SUPPLY AND DEMAND OF PHYSICIANS

Number of doctors in all specialties

Demand for physicians

Shortage
91,500

Supply of physicians

1,000,000 — 900,000 — 800,000 — 700,000 — 600,000 — 500,000

2008 2010 2012 2014 2016 2018 2020

Source: Association of American Medical Colleges.

The U.S. Department of Health and Human Services estimates that the physician supply will increase by only 7 percent by 2020. Meanwhile, health reform will add an estimated 32 million people to the ranks of the insured. By 2020 there also will be a 36 percent increase in the number of Americans over age 65, the age group that consumes the most health care. The 2020 physician shortage is expected to exceed 90,000.

that physician practices will vanish because of market forces and the new law's effects.

Health reform's newly insured will be clamoring for physician services, which will become increasingly scarce because supply is not expanding with demand. The federal government soon will penalize physicians who do not use electronic health records, an expense and service disruption that many physicians cannot afford. Many solo practitioners or small practices are banding together, selling themselves to hospitals or simply going away.

Some see primary care in a death spiral. Because it is so challenging and relatively underpaid, few medical students choose that route. This places greater pressure on existing practices, forcing even more to drop out. Primary-care doctors have little bargaining power. Their reimbursement from Medicare and Medicaid has remained relatively flat over the past decade, and private insurance plans have followed suit.

Even though the workload is expanding, physicians are slowing the speed of the treadmill. The average workweek decreased from 55 hours in 1996 to 51 hours in 2008. That is the equivalent of losing 36,000 doctors in a decade. The financial incentive to work harder, they say, is simply not there.

Only 1 out of 4 say they will work as hard as they always have in three years. The remainder say they will cut back their hours, retire or seek nonclinical employment. The recession has prompted many to delay retirement. The health-care industry experienced the largest decline in retirement rates of all economic sectors. In 2009-2010, about 1.5 percent of full-time workers retired, compared with 4 percent in 2004-2007.

The burden of a physician practice

Qliance, a Seattle-based primary-care practice, has not accepted insurance reimbursement since 1997. Its 13 salaried physicians serve 4,500 patients who pay a flat monthly "subscription fee" for unlimited visits. Dr. Garrison Bliss, chief medical officer, said the business model works well, because 40 to 50 percent of reimbursement to a typical primary-care clinic goes toward billing and collections.

- Increases temporarily Medicaid payment rates to equal those of Medicare for primary-care physicians for 2013 and 2014. Medicare rates typically are about 20 percent higher than Medicaid's.
- Provides a 10 percent reimbursement bonus to primary-care physicians and surgeons who practice in federally designated workforce shortage areas for Medicare from 2011 to 2015.

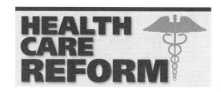

Doctor

- Creates a workforce advisory commission to establish a national strategy to address anticipated shortages of physicians and nurses. Effective in 2010.
- Establishes funding to create training programs for medical homes, team management of chronic disease, and integration of physical-health and mental-health services. Effective in 2010.
- Seeks to boost physician workforce by about 3,500 through 2020, through grants and redistribution of medical residency programs. Effective in 2010. (However, the Association of American Medical Colleges estimates that there will be a shortage of about 45,000 physicians by the end of the decade.)

Qliance clinics have two to three times more patient visits than an average clinic, but significantly lower hospitalization and emergency department visits. Garrison said the Qliance model could save the U.S. health-care system $250 billion to $350 billion annually.

The complexity of the health-care system places an enormous administrative burden on physician offices. For example, many economic sectors besides health care devote 100 or fewer full-time equivalent employees (FTEs) to collect $1 billion. By comparison, the median number of physician-office FTEs to collect $1 billion is 770. For a 10-physician practice, those extra FTEs cost $250,000 annually.

Physicians have to hustle to cover their costs. Laurie Green, a San Francisco obstetrician-gynecologist, told *The Wall Street Journal*, "I live my life in seven-minute intervals." She estimated that she needed to earn $70 every 15 minutes to cover her office overhead.

The average physician spends nearly three weeks per year dealing with health plans. Another 23 more weeks of nursing staff and 44 more weeks of clerical staff are spent on insurance claims.

Commercial health plans are difficult to deal with, but at least they represent revenue that usually is not subject to arbitrary reduction. The average physician practice relies on Medicare for about 25 percent of its revenue. That revenue source is at risk every year because of the sustainable growth rate (SGR), established in 1997 to keep Medicare from growing faster than the overall economy. The SGR formula factored in the rising number of people on Medicare. However, the per-beneficiary costs rose at a faster rate than the economy. When that happens, the federal government is supposed to cut payments across the board to control costs. Every year since 2002, Congress has blocked these cuts. The proposed rate cut to satisfy the SGR would have been 25 percent if Congress had not stepped in again in January 2011. The proposed rate cut will continue to rise until Congress fixes the formula. If ever followed again, physicians undoubtedly would abandon Medicare in droves.

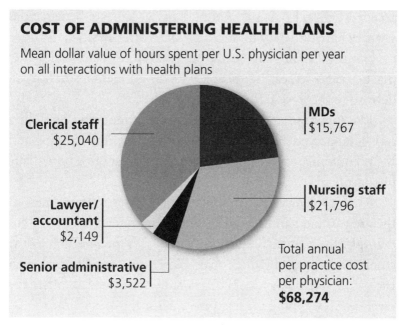

COST OF ADMINISTERING HEALTH PLANS

Mean dollar value of hours spent per U.S. physician per year on all interactions with health plans

Clerical staff
$25,040

MDs
$15,767

Nursing staff
$21,796

Lawyer/ accountant
$2,149

Senior administrative
$3,522

Total annual per practice cost per physician:
$68,274

Source: Casalino LP, et al. *Health Aff.* 2009;w-533-w543.

Dealing with multiple insurance plans represents a burden of time and money for the typical physician practice. *Health Affairs* journal researchers based the estimates in this chart on data from nearly a half-million office-based physicians.

Cutting reimbursement does nothing to improve health-care delivery. Physicians try to offset these cuts by working harder: seeing more patients and providing more services. However, that only goes so far. The Congressional Budget Office estimates that physicians can only make up about 25 percent of fee cuts by working harder and doing more. The patients are negatively affected as well. Physicians spend less time with them, and may provide services that are not necessary.

Physicians have been gradually withdrawing from Medicare and Medicaid for years. For example, two-thirds of Texas physicians say they will accept Medicare patients and 42 percent will accept Medicaid patients. About 1 in 3 Medicare beneficiaries say they have difficulty finding a primary-care physician. As these programs inevitably are cut or fail to keep up with health-care practice expenses, care for people with government insurance will devolve to the lowest-cost provider.

Doctors have attempted to increase revenue by providing services that were once the domain of the hospital. Imaging and X-ray equipment represent a sizable investment but a potentially big payoff.

The problem is that this allows doctors to refer business to themselves, and tempts them to use the equipment too much. For example, the Deficit Reduction Act cut fees for imaging. While costs were reduced by more than 12 percent for each individual use of the technology in 2007, doctors attempted to offset the revenue loss by using the equipment far more than before.

An analysis of physician office self-referrals showed higher patient costs, without improving outcomes in most cases.

There are laws that prohibit physicians from referring patients to freestanding imaging centers in which they have ownership stakes. However, what is called an "in-office ancillary services exception" allows them to install the equipment in their offices. The original reason for the exception was same-day consumer convenience.

So much for good intentions. An analysis of 2006 and 2007 Medicare data showed that about 3 out of 4 X-rays were performed the same day. However, only 15 percent of more-advanced procedures, such as magnetic resonance imaging, were done the same day. Apparently it is inefficient to keep expensive equipment idly standing by for same-day appointments, so they were booked in advance for the maximum use of labor and equipment.

The worsening physician shortages

The U.S. has about the same number of physicians per capita as other industrialized nations. However, the U.S. has far fewer primary-care physicians. They make up about 50 percent of the physician workforce in most other developed nations, compared with 35 percent in the U.S.

This is reflected in the time it takes to see a doctor. A study of 11 industrialized nations found that 80 percent of Americans could get in to see a specialist within four weeks. Only Germany had a better rate. However, only 57 percent of Americans could see a primary-care doctor the same day or the next day. That compares with 93 percent in Switzerland and 70 percent in Great Britain, whose system is often erroneously branded as "socialized medicine." The shorter supply of primary-care doctors—the ones you need in a hurry—means slower service in the U.S.

The number of U.S. specialists per capita has risen dramatically since 1965, while the ratio of primary-care physicians has remained relatively constant. The outlook is for more of the same: greater scarcity of primary care and a growing supply of specialists.

Massachusetts reformed its state health-care system in 2006, giving the nation a glimpse of what is to come when access to health insurance is expanded without expanding the supply of care. The average wait for a non-urgent appointment with an internist rose from 17 days in 2005 to 48 days in 2011. Less than half of family physicians there are accepting new patients, compared with 70 percent four years ago.

The primary-care workload is expected to increase by nearly 30 percent between 2005 and 2025. A number of factors feed this demand, including a growing population, a flood of baby boomers becoming Medicare beneficiaries and acquiring medical conditions as they age, and 32 million more Americans with Medicaid or subsidized insurance.

However, the supply of primary-care physicians is expected to rise by only 2 to 7 percent. Three out of 4 physicians say they already are at or over capacity. The math screams that there will be a crisis of health-care access in the next 15 years. Expect longer waits for appointments, shorter physician visits, greater use of nonphysicians for routine care, and higher prices.

The U.S. trains about 16,000 doctors a year. The nation would have to increase that number by 6,000 to 8,000 annually for 20 years to meet expected demand.

This was an intentional shortage. The Council on Graduate Medical Education (COGME) estimated in 1994 that there would be a surplus of specialists — up to 165,000 too many by the year 2000. As a result, Congress decreased its financial support for specialty physician training in 1997. The number of residency slots was capped — and remains that way today.

COGME has since reversed course and now estimates there will be a shortage of 96,000 doctors by 2020. Even though medical schools are increasing enrollment to meet future demand, residency slots remain frozen. Medical school graduates need to complete a residency to become a doctor. The Balanced Budget Act of 1997 froze the number of Medicare-supported residency positions at 1996 levels. The original health-reform legislation sought to increase the number of slots. However, the increase was eliminated to lower the overall cost of the legislation.

A crisis of care already exists in many pockets of America. About 1 in 5 Americans lives in a primary-care shortage area. The problem is especially acute in rural and low-income areas.

Physicians tend to cluster in areas where supply is already high rather than where the need is greatest. About 80 percent of new physicians in the 1980s and 1990s did this. They like affluent areas with well-insured patients, high-tech hospitals and civic amenities that offer a better quality of life. These high-income enclaves are also home to the nation's healthiest people.

There is no rescue in sight. Only 1 out of 14 of today's medical students want to be a primary-care physician. Primary-care physicians earn two to three times less than specialists. For example, a primary-care physician will earn $2 million to $3 million less than a cardiologist over a career.

Sen. Tom Coburn, R-Okla., is a physician who points the finger at the federal government for perpetuating the disparity in pay and fostering the primary-care shortage.

In a 2010 interview, Coburn said, "It's important to keep in mind that the federal government has mandated the doctor shortage. When the payment differential between primary-care doctors and specialists averages about 300 percent, and that payment is based on Medicare rates, the result is a Medicare-created primary-care doctor shortage."

The health-reform law modestly increases Medicare and Medicaid rates for physicians. This may encourage more physicians to take patients with government insurance, although the initial response among doctors was lukewarm at best.

The medical home: Solution or fool's gold?

Health-care experts are placing a lot of faith in what is called the patient-centered medical home (PCMH). The term is off-putting to some because it sounds like "nursing home." However, it is simply a physician's office organized in a different way.

The PCMH recognizes that health care is rarely one doctor treating one patient. It requires a team of health-care providers, educating family members and using community resources. Physicians are more like team leaders, coordinating care with staff members as well as specialists and hospitals. The doctors are rewarded more for keeping their patients healthy and out of the hospital rather than for short face-to-face visits with lots of tests and procedures. Medical homes are usually paid a monthly fee for patients under their care.

The "patient-centered" aspect assumes patients will participate in their own care. They will ask for and receive the care they want and need, and act on the medical advice they are given. The medical home has a number of features that are missing in most doctors' offices: electronic medical records, email communication, remote monitoring of chronic conditions and frequent reminders about preventive care.

There are many strengths to this kind of approach. Physicians have fewer incentives to provide unnecessary care. Participants recognize that most patient transactions can be handled by email or telephone. A Mayo Clinic pilot study found that "e-visits," or care provided over the Internet, made office visits unnecessary in 40 percent of the cases.

A 2010 *Health Affairs* article described the future physician's office, using medical-home principles. The office might treat 100 patients a day. The doctor might be involved with 30 to 40, of whom perhaps 10 would have traditional face-to-face individual appointments. The other patients interacting with the doctor would do so by telephone, email or group appointments. The remaining 60 to 70 patients would be treated by nurse practitioners, physician assistants or medical assistants, who would handle less complex cases and counsel people with chronic conditions on disease self-management. These team members would spend more time—and likely be more effective—than a physician could in a 15-minute time slot.

The typical doctor's office currently is set up to deal with brief illnesses or disease that can be cured mostly by time and medication. It is ill-suited to treat chronic disease, which accounts for about 75 percent of health-care spending. Effective chronic-disease management requires close monitoring and tweaking of treatment to avoid complications that require hospitalization or emergency department (ED) visits, such as heart attacks, stroke or respiratory failure. Medical homes typically have after-hours arrangements for their patients to be able to see a physician or nurse without going to the ED. Less than one-third of doctors' offices have such an arrangement now.

An estimated 40,000 primary-care physicians work in practices set up as PCMHs. That is about 1 out of 8 physicians and pediatricians. Blue Cross Blue Shield of Michigan said it saved $65-$70 million in 2011 working with PCMHs. It paid an extra $7,500 per physician for the year. However, it saved money because better care yielded fewer hospital and ED visits. The doctors also ordered more generic prescriptions because electronic prescribing allowed them to see lists of covered medicines.

Seattle-based Group Health (GH) is an integrated-care organization with its own health plan. It serves 600,000 members and employs about 1,000 physicians in Washington state and Idaho. Using medical-home care principles, GH has been able to improve quality and lower costs. It resulted in 29 percent fewer ED visits and 6 percent fewer hospitalizations, compared with its patient outcomes prior to becoming a medical home. In a survey at its clinic in Bellevue, patients expressed higher satisfaction with their care. More patients received recommended health screening tests, chronic-disease management and medication monitoring, compared with its prior traditional approach.

Paying doctors to keep people healthy seems so logical. However, it will not be widespread until health plans recognize this as customary care. In an Internet survey of 1,000 physicians, two-thirds said they believed the current health-care environment is detrimental to care. Less than 1 in 5 said they could make clinical decisions based on what is best for the patient rather than what health plans would reimburse.

While many physicians agree with medical-home principles, they already are stretched thin and are suspicious of what may be unrealistic expectations and extra effort. All of this is fine, they say, if they are properly paid. The government and health plans do not have a good track record in this regard. Many health-delivery innovations have been oversold, only to be swept away after impatient payers fail to see promised savings in short order. Health care has long been regarded as an expense rather than an investment. Unless that perspective changes, the medical home may never gain traction.

Two major barriers are money and workflow.

Seattle's GH invested $1.3 million at its Bellevue clinic to create its medical home. It had a 50 percent return on investment because its patients were also part of its insurance plan. Because GH treats and also insures its patients, it has an incentive to treat patients in ways that minimize hospitalizations and expensive procedures. Few clinics will be able to have that kind of pay-back. In most cases, the physicians will make the investment while the health plans and patients will reap the savings.

Typical physicians' offices are built around the doctors' hectic routines. They see patients at a frenetic pace and have little inter-action with staff members. Medical homes, by contrast, require doctors to be managers of care teams, something they have not been trained to do and many are uncomfortable with. The current standard is doctor-centered, not patient-centered, care.

Medical homes will be created by highly motivated, well-funded physician groups willing to overcome the barriers to install an unproven business model. Medical homes appear likely to be islands of excellence rather than the standard of care.

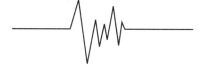

Chapter 21

The Hospital

Reinventing itself by necessity

As government and health insurance plans desperately seek to contain costs, hospital care has become a whipping boy.

Charges can run as high as $18,000 a day. In 2008, two million of the most expensive hospital stays cost nearly $200,000 per person. Days spent in the hospital declined in the 1980s and early 1990s and then stabilized after the federal government changed the way it paid hospitals. Hospitals' portion of health-care costs declined from 43 percent in 1980 to 33 percent in 2009. However, it remains the largest category of health-care spending.

According to the late management guru Peter Drucker, the four hardest jobs in America, in no particular order, are president of the United States, university president, hospital CEO and pastor. Hospitals are under constant pressure to lower costs while improving quality.

The implications of hurried care are reflected in hospital metrics: dismal safety records and high re-admissions, which induce higher costs than if there had been proper initial care. Nonetheless, hospitals are tied with supermarkets as the most trustworthy industry, according to a Harris Interactive poll.

The recession blues

Drucker's observation certainly rings true, given the current health-care climate. The recession has hit the nation's hospitals hard. About 3 out of 4 hospitals treated fewer patients and performed fewer elective surgeries. Nearly all have had to treat more patients who cannot pay.

Hospitals, especially the nonprofits, rely on income from in-vestments and community donations. According to an American Hospital Association (AHA) survey, 90 percent of U.S. hospitals say attracting charitable gifts is becoming more difficult. A similar percentage reported extreme difficulty in securing tax-exempt bonds. Two-thirds have had to delay projects because of difficulty accessing capital markets.

Most hospitals have cut administrative costs and reduced staff. About 1 in 4 has cut services. A financially struggling hospital creates economic ripples. It is often one of the largest employers in town. Hospitals employ more than 5 million U.S. workers, the second largest employer category, behind only restaurants. According to the AHA, they support nearly 1 in 10 U.S. jobs based on the goods and services they buy. Average hospital profit operating margins were 4 percent in 2006, with one-third of hospitals losing money on operations.

There are three kinds of hospitals: nonprofit, for-profit and public.

The primary goal of a nonprofit is to serve its community rather than maximize profits. However, nonprofit health-care organizations must be run like for-profit businesses to sustain themselves. The three main sources of capital are reinvestment of earnings from ongoing operations, philanthropic gifts and tax-exempt municipal bonds. They generally must spend a portion

PRACTICE OWNERSHIP

Ownership of physican practices in United States, in percent

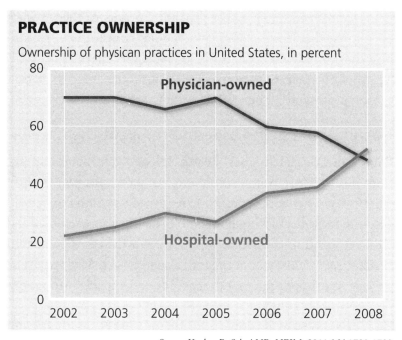

Source: Kocher R, Sahni NR. NEJM. 2011;364;1790-1793.

Hospitals now own more physician practices than physicians do. The trend is accelerating. A September 2010 survey found that three-quarters of hospital leaders planned to increase physician employment by 2013. Hospital-physician consolidation strengthens the organization's market power and tends to raise prices.

of their revenue on charity care and community benefit. Non-profits are exempt from federal and state income taxes, as well as sales and property taxes.

Public hospitals are also nonprofit organizations, owned and operated by local governments. They have an additional revenue source because they can levy taxes. That is critical because many of their patients are either uninsured or have government insurance that reimburses the hospital at less than the cost of care.

For-profit hospitals either distribute profits to their owners or reinvest them in the company. Unlike nonprofits, for-profit hospitals can raise capital in risk-based equity markets.

About 58 percent of hospitals are nonprofit, about 20 percent are for-profit and 22 percent are public hospitals.

Hospitals are being asked to reinvent themselves

Potentially, one of the best health-delivery reforms to emerge from health reform is the accountable care organization (ACO). An ACO is a network of health-care providers willing to be held accountable for achieving measurable quality improvements and reduced spending growth for up to 5,000 Medicare patients. In exchange, an ACO would share the savings with Medicare. The government hopes the model succeeds and spreads throughout the health-care system.

The goal is to improve coordination of patient care and provide an incentive to avoid wasteful services encouraged by fee-for-service medicine.

The most likely ACO configuration would include a hospital, primary-care physicians and specialists. The nation's largest health systems already have these elements under common owner-ship and are best suited to meet the January 2012 deadline for the program's inauguration. The Congressional Budget Office (CBO) estimates that there will initially be 75 to 150 ACOs and that the program will save Medicare about $5 billion by 2020.

However, many are concerned that ACO formation will give large health-care organizations even greater market power (see discussion below).

ACOs may be suffocated at birth because of overbearing regulation. The 429-page document governing ACO creation attempts to thread the needle by encouraging hospitals and physicians to form ACOs without sticking the government with

Hospitals and other health-care providers face a grim outlook for Medicare reimbursement.

The Medicare program pays hospitals and other health-care facilities based on a "productivity adjustment" formula. Under health reform, those payments will grow 1.1 percent more slowly than they would have otherwise—a reduction that compounds over time. The goal is to reduce the government's financial health-care burden and encourage providers to operate efficiently.

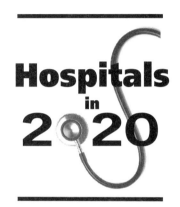

However, Medicare's Office of the Actuary estimates that Medicare reimbursement will be 40 percent below that of private insurers by 2020, and will fall below Medicaid rates. The actuary predicts that those cuts will make 15 percent of hospitals, nursing homes and home health agencies unprofitable by 2020. The actuary's long-term forecast is that about 40 percent of providers will become unprofitable by 2050 because of Medicare's payment cuts.

Richard Foster, chief actuary for the Centers for Medicare and Medicaid Services, said during congressional testimony, "If at some point our payment rates to providers become significantly less than our cost of providing services, they either will be unable or unwilling to provide continued services."

Foster said he expected Congress to phase out the payment cuts around 2020 to stave off the shuttering of unprofitable hospitals.

the tab if the effort fails. The results, many experts say, are meek incentives that do not justify the steep startup costs. Other hurdles include requirements to document 65 quality measures and submit marketing materials for federal editing.

ACOs have two alternatives for a three-year arrangement. Those willing to bear greater risk can earn up to 60 percent of the savings they achieve. However, they will have to repay Medicare for cost overruns. The maximum risk would be 10 percent of what Medicare would have spent on patients if they were not in ACOs.

This so-called two-sided risk may appeal most to established integrated-delivery systems that already operate much like ACOs.

The one-sided risk model allows ACOs to avoid financial risk in the first two years, but they would be eligible to keep only 50 percent of the savings. They would face penalties of up to 7.5 percent in the third year.

Consultant Steven Lieberman, a 30-year CBO veteran, wrote in a *Health Affairs* blog, "The proposed regulation imposes unfavorable economics, unrealistic requirements, high uncertainty and significant risks for ACOs."

The Medicare Physician Group Practice (PGP) demonstration, the model upon which the ACOs were built, was not financially promising. Only half of the 10 participating practices produced savings by the fourth year.

Researchers crunched the numbers from the PGP demonstration and concluded that an ACO with an average of $1.7 million startup costs would have to have an unlikely 20 percent profit margin for the three-year period to recoup costs.

Hospital-physician alignment

Regardless of how reform plays out, the traditional tension between hospitals and physicians is melting out of necessity. Hospitals need physician buy-in as they enhance quality to meet health reform's

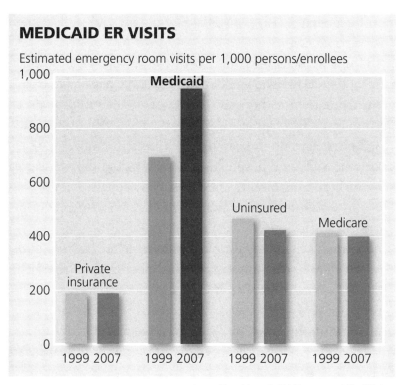

MEDICAID ER VISITS

Estimated emergency room visits per 1,000 persons/enrollees

Source: Tang N, et al. *JAMA.* 2010;304(6):664-670.

Medicaid beneficiaries, not the uninsured, accounted for nearly all of the increase in hospital emergency-department (ED) visits between 1999 and 2007. Health reform will add 16 million recipients to Medicaid. The enrollment increase and growing physician shortages are expected to add to the hospital ED burden.

imperatives. Physicians are abandoning independent practice in droves as they face decreasing revenue and government imperatives for electronic health records.

In many states, hospitals cannot directly employ physicians because legislators fear that hospital executives with profit imperatives might influence physicians to compromise patient care. Therefore, physicians act as independent contractors who autonomously care for patients, using hospital equipment and staff as their "workshop."

Hospitals increasingly have been contracting with "hospitalists," or physicians who work exclusively at the hospital to handle admitted patients. Physicians visiting patients in hospitals are becoming a relic of America's medical past. Many community-based physicians do not mind this, because the travel time between the office and hospital is time they cannot bill. However, they are becoming disengaged with their hospitals. They are less likely to serve on hospital committees or cover emergency-department shifts.

Hospital-physician relationships have pivoted swiftly in the past few decades. Hospitals catered to physicians in the 1970s and 1980s because they competed for referrals. In many ways, physicians were more valued than patients were. Posh physician lounges and prime parking spaces were the norm.

Then the landscape changed and the seeds of mistrust were sown.

The twin threats of Clinton administration health reform and managed care motivated hospitals to buy hundreds of physician practices to create integrated networks. They later unloaded the practices, because both threats shriveled and hospitals could not manage them profitably.

Physicians struck back by investing in outpatient centers and specialty hospitals, siphoning away profitable business. Medical technology became safer, cheaper and less capital-intensive, which encouraged physicians to move their business away from hospitals and into smaller clinics. Outpatient surgeries accounted for two-thirds of all surgeries performed from 1996 to 2006, according to the U.S Centers for Disease Control. Surgeries in freestanding centers tripled while hospital outpatient surgeries were relatively unchanged.

- Requires nonprofit hospitals to conduct community-needs assessments every three years. Also requires a plan to publicize a financial-assistance policy indicating whether free or discounted care is available. Effective in 2012.
- Establishes a trauma-center program to strengthen the capacity of emergency departments and trauma centers. Effective in 2011.

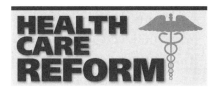

Hospitals

- Allows providers to organize as "accountable care organizations" that, if they meet quality targets, can share in the cost savings they achieve for Medicare. Effective in 2012.
- Reduces annual inflationary adjustments to treat Medicare patients, and reduces Medicare payments for providing uncompensated care by 75 percent. Effective dates vary.
- Penalizes hospitals with excessive 30-day readmission rates and excessive hospital-acquired conditions. Effective in 2012.
- Establishes bonus payments to hospitals based on how well they follow 12 measurements of clinical care and how patients rate their experiences. Effective in 2012.

Physician alignment, or hospitals working collaboratively with physicians, has always been a core strategy for hospitals. Doctors control 70 to 80 percent of hospital admissions. Fewer than 60 percent work exclusively with one hospital.

Physicians by nature are fiercely independent. Most are in solo or small practices, with little outside accountability. The teamwork required in integrated care organizations is a foreign concept. Doctors are highly trained scientists used to having the final say on how they treat their patients. Hospital executives, many of whom lack a clinical background, are much more comfortable with a top-down management style to increase revenue and allocate resources efficiently.

A 2011 study found that hospital quality scores were about 25 percent higher when physicians ran the hospital, compared with those that were not. Scores for cancer care were even higher at physician-run hospitals

According to a 2010 PricewaterhouseCoopers (PwC) survey, 1 of 5 physicians does not trust hospitals. Conversely, 60 percent of hospitals say it is difficult to get information from physicians to improve patient care.

The demands of health reform probably will change the physician-hospital relationship forever. Alignment and engagement need to happen rapidly.

Shrinking Medicare reimbursement will squeeze hospital margins throughout the coming decade. A PwC analysis estimated that, without reform, Medicare rates would have risen by 27.5 percent over that period. Under health reform, the increase will be 11.9 percent.

The Medicare value-based purchasing program will begin paying hospitals based on patient satisfaction and quality of care, reducing payments for those in the bottom 25 percent. An average-size community hospital could lose more than $1.4 million annually if it receives poor quality scores beginning in 2013. Until health reform, there arguably was not a business case for hospitals to stress safety and quality.

Opportunity: The time has come

Under health reform, the most successful hospitals will be those that align tightly with physicians who answer the call for safer, more efficient, effective and patient-centered care.

Physicians are ready to answer that call. The number of hospital-owned physician practices reached 55 percent in 2009, up from 50 percent in 2008 and 30 percent five years ago, according to the Medical Group Management Association.

Merritt Hawkins, a physician-recruiting firm, reported that more than half of physician job searches were for hospitals for the year ending March 2010, compared with 45 percent the previous year and 19 percent five years earlier. The percentage of physicians who own their practices has been declining about 2 percentage points a year for the past 25 years.

According to a 2010 HealthLeaders Media Intelligence Unit report, 3 out of 4 hospital executives said they were getting more employment requests from physicians and they planned to hire more physicians within the next three years. More than 60 percent said they planned to buy medical groups.

More than half of physicians believe they will become more aligned with hospitals, according to the PwC survey. Further, roughly the same percentage wants to align more closely with hospitals to increase their income. This includes two-thirds of cardiologists, whose income was cut significantly by Medicare.

The potential cuts in physician reimbursement from the ever-present threat of the Medicare sustainable growth rate (SGR) are even more frightening to doctors. If implemented, the CBO estimated, the SGR would have fallen more than 21 percent in 2010, and 6 percent in each of the following three years. The cumulative effect would be 40 percent by 2014.

Physicians' income generally has kept pace with inflation despite flat or declining reimbursement because they have increased volume—seeing more patients, shortening appointments. Finite office hours dictate that this is not a sustainable business strategy, and certainly not ideal patient care.

Medicare and commercial outpatient reimbursement generally is higher at hospital-owned facilities, perhaps because they have more market power to command better rates than independent physicians do. Therefore, doctors employed by hospitals can make more for performing the same procedures—and that extra reimbursement could be baked into their compensation.

Demographics favor physician-hospital alignment. Women comprise a growing percentage of the physician workforce. They prefer the financial security and shorter hours of a salaried position. Younger physicians generally shy away from taking on the large debt involved in establishing a practice and seek a greater work-life balance.

The hospital is a dangerous place

In 1999, the Institute of Medicine estimated that nearly 100,000 people suffer preventable deaths and 1 million are injured during hospital care annually. A large-scale study of hospital safety a decade later found little progress despite prevention campaigns, rhetorical outrage and technological advancements.

Even more disturbing, a group of researchers examined care at three sophisticated U.S. hospitals and found 10 times as many mistakes as previously detected. They concluded that 1 out of 3 hospital patients are victims of an adverse event.

A 2009 *Journal of the American Medical Association* commentary bluntly stated, "For years, clinicians considered most harm as inevitable."

Do not expect to see a hospital marketing campaign built around that assertion.

The disregard for patient safety can be infuriating. The U.S. Centers for Disease Control established hand-washing guidelines for clinicians in 1975. A 2010 study found that health-care providers were following the guidelines less than half of the time. One alert health-care blogger noted, by comparison, that in a study of hygiene in U.S. public restrooms, the worst hand-washing rate cited for men's rooms was 65 percent.

Consequently, it is no surprise that the Department of Health and Human Services ripped the nation's hospitals in 2010 for failing to protect patients from potentially fatal infections.

An association of medical professionals specializing in infection control charged that easily preventable bloodstream infections persist because hospital administrators pay too little attention and fail to commit resources to combat them. Those infections strike 80,000 patients annually, killing 30,000 of them. They could be virtually eliminated by hand-washing, sterilizing wounds and using sterilized clothing.

Adverse drug events (ADE) result in higher costs of care and longer hospitalizations. Among hospitals that have conducted ADE studies, the incident rate ranged from 2 per 100 admissions to 7 per 100. The likelihood increases as the patient stays longer in the hospital and takes more medications.

An ADE specifically is harm caused by a drug or by its inappropriate use. This is different from an adverse drug reaction, which is a severe, unpredictable reaction to a properly administered medication. (A "side effect" generally is predictable and usually inconsequential.)

Medication errors can occur at any point in the pharmaceutical-care process—physician order, prescription transcription, dispensing or administration. Computerized medication-order entry has the potential to eliminate an estimated 84 percent of dose, frequency and routing errors, according to the U.S. Agency for Healthcare Research and Quality. Only 17 percent of hospitals have such systems.

Hospitals have a lust for sophisticated diagnostic-imaging equipment and space-age surgical devices. However, they rely on 19th-century technology to chronicle their activities: paper charts and clipboards; pens; overstuffed manila file folders to be shelved and pulled. According to a 2009 study, less than 2 percent of hospitals had fully functioning electronic health-record systems.

A 2007 Institute of Medicine report called medication mistakes the most common overall medical error. It estimated the annual cost of those errors to be $3.5 billion in lost wages, productivity and additional treatment expenses.

One out of 7 Medicare hospital patients is harmed by hospital medical care, at a cost of about $4.4 billion annually. More tragically, those errors contribute to the deaths of about 180,000 patients a year. About 40 U.S. surgeries a week are performed on the wrong person or the wrong body part, despite numerous safeguards.

However, it is not all bad news. There have been major improvements in the use of care backed by scientific evidence by hospitals for heart attacks, pneumonia, surgical care and children's asthma care.

The quality of hospital care is often tied to how well the facility is run. Yale University researchers investigated why there was such a large difference in death rates among people treated for heart attacks. They reviewed 11 hospitals that were rated the best and worst performers by Centers for Medicare and Medicaid Services.

In high-performing hospitals, they found strong organizational values and goals, senior management involvement, staff expertise and involvement during care, good communication and coordination, and superior problem-solving skills. Senior management at low-performing hospitals was disengaged and did not create a system of performance accountability.

Transitions of care

Hospitals release patients as early as possible to minimize care expenses. Health plans and the government determine in advance how much they will pay the hospital based on the patient's condition. There is one price for the entire hospital stay, rather than a charge for every service and supply used. Medicare has a list of about 750 diagnostically related groups of similar medical episodes.

This is a cost-containment strategy. The incentive is to release the patient on or before the reimbursement period runs out. Unfortunately, too many come back for additional care within a month. This may be a penny-wise, pound-foolish situation. Initial costs were minimized but overall costs likely increased. Hospitals are able to bill the government or health plans for another hospitalization.

Hip replacement illustrates the point. In the early 1990s, according to a study in the *Journal of the American Medical Association,* patients spent more than nine days, on average, for surgery and recuperation in the hospital. By 2008, that period was less than four days. The percentage of patients sent directly home decreased from about two-thirds to less than half. The proportion sent instead to rehabilitation facilities doubled. Furthermore, there was a 44 percent increase in the number of patients returning to the hospital within 30 days for further care.

Dr. Peter Cram, the study's lead author, said, "You're really just squeezing a balloon here. If we reduce the length of stay in the hospital, we can save money ... But when we squeeze the balloon on one end to reduce length of stay, other costs pop up on the other end. This is why it's so hard to reduce or contain health-care costs."

A key provision of the health-reform law attempts to reduce 30-day hospital readmission rates by penalizing the worst offenders. As of October 2012, Centers for Medicare and Medicaid Services can decrease payments by 1 percent to hospitals with excessive rates for patients with heart failure, acute myocardial infarction or pneumonia.

One in 5 Medicare beneficiaries was readmitted to the hospital within 30 days, and 1 in 3 within 90 days in 2003-2004. The cost of these unplanned readmissions was more than $17 billion in 2004. Blacks are 43 percent more likely to have unplanned readmissions. The risk is up to 33 percent more likely for those on high-risk medications.

The Joint Commission, which accredits hospitals, studied miscommunication from one caregiver to the next in 10 hospitals. These so-called transitions of care often are the culprit in readmissions. The commission found that handoffs were defective 37 percent of the time. There are 4,000 handoffs a day at a typical hospital, which means nearly 1,500 are mishandled. Those fumbled handoffs are associated with 80 percent of serious medical errors.

Patient satisfaction

Medicare's value-based purchasing will take patient satisfaction into account. Traditionalists scoff at new hospitals that boast hotel-style amenities such as valet parking and high-definition TVs.

However, some experts remind clinicians that such glitz can affect clinical outcomes and certainly improve patient satisfaction.

For example, the Ronald Reagan UCLA Medical Center opened in 2008 to replace a facility damaged in the 1994 Northridge earthquake. Amenities included patient selection of meal choices, massage therapy and magnificent views. The percentage of patients who said they would recommend the facility shot up to 85 percent, about a 15 percentage point improvement.

For many patients, amenities trump quality of medical care. Their physicians are willing to accommodate them. Nearly 1 out of 3 said they hypothetically would honor a patient's request to be admitted to a fancy hospital regardless of clinical quality. Amenities matter because patients are better able to judge atmosphere and creature comforts more than clinical quality.

Hospitals find that adding amenities costs more than improving clinical quality. However, amenities drive more patient volume. It pleases patients, and it is no-brainer marketing.

Consumers are understandably confused about how to research hospital quality. Researchers compared five websites to determine their level of agreement on rankings of hospitals for diagnoses. All used different measures, inconsistent definitions and staggered reporting periods. Predictably, they failed to agree, undermining their consumer value.

The ratings may not even matter. A study of nearly 230,000 Medicare patients who had one of six surgeries in low-rated hospitals showed that they did just as well as patients who were treated in the best hospitals, as rated by the CMS Hospital Compare website.

Overall, hospital patients are unhappier than they were in 2004, with an American Consumer Satisfaction Index of 73 out of 100. Emergency departments (ED) were even worse, at 54.

Emergency department traffic jam

N. R. Zenarosa, a physician and executive at a Dallas-based ED physician outsourcing firm, calls the ED "the de facto access point for the uninsured or those without health-care knowledge."

Even though EDs employ about 4 percent of the nation's physicians, they treat more Medicaid beneficiaries and uninsured than the rest of U.S. physicians combined. Physician offices are open about 45 hours a week, and getting a timely appointment is difficult. The ED never closes and cannot turn away anyone. EDs handle 28 percent of first-contact non-emergency care in the United States, compared with 42 percent in doctors' offices.

From 1997 to 2007, ED visits per 100,000 population increased at twice the rate of U.S. population growth. Medicaid patients accounted for a large proportion of the increase, because many of them cannot secure a timely appointment with a physician. Health reform will add about 16 million to the Medicaid rolls, undoubtedly jamming the ED even more.

Despite the increased patient load, the number of EDs has declined 25 percent in urban and suburban areas in the past 20 years because many are money-losers for hospitals and are difficult to staff. ED traffic increased by 35 percent during that time.

The average waiting time for patients in the ED has grown by more than 30 minutes in the last decade, to an average of more than four hours.

What market power can mean

Patients love to talk about their hospital bills. The $5 aspirin and $3 towel-use fee are great conversation starters. For most people, those stratospheric prices are ultimately discounted to amounts negotiated by health plans, and patients submit a relatively small co-payment.

Those negotiated prices can differ significantly between hospitals for the same service. The technical term is price discrimination. In reality, the prices reflect the annual power struggle between insurance companies and health-care organizations.

One of the least-recognized causes of medical inflation is hospital market power. Hospitals with dominant market share and "must-have" health-network star status can negotiate highly profitable rates. Conversely, in areas with few health plans and many hospitals, there is less market power and the institutions must accept smaller rate increases.

With a wave of hospital mergers from 1990 to 2003, about 90 percent of metropolitan-area hospitals acquired what the Federal Trade Commission (FTC) considered excessive market power. The mergers lifted prices by as much as 40 percent over what they would have been without the mergers, according to the FTC.

According to an investigation by the Massachusetts attorney general, the state's insurance companies paid some physicians and hospitals twice as much as others in the same market for the same services and no better quality. The report attributed the higher prices to the fact that providers can dictate what they care to charge.

Robert Blendon, a Harvard professor of health policy and political analysis, told Kaiser Health News: "There is a chance that you could arrive (in Massachusetts) 10 years from now and there are three organizations to negotiate with, and every physician and hospital is affiliated with one of them. There are mergers, consolidations, groups merging with larger groups, so when negotiations come, there are going to be very large players, even larger than the systems that most people envision."

Market power also allows more cost-shifting. For many hospitals, Medicare and Medicaid reimbursement is less than the cost of care. They typically compensate by charging commercial insurance companies more. On average, that rate is nearly 30 percent more than what Medicare pays. But hospitals with market power can exceed that differential.

However, the health plans flex their muscles as well. Nearly half of U.S. metropolitan areas have one insurer with 50 percent or more market share, according to an American Medical Association survey.

Both sides are increasingly concentrated among a few companies, so it is becoming a titanic market-to-market struggle behind closed doors. For consumers, the unlikely heroes are the often-demonized insurance companies. When they dominate, prices for care are more moderate.

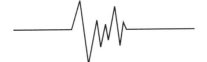

Chapter 22

Pharmaceuticals
Industry at a crossroads

The pharmaceutical industry is facing a crossroads. For decades, it lived off what it called "blockbuster" drugs: patented medications aimed at broad populations with chronic conditions. However, the patent-drug gravy train appears headed for the horizon. Cheaper generics now account for more than 3 out of 4 U.S. prescriptions.

The heyday of the pharmaceutical industry was 1935 to 1955. More drugs that proved effective were created during that period than in all of previous history. Vitamins, tranquilizers, antihistamines and antibiotics such as penicillin all came about during this period. Drugs that conquered polio and tuberculosis also debuted.

By comparison, only 7 of the 78 new drugs approved by the Food and Drug Administration (FDA) in 2002 were innovative, meaning they contained active ingredients that improved upon existing medicines. The rest were so-called "me too" drugs that replicated existing drugs.

Prescription drug spending in 2010 increased an anemic 2.3 percent, which was the second-smallest annual increase in 55 years. The smallest was 1.8 percent in 2008, when a wave of widely used medicines became available as generics. Spending on generics rose by nearly 22 percent in 2010, while spending on the more expensive branded drugs declined slightly. Generics on average cost about one-quarter of the retail price of branded medications.

The recession certainly was a factor. A 2010 decrease in physician-office visits contributed to the weak growth, as 3.4 million fewer patients started new treatment for chronic conditions. Medicines for chronic conditions account for about half of drug spending.

Nevertheless, it is difficult to feel sorry for pharmaceutical companies. The U.S. has become a drug-addled nation, reaching for the pill bottle at an alarming rate. The number of prescriptions grew by 39 percent from 1999 to 2009, while the U.S. population grew 9 percent. Spending on drugs in that decade more than doubled, even after accounting for inflation, and is now six times greater than in 1990.

One factor that fueled the trend was the rise of pharmaceutical insurance benefits. In 1990, consumers paid for two-thirds of drug costs out of pocket. By 2000, that dropped to one-third. Consumers were more insulated from the effects of greater volume and prices.

Nearly 9 out of 10 people over age 60 use at least one medicine and more than 2 out of 3 take five or more. About half take a cholesterol-lowering prescription medicine, which is twice the rate of a decade earlier.

The prescription-drug habit has spread to the younger set. The growth in use of prescription drugs by children was four times greater than for that of the overall U.S. population in 2009. About 1 in 4 children ages 10 to 19 take medication to control a chronic condition—especially asthma or Type 2 diabetes.

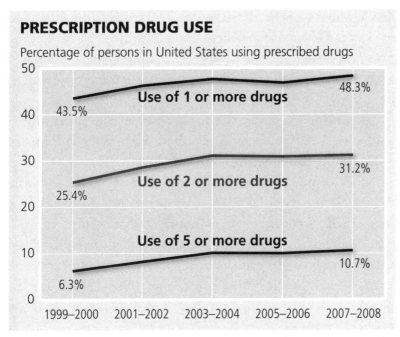

Source: National Center for Health Statistics; Medco.

The use of prescription drugs rose steadily over the past decade. Specifically, 9 out of 10 Americans 60 and older use at least one prescription drug in a given month, more than three-quarters used two or more, and more than one-third used at least five. More than one-quarter of children under 19 take medication for chronic conditions.

Among developed nations, the U.S. spends more on prescription drugs per capita because of higher prices for similar medications and a more expensive mix of drugs. Americans also spend more out of pocket and are less likely to be able to afford the drugs their physicians say they need.

U.S. drug prices are as much as 25 percent higher than those in European nations for the same drugs. Many Americans believe that higher U.S. prices essentially underwrite the research and development costs for drug companies. However, the difference in price largely is due to other nations directly negotiating drug prices on behalf of their nationalized health systems. The U.S. government does not directly negotiate drug prices on behalf of its citizens.

According to Express Scripts, a pharmaceutical mail-order company, U.S. drug consumers will waste $1.2 trillion, or $3,722 per person, between 2010 and 2014. That is $1 out of every $3 spent. The company blames the waste on patients who do not use the cheapest sales outlet or the least expensive drug mix, as well as patients who do not heed doctors' orders.

A more difficult problem to address is that prescribed drugs work for only about half the patients. That is a lot of trial and error, as well as enormous effort, expense and waste for the health-care system. Moreover, if a drug does not work, it can only do harm.

The costs are significant

The cost of brand-name prescription drugs rose nearly twice as fast as that of other medical goods and services for the past four years, despite the fact that they are losing market share.

Medical bills and illness were a factor in nearly 2 out of 3 personal bankruptcies in 2007, up from 46 percent in 2001. Drugs were the largest expense in 1 out of 5 of those bankruptcies. On the surface, it would seem counterintuitive that the cost of drugs could make that big a dent in a household budget. However, AARP estimates that the average annual cost of treatment with a branded specialty drug is 100 times as great as with a generic: $34,550 compared with $310.

Medicare Part D began offering prescription-drug coverage to seniors in 2006 to help those who could not afford the cost of their medication. Before the benefit began, 58 percent of the

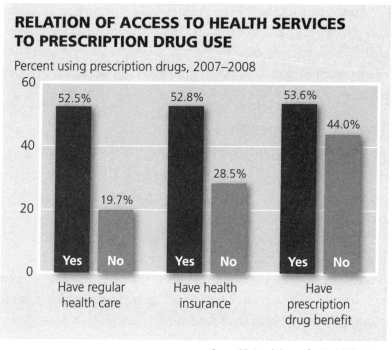

RELATION OF ACCESS TO HEALTH SERVICES TO PRESCRIPTION DRUG USE

Percent using prescription drugs, 2007–2008

Source: National Center for Health Statistics.

People use more medication if they have a regular source of health care, health insurance and prescription-drug insurance benefits.

elderly had limited drug insurance coverage. The study on the benefit's effects found that spending on nondrug medical expenses who had limited coverage was 10 percent lower than if the drug benefit had not existed. The average savings was $1,200, primarily because prescription-drug use allowed seniors to avoid hospitalization or nursing-home care.

The so-called "doughnut hole," or gap in coverage, closes by 2019 because of health reform. Because of that, Fidelity Investments estimates a 65-year-old couple retiring in 2011 would need $230,000 to pay for medical expenses during retirement, which is an 8 percent decrease from the previous year.

However, there have been unintended consequences of Medicare Part D. The price of popular brand-name drugs sold to the elderly with chronic conditions rose more than 41 percent after the program began, compared with the Consumer Price Index increase of about 13 percent.

The ascent of generics

However, worldwide sales of brand-name prescription drugs could be cut in half by 2015 as lucrative brands lose patent protection. Generics generally capture 80 percent of a brand-name's volume within six months.

Patients are driving the trend toward generics. About 1 in 4 physicians say the patients ask for them or prefer them. And 1 in 5 physicians say they always prescribe generics if they are available.

Surprisingly, just over half of physicians believe generics are clinically equivalent to the brand names they replace. That speaks loudly to the ability of pharmaceutical companies to persuade doctors that equivalent chemical compounds are somehow not equivalent. The FDA requires generic drugs to have the same amount of the same active ingredients of the brand names they replace and to be of equivalent quality.

Some patients are just as skeptical. A Consumer Reports poll found that 22 percent believed generics were not as effective. An equal number said generics had different side effects, despite FDA assurance on its website that generics have the same risks and benefits. In addition, 16 percent said generics were not as safe as brand-name drugs.

Generic drugs saved the health-care system more than $824 billion between 2000 and 2009. The 2009 savings *per day* was $383 million. In fact, a poll of drug-consuming households found that nearly half of the respondents considered branded prescription drugs "luxury purchases."

Two-thirds of consumers do not know how much their medications will cost until they show up at the pharmacy counter. People take extraordinary measures to be able to afford their medication. About 1 in 4 use potentially dangerous practices to save money, such as failing to fill a prescription, skipping doses, using expired medicine, splitting pills or sharing medicine. About the same number reduce their spending on clothing, cut back on groceries or use credit cards more often. About 15 percent postpone paying bills.

Polypharmacy

The consumption of all these drugs inevitably has created problems for the health-care system.

The drug-induced deaths of Michael Jackson and Anna Nicole Smith are high-profile examples of larger problems. In 2008, 1.9 million people were hospitalized because of adverse drug events (ADEs), which is more than a 50 percent increase from 2004.

That does not include the 838,000 treat-and-release emergency-department patients affected by ADEs, a number that doubled from four years earlier. More than a third of those were for misuse of prescription painkillers.

The 28,000 prescription overdose deaths in 2007 are five times more than in 1990. Most of those deaths have been from painkillers. The Obama administration has called the current prescription overdose epidemic worse than those of crack cocaine in the 1980s and heroin in the 1990s. The White House launched an anti-abuse plan in April 2011 to cut the rate of abuse by 15 percent in five years.

A study at Pennsylvania-based Geisinger Health System found that more than one-third of patients treated for chronic pain with painkillers met the criteria for addiction. Between 20 and 40 percent of U.S. adults have persistent pain that lasts more than six months.

Seven out of 10 who abuse prescription painkillers got them from a relative or friend. However, physicians have been quick to reach for the prescription pad when patients complain of aches and pains. Spending on prescription painkillers tripled from 1996 to 2006.

The elderly have a particularly difficult time juggling multiple prescriptions. Researchers examined prescription use by people with chronic heart disease, using CVS Caremark data. Patients filled prescriptions for an average of 11 medications during a 90-day period. One in 10 used 23 prescriptions during that period. Each medication a patient takes causes an average of 10 percent additional adverse drug events in a hospital setting.

Dr. Jerry Avorn, in a commentary in the *Journal of the American Medical Association*, said, "The use of medications in older patients is arguably the single most important health care intervention in the industrialized world."

However, the Harvard professor listed a number of factors that hamper medication management in the elderly. The fragmented health-care system causes patients with several chronic conditions to see multiple prescribing physicians, most of whom do not communicate with each other. That, Avorn said, creates "pharmacological chaos."

Clinical drug trials rarely include many over 80 years old, so safety and side effects are less well known among that group. This population may metabolize drugs differently than younger patients and may experience more side effects. Overmedication, also called "polypharmacy," can increase the risk of falls, cognitive decline and depression. All of that, of course, calls for more prescriptions.

Taking so many drugs is complicated. According to one study, only 15 percent of older adults could consolidate seven drugs into four doses a day correctly. People with less formal education performed even more poorly.

Satisfying the customer

Direct-to-consumer (DTC) pharmaceutical advertising quietly came into existence in 1985. It expanded rapidly in 1997, when the FDA eased restrictions. The only other nation that allows DTC advertising is New Zealand.

Pharmaceutical companies defend DTC marketing as providing important health information to patients. Critics say the industry creates diseases and then fills the artificial need with products of dubious value.

In marketing parlance, this is known as "condition branding." Marketing executive Vince Parry calls it "the creation of medical disorders and dysfunctions." In a revealing magazine article in *Medical Marketing & Media*, Parry says the marketing strategy is to elevate the importance of a condition, reduce its stigma and create the illusion of an unmet need.

Parry was instrumental in launching Viagra in 1998 by redefining impotence as "erectile dysfunction" to give an artificially scientific password for an embarrassing conversation between patient and doctor. Viagra used several celebrities, including former presidential candidate Bob Dole, to lift the stigma and give impotence a disease-like aura.

Condition branding has given life to many syndromes and "-isms" that were once simply functions of aging or life: baldness, overactive bladder, panic attacks, and sadness rebranded as depression. James Goodwin, a Texas geriatrician, attacks what he calls the medicalization of aging, which transforms the natural progression of life into discrete, treatable conditions.

"With medicalization," he wrote in the *New England Journal of Medicine*, "the role of physicians has become so expanded and technologized, that we fail at our most important task—providing relief from suffering ... The challenges of very old age are spiritual, not medical. The appropriate role of that physician is as counselor or helper, not as scientific expert."

DTC advertising tripled between 1995 and 2007. Consumer response to ads accounted for about 20 percent of growth in prescription drug expenditures during that time, with price increases accounting for the remainder.

Drug makers spent $4.3 billion in 2009 on consumer advertising. They dominate the airwaves during network news shows and represent an important source of advertising revenue for struggling newspapers and magazines. However, they spent about 50 percent more—$6.6 billion—on promotions aimed at doctors.

It all seems to be working. According to a Consumer Reports poll, about 20 percent of respondents said they asked their doctors about a medicine they had heard about from advertising. They said nearly 60 percent of their doctors accommodated them by writing prescriptions.

Patients are clearly uncomfortable with drug-company influence over doctors. In a separate Consumer Reports poll, about 70 percent said they believe drug makers have too much control over physician prescribing habits. Their suspicions are not unfounded.

The number of U.S. pharmaceutical sales representatives nearly doubled between 1996 and 2005, while the number of physicians rose 26 percent. However, the number of representatives is expected to shrink to 75,000 in 2012 from a peak of 102,000 in 2007 because it is an increasingly ineffective sales method. Only 20 percent who enter a physician's office are able to meet with the doctor personally. One out of 4 physicians works in a practice that refuses to see drug representatives.

Those who can see doctors come armed with very specific data. They know the brands and amounts each physician prescribed, culled from information purchased from data brokers. They use the information to tailor the sales pitch, often grilling doctors about why they prefer a competitor's brand to their own. Vermont, New Hampshire and Maine have passed state laws limiting pharmaceutical-company use of prescription records for marketing.

People are suspicious of drug companies. A Harris Interactive poll showed that only 11 percent of consumers considered pharmaceutical companies generally honest and trustworthy and 46 percent believed they should be more regulated—barely ahead of how people regarded tobacco companies and health insurers.

The Internet has become an important sales channel for pharmaceutical companies. About 100 million consumers sought drug information online in 2009, which was triple the number five years earlier. About half of those use video on pharmaceutical-company websites. Websites discussing oral contraceptives and erectile-dysfunctional drugs are among the most popular sites in terms of traffic.

The Internet also has become an enormous source of bootleg drug sales. One in 6 Americans have purchased drugs online without a prescription—and do so at their own peril. Illegal online drug sellers often sell counterfeit or unapproved medications.

However, consumers rate pharmaceutical TV advertising as more balanced and fair than online ads. Apparently that is because 8 out of 10 consumers notice risk and benefit information on TV more than they do in advertising online or in magazines.

Those instincts are dead on. John Santa, director of the Consumer Reports Health Ratings Center, calls the Internet "shark-infested waters" as a source of pharmaceutical information.

"Brand drug makers have so much money and are so smart that it is very difficult to find information online that they do not influence heavily. In my mind, unless you are very careful and already well informed, you should assume whatever you read on the Internet is coming from a drug company," Santa said.

When it comes to satisfying customers, independent pharmacies are the winners. Chains such as Health-Mart, The Medicine Shoppe and Bi-Mart beat big-box retailers such as Target, Wal-Mart and Sam's Club as well as major chains Walgreens and CVS. According to a Consumer Reports survey, they committed fewer errors, were more responsive at the pharmacy counter, had medicine ready when promised more often and had more accessible pharmacists. A J.D. Power survey indicated that the convenience of the prescription and pickup process and condition of the store were more important to consumers than price.

Drug adherence

Former Surgeon General C. Everett Koop famously remarked, "Drugs don't work in patients who don't take them."

Alternatively, as the National Council on Patient Information and Education puts it, "Lack of medication adherence is America's other drug problem and leads to unnecessary disease progression, disease complications, reduced functional abilities, a lower quality of life, and even death."

Medication adherence refers to whether patients take medicine as prescribed. Lack of adherence takes many forms. People abandon prescriptions at the pharmacy counter, split pills, skip doses, take the wrong number of pills or take them at the wrong time of the day.

About half of chronic-disease patients in the developed world do not take their medicines properly, and the rates are even worse in developing nations. The result is more than $100 billion in avoidable hospitalizations annually. Poor adherence to blood-pressure medicine kills 90,000 Americans annually, according to one study.

The New England Healthcare Institute (NEHI) estimates that the cost of drug-related injury and illness, including poor adherence, represents about 13 percent of total health-care expenditures. Adherence is lower for people with chronic conditions. They also are the most vulnerable from not taking their medicine consistently because flare-ups can result in emergency department visits, or even death.

For example, 1 in 4 patients who had been hospitalized for an acute stroke stopped taking their prescribed medication within the next three months. Many did not understand why they were taking the drugs, or their side effects.

Death rates for diabetes and heart-disease patients who did not take their medicine consistently were nearly double those of patients who complied with their prescription therapies. Diabetes patients with low compliance have about twice the annual health-care costs that they would if they took medication properly. The biggest barriers are confusing regimes, forgetfulness and high costs. If patients take their medicine less than 80 percent of the time, they are at twice the risk of recurring symptoms and hospitalization. On the other hand, medication adherence leads to lower use of the health-care system and lower overall costs despite increased spending on drugs.

About 3 percent of patients simply do not show up at the pharmacy counter to collect their prescriptions because of cost. The rate is especially poor for new prescriptions: One out of 4 is not picked up. At a processing cost of $5 to $10 per prescription, this abandonment costs the U.S. health-care system nearly half a billion.

Another reason patients do not take prescriptions properly is the awful execution of drug-information fliers. The instructions accompanying prescriptions can run several pages long, with microscopic print, incomprehensible legalese and jargon. Important consumer information is often buried among mounds of useless information, and instructions are tossed.

Patients who take their medications properly improve health outcomes and reduce health-care costs. For health-care providers, there are no incentives or direct reimbursement to help patients do so. Accountable care organizations and patient-centered medical homes, which will be reimbursed for keeping people healthy and coordinating care, may have those incentives.

Medication adherence is about 80 percent when patients can discuss their treatment with their physicians. Positive, respectful communication can help mitigate low health literacy, language barriers and cognitive decline. Patients and their families who understand their illnesses, know what to expect from treatment and understand a medication's importance are more likely to be adherent. Unfortunately, only 1 out of 4 people recently discharged from a medical service could list their medications, and even fewer knew the potential side effects.

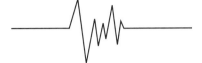

Chapter 23

End-of-Life Care
Quality of death

"Patient-centered" marketing rhetoric from health-care providers rings hollow when it comes to end-of-life care. The most important issues to any patient are how to live and die. The U.S. health-care system does a good job enabling the former, and an awful job with the latter.

A humane health-care system would help patients and their families understand a terminal illness and make informed decisions about care. In many cases, quality patient care means withdrawing the burden of treatment rather than vainly imposing aggressive and undignified interventions. Too often, though, the patient has not been given a say about either option.

Nearly everyone talks about improving quality of life. Few think about striving for quality of death. Despite its inevitability, the subject is often taboo. In a 2009 survey of people over 50 years old, nearly half said they had not thought about end-of-life care and 90 percent said they had not documented their wishes.

More than 80 percent of U.S. adults die from a protracted illness such as cancer, heart failure or Alzheimer's Disease. A similar percentage do not want to be hospitalized when they are dying, according to the Dartmouth Atlas Project.

For people who die suddenly and unexpectedly, a "quality death" is not an issue. Modern medicine, however, can keep death at bay, often at the cost of a painful existence. Quantity of life trumps quality of life.

In a moving account of end-of-life care in *The New Yorker*, physician Atul Gawande wrote that patient surveys indicate the top priorities of patients with terminal illnesses are avoiding pain, being with family, being mentally alert and not being burdensome to others.

"Our system of technological medical care has utterly failed to meet these needs," he wrote. "The hard question we face is ... how we can build a health-care system that will actually help dying patients achieve what's most important to them at the end of their lives."

The goal of palliative care is to help families understand treatment options. Care typically begins with a discussion of what a patient with a terminal illness wants out of his or her remaining life. Besides medical care, palliative care can also include legal, religious, insurance and advance-directive issues. Once the patients and their families express their wishes, palliative-team members can guide them toward reaching their goals.

Palliative care is about managing symptoms—such as pain, nausea, insomnia, loss of appetite—that accompany disease or treatment. Unlike hospice, palliative care can be employed while attempting to cure a disease.

One out of 4 patients experience significant and needless pain during their last two years of life. In the last six months, the number rises to nearly 50 percent. The biggest contributor is arthritis.

Palliative care is a relatively young medical discipline. The American Board of Medical Specialties officially recognized it in 2006. In a recent survey, less than one-quarter said they were familiar with the term.

The American Society of Clinical Oncology (ASCO) has established a goal of integrating palliative care into its model of comprehensive cancer care by 2020.

The swelling ranks of the U.S. elderly population inevitably will increase the prevalence of cancer. Even though the U.S. has one of the best cancer-cure rates in the world, nearly half of all cancers still result in death. That death rate essentially has remained flat for the past 30 years.

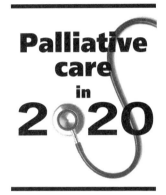

Palliative care is available at every U.S. cancer center. However, patients often are placed in the program too late to reap its full benefits. Some oncologists believe a palliative-care referral will destroy a patient's hope. Unlike with hospice, patients can receive cancer treatment and palliative care simultaneously. Palliative care can ease the often-painful symptoms caused by the condition and its treatment. For patients, maximizing comfort is nearly as important as fighting the disease.

A 2009 study of cancer patients found that palliative care improved patient satisfaction and eased pain, fatigue, nausea, insomnia, anxiety and depression. It also increased appetite.

Many people—including some physicians—confuse palliative and hospice care. Non-hospice palliative care addresses symptoms regardless of prognosis. Hospice is a subset of palliative care those who are believed to be in their last six months of life. Some fear health-care providers will not try as hard to cure them if they ask for palliative care. Others believe hospice is a "place" rather than a form of care that can be delivered in various locations.

Hospice care depends on a physician's estimate that a patient will live no longer than six more months. However, care will continue after that time as long as the physician and hospice caregivers certify that the patient's condition is terminal.

Both palliative and hospice include care given by a multi-disciplinary team that may include physicians, nurses, social workers, chaplains and others. The diversity of care underscores the fact that end-of-life treatment extends beyond the physical to include psychological, spiritual and emotional needs.

According to the Worldwide Palliative Care Alliance, more than 100 million people annually could benefit from palliative or hospice care. Yet less than 8 percent have access to it.

However, end-of-life care is growing rapidly in the United States. The percentage of heart-failure patients using it more than doubled from 2000 to 2007, to about 40 percent. The number of palliative-care programs in U.S. hospitals doubled during the same period, to nearly 1,500—including 80 percent of hospitals with 300 or more beds. Despite greater availability, use of palliative care by physicians is low. They tend to view it as the opposite of curative care, rather than a companion therapy.

Hospice is equally underused. Physicians are often unrealistic about how long a patient will live. A Harvard researcher found that 2 out of 3 doctors overestimated survival time. The average estimate was 530 percent too high.

Physicians also equate suggesting hospice with "giving up." The American Society of Clinical Oncology had to issue a policy statement in January 2011 to urge oncologists to speak candidly with incurable patients about end-of-life treatment options. Fewer than 40 percent do so.

Palliative and hospice care inevitably will become better-accepted clinical tools in the coming decades. Medicare increasingly will buckle under the economic strain of a rapidly growing elderly population. American medicine traditionally has delivered aggressive, expensive care in the last year of life, even if it is futile and unwanted.

According to one study, half of patients were in moderate to severe pain in the last three days of life, and 38 percent spent more than 10 days at the end of life in the intensive-care unit in a coma or on a ventilator. One-third of families lost most or all of their savings because of a terminal illness.

The folly and waste of such practices will become less acceptable. As people grow more aware of alternative treatment options, end-of-life care may or may not become less expensive. Nevertheless, it certainly is more humane and patient-centered.

Palliative care: Advantages and challenges

Palliative care offers multiple benefits. Pain can slow the healing process. It extends hospital stays, prolongs needless suffering and erodes a patient's capacity to adhere to prescribed treatment.

A 2008 *Journal of Palliative Medicine* study measured the impact of palliative care on patient satisfaction, clinical outcomes and cost of care for six months after being released from the hospital. Patient satisfaction was higher, more advance directives were completed, fewer intensive-care unit (ICU) admissions were necessary and medical costs were lower compared to patients with life-limiting illnesses not in palliative care. Patient satisfaction stems primarily from palliative care's patient-centered approach, which incorporates personal values and preferences.

This is in contrast to the usual intensive care many patients receive regardless of their preferences. More than half of Medicare spending on beneficiaries in their last two years is for hospital costs. About 25 percent of total Medicare costs is spent for patients in the last year of life. Most of those expenses are for hospitalizations, including readmissions and ICU stays. One out of 5 cancer patients are still receiving chemotherapy in the last two weeks of life.

Patient satisfaction with hospital care is inversely related to intensity of care. It falls in direct proportion to higher spending, greater use of resources and intrusive care.

Early palliative care can actually extend life. A 2010 study found that people with lung cancer who received the care lived three months longer, compared with those receiving standard care. Those with lung cancer can expect to get only two or three additional months of life at most from chemotherapy.

Despite its advantages, there are several barriers to widespread use of palliative care. Physicians are trained to save lives, even if it requires aggressive measures. It is often not clear at what point a condition becomes inevitably terminal. For many physicians and their patients, palliative care represents a surrender of sorts. Aggressiveness is the default approach to end-of-life care in the U.S.

An intensive battery of procedures and tests is paid for by Medicare and private insurers without questions. Reimbursement for palliative care is less certain. Medicare and private insurers pay for some palliative care, but the billing can be less comprehensive and more complicated than for standard hospital care, and physicians may consider this too burdensome. Customarily, most health plans do not pay for time-consuming care coordination and shared decision-making.

To counter these barriers, Governor David A. Paterson signed into law the New York Palliative Care Information Act, in 2010, which requires physicians to offer terminal patients and their families information about prognosis and options for end-of-life care. New York State's medical society opposed the law because they believed the government was intruding on the physician-patient relationship.

Palliative care is not necessarily intended to be less expensive care, but that often is the result. A hospitalized palliative-care patient costs $279 to $374 less a day. There are significant reductions in pharmacy, laboratory and ICU costs. The average annual savings of a palliative-care program is $1.3 million for a 300-bed community hospital and $2.5 million for an average academic medical center.

In a study of Medicaid patients in four hospitals in New York state, patients who received palliative care cost $6,900 less during a hospital stay compared with those who received standard care.

In Spain, a 2006 study found that a shift to palliative and at-home care and away from traditional hospitalization saved 61 percent.

Hospice: It is care, not a place

The magazine *Modern Healthcare* held a "tournament" in 2011 to determine what "one person, event, organization or innovation had the biggest impact on the health-care delivery system in the past 35 years." Hospice was "seeded" No. 12 at the beginning of voting. It was the landslide winner, beating out the Institute for Healthcare Improvement by a 3-to-1 margin.

Hospice care focuses on caring rather than curing. Most hospice care is provided in the patient's residence. However, it is also available in hospice centers, some hospitals and long-term-care facilities.

Hospice caregivers use a variety of alternative therapeutic techniques to comfort patients. They use massage, group therapy, music therapy and pet therapy and guided imagery to supplement traditional pain-relief tactics.

Nearly 1.5 million patients were treated in hospice programs in 2008, compared with only 25,000 in 1982 when it first became a Medicare benefit. It is also covered by Medicaid and most private insurance plans. The average length of time in hospice is about 21 days. The National Hospice and Palliative Care Organization estimates that nearly 40 percent of 2008 U.S. deaths were in a hospice setting.

The three leading causes of death in hospice programs— cancer, Alzheimer's disease and kidney disease—also are the easiest to predict remaining life expectancy, and they impose the greatest burdens on family caregivers.

Hospice care remains largely a white, upper-class and upper-middle-class phenomenon. Evidence indicates minority-group members generally are suspicious of the health-care system and are less open to the idea of withholding curative care. Many have had to forgo medical care most of their lives and have a different view of what it's like to have nature take its course. A survey of more than 4,000 newly diagnosed cancer patients found that 80 percent of blacks said they were willing to exhaust their resources to extend life, compared with 64 percent of Hispanics and 54 percent of whites.

As with palliative care, hospice sometimes prolongs life. In a 2007 study, hospice patients survived nearly a month longer than non-hospice patients with comparable conditions did. Hospice care improved survival in 4 of 6 disease categories. The largest difference was for congestive heart failure, where average survival rose from 321 to 402 days.

Nonetheless, it is difficult for some patients to choose hospice because forgoing medical care seems like accepting a death sentence. However, research shows that patients who choose hospice care do not die faster than those who do not.

In a pilot test, Aetna allowed a group of policyholders with a life expectancy of less than a year to receive hospice care without abandoning medical care. The number of patients who chose hospice shot up to 70 percent from 26 percent. The cost of care for these patients was 25 percent less, despite the concurrent care. They visited the emergency room half as often as non-hospice patients with life-limiting conditions. Their hospital and ICU use dropped by two-thirds.

For Medicare patients, hospice care saves an average of $2,309 per patient. A 2007 study found that Medicare costs would be lower for 70 percent of hospice recipients if such care were provided earlier. Cost of care was less expensive for cancer up to 233 days and non-cancer cases up to 154 days. Thereafter, hospice costs more than conventional care. However, the authors said, "More effort should be put into increasing short stays as opposed to focusing on shortening long ones."

For example, a study of men with advanced prostate cancer showed that about half eventually turned to hospice care but often waited until a week or two before death to enter the program. Brief hospice care delivers far fewer benefits.

More than two-thirds of hospice patients receive the services at home. However, a growing number of freestanding facilities are sprouting to meet demand. Construction of new hospice centers has increased by more than 40 percent since 2000. Nearly every U.S. citizen lives within 60 minutes of a hospice center, and 88 percent live within 30 minutes.

According to a 2010 study, the length of time that nursing-home patients are in hospice has doubled in the past decade, from 46 to 93 days. The study speculated that the increase was associated with a 50 percent growth in the number of nursing-home hospice programs. Medicare pays nursing homes far more for hospice care than the facilities would receive for standard care from Medicaid. The Medicare Payment Advisory Commission has recommended that standards for hospice certification be strengthened to ensure nursing-home programs are qualified to provide care.

Presumptuous and aggressive care

The Dartmouth Atlas Project systematically tracks aggressive end-of-life care as part of its ongoing research on regional Medicare spending. The project compared data from 2003 and 2007. The good news: Researchers found that patients spent slightly less time in the hospital and received more hospice care in 2007. The bad news: The intensity of care for those in the hospital increased.

The average number of hospice days rose from about 12 to more than 18. However, the number of chronically ill patients treated by 10 or more doctors in the last six months of life rose from about 30 to more than 36 percent.

Minorities are more likely to receive the latter kind of care. Besides choosing hospice less often than whites do, they live in urban areas where more medical interventions are available and used. For example, whites on Medicare spent about $20,000 during the last six months of life, compared with nearly $27,000 for blacks and nearly $32,000 for Hispanics.

Of course, it is often the wealthiest who spend the most to cling to life and ease the pain. The average patient spends about $11,600 out of pocket in the last year of life. But those in the top 10 percent of wealth spend an average of nearly $30,000, and the top 1 percent spent more than $94,300. Expensive home modifications, high-end nursing homes and various helpers and handlers can run up quite a tab.

Some economists, including Nobel Prize winner Gary Becker, defend such spending. They correctly point out that you cannot take your money with you. The issue becomes murkier, however, when such care is heavily subsidized by government insurance.

Religious beliefs also play a part. Many terminally ill patients rely on their religious faith to help them cope, and are more likely to receive aggressive care in the last week of life. They tend to believe it is in God's hands—not the doctor's or the patient's—to determine when death will come. They often see the fight for life as a collaboration with God to overcome illness, and they feel a religious purpose in enduring invasive and painful therapy.

On the other hand, physicians who say they are not religious are twice as likely to make recommendations that may end a person's life, compared with physicians who say they are religious. The most religious physicians are much less likely to discuss end-of-life decisions with their patients. Unfortunately, patients rarely know how these views bias a physician's outlook and advice.

Americans strongly believe that patients have the right to decide whether they want to be kept alive. Nearly 3 out of 4 say there are circumstances in which patients should be allowed to die. There are deeper divisions over legalizing physician-assisted suicide. About 46 percent favor such laws, while 45 percent oppose them.

Communication is critical

End-of-life discussions between patients and physicians often are uncomfortable. Patients who have such discussions are more likely to accept their illness as terminal and choose pain relief over life-extending therapy. They are also more likely to complete advance directives and three times more likely to enroll in hospice.

Ironically, patients are less likely to suffer emotional harm or an increase in severity of depression if there is a frank discussion about their prospects.

However, not all physicians and nurses are suited for these discussions. At 12 hospitals in the Seattle area, a program to teach providers how to communicate with families of terminal patients failed to improve family satisfaction. Researchers admitted that it was difficult to change the behavior of busy clinicians.

Even when done skillfully, the physician's message is not always taken at face value. Family members often take a more optimistic view of the patient's prognosis than physicians do, even when they a given a specific time estimate of remaining life or chances of survival.

Documents known as advance directives take the guesswork out of figuring out a patient's wishes and values. They are legal documents that establish guidelines for which treatments patients wish to receive—or not receive. They also may designate who will make treatment decisions for them if they are incapable. They include a living will, which can include choices regarding do-not-resuscitate orders, artificial breathing and feeding, and organ donation. A durable power of attorney designates someone to make end-of-life decisions on your behalf if you are unable to do so.

More than 1 in 4 elderly patients were incapable of making end-of-life decisions. Those with advance directives nearly always got the treatment they wanted. Notably, of those who had directives, only 2 percent wanted aggressive end-of-life care, according to a *New England Journal of Medicine* study.

Some experts say advance directives do not adequately cover the variety of situations that arise. Some prefer a more detailed document known as physician orders for life-sustaining treatment (POLST), used in a handful of states but spreading rapidly. POLST offers the ability to detail preferences regarding a much wider range of treatments.

A barrier to completing advance directives is that most are laden with legalese that most people do not understand. Researchers evaluated the documents in all 50 states and found they were written at or above a 12th-grade reading level. Unfortunately, 40 percent of Americans read at an eighth-grade level or lower.

In 2008, Congress added discussion of directives to the initial "Welcome to Medicare" preventive exam. The comprehensive exam is free in the first 12 months for new beneficiaries. The 2009 health-reform effort to reimburse physicians for these kinds of discussions at any time spawned the famous and fatuous "death panel" demagoguery. Readers of PolitiFact, a fact-checking website, overwhelmingly anointed "death panels" the 2009 "Lie of the Year."

When people are asked to imagine themselves incompetent and with a poor prognosis, more than 70 percent say they would refuse life-sustaining treatment. Only 1 in 8 nursing-home residents want aggressive end-of-life care, even though that is what they get if their wishes are unknown.

The medical community in La Crosse, Wis., has made a commitment to ensuring that patients complete advance directives. As a result, 96 percent of its residents die with such forms filled out. The cost of care at the local hospital in the last two years of life is about $18,000, compared with the national average of $26,000.

Advance directives also lift the emotional burden off loved ones responsible for making care decisions. Family members unaware of patients' wishes take nearly two weeks longer to decide to withdraw medical care. That can become expensive. The cost of care in the last week of life is 55 percent higher for those who have not had these discussions.

Part 5

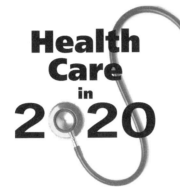

Conclusion

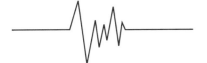

Chapter 24

Final Thoughts

With the nation in such dire financial straits, health care has a budgetary target on its back. Medicare and Medicaid are expected to account for 40 percent of the projected growth in federal spending by 2020. Health-care costs are expected to consume 20 percent of the nation's gross domestic product by the end of the decade.

The "we must control health-care costs" mantra emanating from Washington and state capitals has yet to move beyond rhetoric or wishful thinking. For medical costs to be truly controlled, Americans would need to be more comfortable with government regulation and more cautious use of medical technology. Patients would have to clean up their act by paying closer attention to their health and becoming more engaged and savvy medical-care consumers. Providers would have to set aside their financial self-interests—or sound business practices, depending upon your perspective—for the nation's fiscal well-being. None of these things is likely.

Most Americans have accepted that health-care costs are paid with a blank check despite a limited budget. The polls reflect this. Most oppose cutting or tinkering with Medicare and Medicaid.

Even 70 percent of Tea Party members consider Medicare a sacred cow.

The health-care debate generally has not been about controlling costs. It has been about to whom costs should be shifted: from the federal government to the states; from government insurance programs to private insurers; from employers to employees.

Controlling costs would require the cooperation of powerful health lobbies. They will fiercely protect their turf. Health-care industries—hospitals, physicians, medical-device makers, pharmaceutical companies, health plans—arguably have become the most powerful advocates in Washington. That is to be expected from an economic sector that represents nearly one-fifth of the nation's economy.

In a report called *The New Gold Rush*, the consulting firm PricewaterhouseCoopers noted that more than three-quarters of the Fortune 50 either are in the health-care industry or have health divisions. Less than a quarter of those are traditional health-care companies. These enormous, nontraditional market entrants provide added political muscle.

The sector grew stronger as the rest of the nation grew weaker during the most recent recession. According to the Bureau of Labor Statistics, the recession resulted in a loss of 8.4 million jobs. Meanwhile, health-care employment grew by 732,000.

From 1990 to 2009, the U.S. workforce expanded by 16 percent. The health-care workforce grew by 65 percent. Nearly 1 out of 3 U.S. adults either work in health care, previously worked in health care or want to do so.

What will health care look like in 2020?

Uncertain reform

Certainly anything can happen to derail the health-reform law before 2019, when it is implemented completely. Moreover, it will

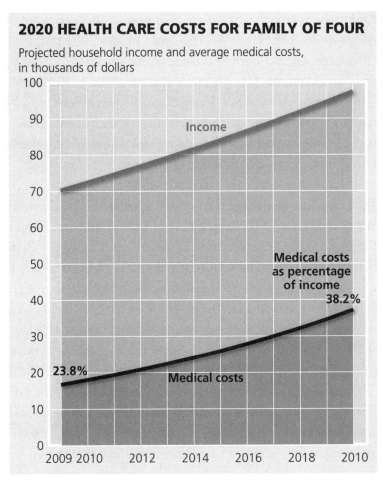

2020 HEALTH CARE COSTS FOR FAMILY OF FOUR

Projected household income and average medical costs, in thousands of dollars

Author's calculations based on historical Milliman Medical Index trends.

Assuming current cost and wage-increase trends continue, median annual household income in 2020 is projected to be $97,385 and annual health costs will be $37,181, or 38 percent of income. The employee share of that is expected to be 45 percent, or $16,731. By 2020, out-of-pocket health-care costs are expected to exceed 17 percent of household income for a family of four. This projection is based on the last five-year average of 7.5 percent annual medical cost growth and 3 percent annual wage increases. A rule of thumb is that health-care costs become a financial burden at 10 percent of household income.

certainly be tweaked as the inevitable unintended consequences present themselves. However, the smart money is betting that it will emerge largely intact by the end of the decade.

According to the Congressional Budget Office (CBO), repealing the law would add $210 billion to the deficit between 2012 and 2021. Opponents would have to overcome that financial hurdle, as well as offer a credible alternative that would cut the rate of uninsured Americans nearly as much as the new law does.

The tougher sell of repeal by Republicans would be the collateral damage. Insurance companies again would be allowed to deny people coverage because of pre-existing conditions, impose lifetime limits on coverage and charge discriminatory rates based on age and gender. The CBO estimated the uninsured rate for nonelderly U.S. adults would be about 17 percent, or roughly what it has been in recent years.

Even if a Republican president and GOP-dominated Congress are elected in 2012, they are unlikely to stand up to powerful health-care interests. Health reform may often be referred to as "Obamacare," but it was shaped by the health-care industry. Health-care providers and insurers like the individual mandate because it expands their markets with newly insured, healthier participants. The law also significantly reduces uncompensated care. It slowly closes the Medicare coverage gap, also known as the "doughnut hole," which should lead to increased sales for pharmaceutical companies.

Although polls show Americans are split in their attitudes toward the law, health reform is likely to gain support throughout the decade as its programs affect more people. However, people's expectations may be unrealistic. If they expect inexpensive insurance on the exchanges with robust benefits and myriad choices, they will be disappointed. The coverage tiers with the most affordable premiums will have steep out-of-pocket costs.

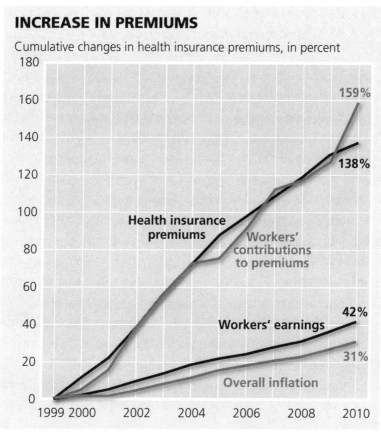

INCREASE IN PREMIUMS

Cumulative changes in health insurance premiums, in percent

Source: Kaiser/HRET Survey of Employer-Sponsored Health Benefits, 1999-2010.

Employee-sponsored health-insurance premiums have grown significantly since 1999, and the employee share of those premiums has grown at almost the same rate. On a percentage basis, both have grown more than three times faster than workers' salaries and general inflation.

For example, the "Silver Plan" will be the second-lowest benefit category. It will have a standard major-medical plan deductible of $1,000 and will pay for 70 percent of anticipated medical costs. A family of four with a household income of $65,000 a year will pay $6,175 in premium costs.

Health-policy experts who supported the law have faith that it will be able to corral costs. To borrow a football analogy, that belief likely is a Hail Mary pass. Harvard economist David Cutler believes the Obama administration must move quickly on testing and rolling out Medicare demonstration and pilot programs that encourage more cost-efficient care. According to Cutler, the typical 5-to-10-year timetable for such experiments must be cut to a year or less to alter the cost-increase trajectory as swiftly as possible.

Cutler also believes providers must respond to incentives to save money and improve quality of care. The federal government is expecting health-care providers to embrace electronic medical records, to work as teams and to figure out how to operate efficiently—when it is much more profitable to be inefficient by providing more care than necessary.

All of this is asking the federal government and the health-care industry to be nimble organizationally and act with a sense of urgency—a strength of neither institution.

There already are several early signs that change will not come easily.

- The patient-centered "medical home" requires a significant financial commitment and change in how care is delivered. The model relies on enhanced primary care, a greater reliance in non-physician staff members, and new payment methods. A survey of more than 1,300 physician practices found that only 20 percent of medical-home processes were being employed.
- Electronic health records are considered critical to tracking population health and care quality, and to qualifying for payment bonuses under new health-care delivery models. Through mid-May 2011, however,

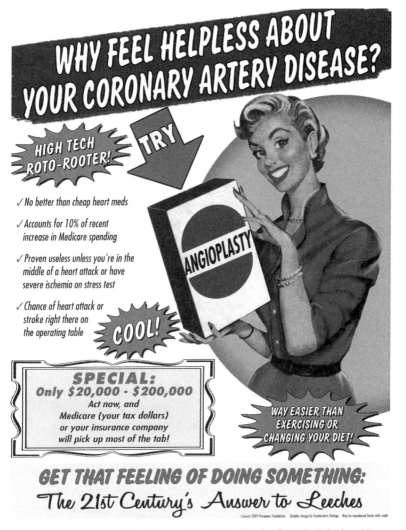

Source: Parsemus Foundation. Graphic design by Federskirts Vintage.

This Parsemus Foundation poster on angioplasty raised the ire of cardiologists who found the satire unfair. However, recent research found that angioplasty and stents are used commonly in circumstances that violate guidelines established by the American Heart Association and the American College of Cardiology.

fewer than 2 percent of eligible hospitals and physicians had met the federal government's standards to earn reimbursement.

- A cornerstone of health reform's health-care delivery reform is accountable care organizations (ACOs). They are networks of primary care-led physician and hospital organizations. Each network agrees to provide coordinated care for at least 5,000 Medicare beneficiaries. The ACOs would qualify for bonus payments if they meet quality and cost targets. The American Medical Group Association, which represents several hundred health-care organizations and includes some of the nation's best candidates to become ACOs, rejected the model and called it "overly prescriptive, operationally burdensome, and the incentives are too difficult to achieve to make this voluntary achievement attractive."

- A health-policy mantra is to move toward a system that pays physicians for keeping people healthy rather than performing as many procedures and tests as possible. But Merritt Hawkins, a physician search and consulting firm, said 3 out of 4 of its 2010 physician job searches included performance bonuses. Of those bonuses, about 90 percent were for "fee-for-service style volume."

Regardless, many are keeping the faith. Brookings Institution economist Henry Aaron spoke for many health-reform supporters when he said that it "contains, at least in embryonic form, virtually every idea for cost control that any (health-care) analyst has come up with ... The most practical cost-control strategy that is now available to Congress is to accelerate the implementation of these provisions, not stymie them."

Bad habits

Americans with risky health behaviors cannot expect the medical system to patch them up when their bodies begin to falter after decades of carelessness. Such efforts are expensive and too often ineffective.

The most effective way to cut health-care costs is to use less health care. The research of Dee Edington, a University of Michigan professor who has been studying workplace health for decades, shows the correlation between disease and health-care costs. As risks rise, so do costs. As they fall, so do costs.

Americans can control most of this spending. A significant percentage of disease—especially chronic conditions—is self-inflicted. For example, a 2004 study found that lifestyle changes could prevent at least 90 percent of heart-disease cases. Nearly 4 out of 10 U.S. deaths are attributable to four behaviors: tobacco use, diet, physical inactivity and alcohol abuse.

When they do need treatment, patients are not holding up their end of the bargain. Only half take medication in the prescribed doses. About half did not take referral advice, three-quarters did not keep follow-up appointments, and about half of those with chronic illnesses abandoned regular medical care within a year.

Forty years ago, Americans could expect to live slightly longer than Western Europeans. Americans on average now live about 18 fewer months than those in nations such as France, Denmark, Germany, Spain and Italy.

Researchers at Harvard, the RAND Corp. and the University of Southern California have concluded in a joint study that Americans begin falling behind in life expectancy around age 50. After adjusting for U.S. income inequality, they concluded the life-expectancy disparity would disappear if the U.S. could lower middle-age obesity and obesity-related chronic diseases such as high blood pressure and diabetes to European levels. Doing so would save the health-care system about $1.1 trillion, after adjusting for inflation, by 2050. The Medicare and Medicaid portion of those savings would be $632 billion.

The lifestyles of older Americans have become increasingly unhealthy in the past two decades. Consumption of fruits and vegetables among that group has declined by nearly half. The percentage who worked out at least 12 times a month has declined. Only about 5 percent of U.S. adults exercise vigorously on any given day.

Even those who have acquired heart disease, high blood pressure or diabetes are no more likely to change their habits than those without the conditions. Nearly half of smokers who survive a heart attack are still puffing away a year later. Most overweight heart-attack survivors do not lose weight or give up junk food. One out of 5 patients diagnosed with lung cancer continue to smoke. A study of 9,000 cancer survivors found that only 1 out of 20 were consuming at least five fruits and vegetables daily, engaging in regular physical activity and refraining from smoking.

The health-care system has its own bad habits to address. Many patients do not get the recommended care. Doctors write prescriptions because it is easier than extended discussions with patients. Hospital readmissions are frequent because patients are hustled out the door. A 2010 study found that health-care providers were following evidence-based guidelines less than half of the time. Doctors order redundant tests recently performed by other doctors. People are given aggressive end-of-life care against their wishes.

Changing bad habits costs little, can generate enormous savings and extend healthy life.

Too few doctors

This is shorthand for "too few health-care providers." It is going to get ugly. Nearly 9 out of 10 health-care opinion leaders say they are concerned or very concerned about the nation's supply of primary-care providers, according to a Commonwealth Fund survey. Shortages will extend to some specialty physicians as well.

Take a peek at Texas health care in 2020.

Demand has been artificially suppressed because of the state's top-ranked uninsured rate, the highest among 50 states. According to the Centers for Disease Control and Prevention, nearly 32 percent of nonelderly adult Texans were uninsured in 2009. They generally only see a physician when they have to.

By 2014, expanded Medicaid, insurance exchanges and the individual mandate are expected to push the state's uninsured rate well below 10 percent.

The demographics are daunting.

The number of residents with health insurance will grow by half, or about 9 million people. The Austin-based Center for Public Policy Priorities estimates the health-reform law will insure about 4.5 million more Texans. The state demographer projects Texas will also grow by about 5 million residents in this decade. At least 90 percent of them, or another 4.5 million, will also be insured.

The population will be older and sicker. Demographers say more than 97 percent of the states will be minority groups members, who typically have poorer health. The youngest baby boomers turn 50 in 2014, an age beyond which about 80 percent have at least one chronic condition. The Federal Reserve Bank of Dallas predicts both factors "will dramatically affect the health care industry in Texas." The Fed expects that increases in doctor visits, hospital and nursing care will exceed the rate of population growth. There will be a surge in care around mid-decade. Research indicates that an uninsured adult who then gets coverage incurs an extra $1,600 in expenses because of previously unmet medical needs.

There will not be enough doctors and nurses. Nearly 40 percent of doctors are 55 or older. About 22 percent of Texas physicians will reach retirement age in the next five years. About one-third of nurses are 50 or older, and more than half of those want to retire before 2020—creating a shortage of perhaps 71,000 in Texas. Health economist Peter Buerhaus predicts a national shortage of 100,000 physicians and 300,000 nurses by 2020. Texas has 212 physicians per 100,000 residents. The rate has been stable because the state's 2003 medical-malpractice reforms have attracted thousands of out-of-state doctors. That has allowed the state to keep up with population growth. But it will be insufficient in the future.

Traditional primary care will become scarce. Massachusetts has had universal health-insurance coverage since 2006. The percentage of family physicians who no longer take new patients increased from 30 to 40 percent from 2007 to 2009, according to a state medical society survey. Those accepting new patients impose an average of 44 days' wait for an appointment. Ominously, Massachusetts has more than twice as many physicians per capita as Texas.

Already-jammed emergency departments (EDs) will become even more crowded with nonurgent cases. The ED supposedly dominated by patients who are uninsured is a myth. Fully insured Massachusetts residents use the ED at a rate 40 percent greater than that of the U.S. as a whole. Medicaid patients use the ER twice as much as the uninsured, and three times more than the privately insured. The reason: They do not want to—or cannot— wait to see the doctor.

By 2015, Texas medical schools plan to increase enrollment by 30 percent. The Texas legislature increased its funding for residency programs in 2009. However, these efforts are paltry compared with the need. Health reform fixed the health-insurance problem. However, insurance is useless if timely care is unavailable. Texas has the most to gain by insurance expansion. It also will experience the greatest aftershock from the resulting demand.

Health reform will create a different kind of rationing. Before the law, the primary method of rationing was lack of insurance. People without insurance generally avoid the health-care system until care is absolutely necessary. Once the law fully rolls out, the U.S. will have what health economist John Goodman calls rationing by waiting. The effect of the demand created by 32 million newly insured patients without a concurrent increase in provider supply is grossly underappreciated. It will be fully appreciated by 2020.

Skyrocketing costs

The elephant in the room is the fact that Medicare and Medicaid essentially are paid with a blank check. The federal government sets the price it will pay for medical services, but places no limit on the volume of those services. The result: Services, especially high-priced procedures and tests, have multiplied without a concurrent improvement in population health.

Few health-care services are denied, regardless of whether there is evidence that they are effective, because policymakers do not want to be accused of rationing care. Unlike with the rest of the federal budget, the government passively pays the bill and allows others to determine its size.

There is no health-care "budget" in the sense that government allocates a certain amount of money it will spend, and no more. Instead, policymakers allow health-care providers to determine "medical necessity" without restraint. Abdicating this oversight often encourages expensive treatment that does not benefit patients and is an outrageous waste of taxpayer money.

Take angioplasty, used to open narrowed coronary arteries and usually involves placement of a tiny metal tube called a stent to prop open arteries. It is highly effective for people who have just had heart attacks. However, a 2006 landmark study established that performing the procedure in patients more than 24 hours after a heart attack had no benefit. In 2007, the American College of Cardiology and the American Heart Association issued guidelines saying that the procedure "should not be performed" in those circumstances.

Yet more than half of patients who survive a heart attack for more than 24 hours have angioplasty afterward—a rate that essentially remained unchanged between 2005 and 2008, according to a 2011 study. According to the study's findings, about 50,000 Americans annually are receiving this unneeded procedure, at a cost of $20,000 each. Although the study was not specific on this point, Medicare undoubtedly was picking up a significant portion of the tab.

Cardiologists attempt to defend the procedure with non-clinical justifications, speaking vaguely of malpractice fears and the virtues of clear arteries. Why are taxpayer dollars being spent on scientifically baseless, even potentially dangerous, medical procedures? The Parsemus Foundation poster on angioplasty (see page 345) captures the absurdity of the situation.

Health reform potentially did a great service to medicine and American taxpayers by creating the equivalent of a U.S. Preventive Services Task Force (USPSTF) for treatments and procedures. The

USPSTF evaluates the latest scientific evidence on the effectiveness of about 200 clinical preventive services, including screening, counseling and medications. It assigns grades from A to D. The health-reform law dictates that nearly 90 million Americans with employer or individual insurance—as well as Medicare—will not have to pay a deductible or co-payment for services the USPSTF has graded A or B.

The law created the Patient-Centered Outcomes Research Institute (PCORI), which is designed to evaluate existing research and sponsor new research to evaluate comparative effectiveness and quality of medications and treatments. The federal government included $1 billion in the 2009 federal stimulus bill for comparative-effectiveness research.

The New England Healthcare Institute, which represents a broad array of health-system stakeholders, has called on PCORI to be a "highly visible champion" for publicizing and disseminating the research. Critics have charged that PCORI somehow will ration care. However, its role should be aimed squarely at identifying, and encouraging government insurance programs to stop paying for, the estimated 30 percent of medical care that has no benefit.

Two physicians, who also are former Medicare officials, have suggested that the government give expensive new treatments three years to prove they work better than cheaper alternatives. If not, their reimbursement would be cut to that of the cheaper treatments. In other words, payment for proton beam therapy discussed in Chapter 17 would be cut in half if it did not justify its higher price. Private insurance plans such as Aetna and Cigna have experimented with similar policies.

Health economist Goodman has urged the greater use of health savings accounts to pay for purely discretionary care such as uvula removal to cure snoring, in vitro fertilization and testosterone supplements. Insurance coverage of such treatments encourages excessive use and higher prices. He points out that treatments costs fall for discretionary medical care that is generally not covered by insurance, such as Lasik and cosmetic surgery.

Health reform will not have an appreciable effect on aggregate national health-care spending, according to the office of the chief Medicare actuary. Its report undercut the arguments of both reform's harshest critics and its most ardent supporters. Yearly spending is predicted to grow from about $2.5 trillion to $4.6 trillion by 2019, which would be an annual increase of 6.3 percent.

The annual Milliman Medical Index (MMI) measures the total cost of health care for a typical family of four covered by a preferred provider organization (PPO). A PPO usually is the most generous employer-sponsored insurance plan that offers the deepest discounts in exchange for using a designated network of health-care providers. MMI calculates how much employers subsidize employee premium costs, how much employees contribute to the cost of the premiums and how much employees pay for deductibles and co-payments at the time of service.

In 2009, the median annual household income for a family of four was $70,354 and household health-care costs were $16,771, or 24 percent of income. Families paid $6,284 of that amount. Assuming current cost and wage-increase trends continue, by 2020 median annual household income is projected to be $97,385 and annual health costs will be $37,181, or 38 percent of income. The employee share of that is expected to be 45 percent, or $16,731.

A common rule of thumb is that health-care costs become a financial burden when out-of-pocket costs reach 10 percent of household income. By 2020, those costs are expected on average to exceed 17 percent for a family of four.

Reform likely will dominate health-care headlines throughout this decade. However, the larger story will be this growing household burden. The average deductible for PPOs is $1,200. Enrollees of consumer-directed health plans (CDHPs), with much higher deductibles, have been growing by 2 percentage points a year. If that trend continues, about one-third of U.S. workers with employer-sponsored insurance will have CDHPs by 2020. High-deductible plans will become the norm. Free-market economists have long advocated giving patients more "skin in the game" to discourage overuse of medical services and to encourage providers to compete for business. The health-care marketplace is headed there by default.

Beyond 2020

The best way for government to cut health-care costs is to stop paying for medical care that has little or no proven benefit. Rationing medical care implies withholding needed care. But refusing to continue paying for medical care that has no benefit is not rationing. It is about setting rational budgetary guidelines. Research shows that health-care providers are very responsive to reimbursement changes. If they are no longer paid for specific services, many stop performing them. This also protects patients, because medical care without benefit is, by definition, harmful.

Government's knee-jerk reaction to escalating health-care costs has been to cut, across the board, payments to doctors and hospitals. Continuing to follow this course will backfire. Fewer doctors will participate in government insurance programs, or will be able to stay in business because reimbursement does not cover office overhead. Indiscriminate payment cuts will lead to reductions in access, quality and service.

If health-care costs continue their trajectory, expect intrusive government regulation between 2020 and 2030. The two most likely forms will be a single-payer system or an all-payer system.

The state of Vermont is preparing to launch a single-payer system in 2015. The publicly financed insurance is designed to achieve universal coverage and to control costs. Vermont expects to cut health-care costs by 25 percent annually, compared with current costs. The system also is projected to reduce household and employer costs by $200 million, create 3,800 jobs and boost the state's economic output by $200 million. If Vermont achieves these numbers, other states and the federal government certainly will take notice.

Government has the ability to cut costs by wielding its purchasing power to negotiate the lowest prices for medication, physician fees and hospital services. For example, Medicare or Medicaid paid for about one-third of the $300 billion Americans spent on prescription drugs in 2010. Government historically has chosen not to use its buying power to lower costs. That may not be a tenable long-term position.

A single-payer system is what economists call a "monopsony." It means that demand comes from one customer. That is in contrast to a "monopoly," when there is only one or a limited number of suppliers. Theoretically, a single buyer can push the price of a good down to near the cost of production.

What would be the effect of a federal single-payer system? The Commonwealth Fund commissioned the Lewis Group to estimate the impact of the America Health Care Act, introduced in 2009 by Rep. Pete Stark (D-Calif.). The proposal would have enrolled every American in a Medicare-style public plan at birth. Employers either would have covered their employees or paid into the public plan. According to the Lewis Group, the plan would have saved $58.1 billion in national health spending in 2010. True, the federal deficit would have increased by about $189 billion and employers would have paid about $62 billion in that year. However, state and local governments would have saved about $84 billion, and households would have saved about $225 billion.

Another alternative is an all-payer system, which has been used by Maryland to set hospital prices since the 1970s. In an all-payer system, each hospital charges the same price to all buyers for an emergency-room visit or appendectomy. In Maryland, a board establishes rates for individual hospitals based on local wages, amount of charity care and the severity of patient cases. State officials calculated that state regulation of hospital rates has saved $40 billion since 1976. If all states used a similar system, the savings would have been at least $1.8 trillion, according to Maryland officials.

A more market-based version would have associations of insurers negotiate with each provider to establish prices. Under the current system, each insurer negotiates with each provider individually. Pooled negotiating power likely would result in lower prices and offset the market power of monopoly health-care providers. It would also enable greater price transparency and streamline the billing process.

In a 2010 Commonwealth Fund survey, a majority of U.S. health-care leaders said they favored either all-payer rate setting or a negotiation process on behalf of all payers.

Concluding thoughts

As much as patients and providers complain about the dysfunctional U.S. health-care system, they are not ready to change it significantly, despite opinion polls to the contrary. Patients generally are happy with their doctors and their insurance plans. Providers generally are uncomfortable with changes in government reimbursement, which are rarely in their favor. Policymakers know tinkering with health-care funding—especially Medicare—can be politically toxic.

The public-health battlefield is littered with well-meaning but ineffective calls for a variety of interventions. The U.S. Surgeon General and the Institute of Medicine produce tomes with lofty goals that get heads to nod, and then are promptly forgotten.

Health care in 2020 will present a very different landscape. It will have been driven by the consequences of health reform, the prospect of unbridled costs and an increasing shortage of health-care providers. There is no single solution to combating these forces. However, this book has outlined a number of efforts that are good medicine as well as being cost-effective: improving chronic-disease management; humane end-of-life care; shared decision-making by physicians and patients, workplace wellness programs and reorienting financial incentives toward quality and care efficiency rather than volume.

Measures like these must be put in place. We have little time to lose.

Notes

Chapter 1. Health Care in 2020

Page 3 The Congressional Budget Office ..." The budget and economic outlook: Fiscal years 2011 to 2021. Congressional Budget Office. cbo.gov/ftpdocs/120xx/doc12039/01-26_FY2011Outlook.pdf January 2011. Accessed July 25, 2011.

4 "If the price of gasoline ..." Kendall DB. Improving health care—by "spreading the Mayo" (the Mayo Clinic Model, that is). Democratic Leadership Council website. dlc.org/print.cfm?contentid=254811. January 15, 2009. Accessed July 28, 2011.

4 "Donald Berwick ..." Berwick DM, Nolan TW, Whittington J. The triple aim: Care, health, and cost. *Health Aff.* 2008;27(3):759-769.

4 "When Berwick assumed his role ..." Fleming C. Berwick brings the "triple aim" to CMS. Health Affairs blog. healthaffairs.org/blog/2010/09/14/berwick-brings-the-triple-aim-to-cms/. September 14, 2010. Accessed July 25, 2011.

5 "That tension is highlighted ..." Kissick W. *Medicine's Dilemmas: Infinite Needs Versus Finite Resources.* New Haven: Yale University Press; 1994.

5 "Sharon Kaufman ..." Kaufman S, Max W. Medicare's embedded ethics: The challenge of cost control in an aging society. Health Affairs blog. healthaffairs.org/blog/2011/03/28/medicares-embedded-ethics-the-challenge-of-cost-control-in-an-aging-society/March 28, 2011. Accessed July 28, 2011.

5 "Bioethicists Daniel Callahan ..." Callahan D, Nuland SB. The quagmire: How American medicine is destroying itself. *The New Republic.* May 19, 2011. Accessed July 28, 2011.

6 "A 1994 Harvard study ..." Brownlee, S. *Overtreated: Why Too Much Medicine Is Making Us Sicker and Poorer.* New York: Bloomsbury USA; 2008.

6 "Americans generally are happy ..." Saad L. American's ratings of own healthcare quality remain high. The Gallup Poll. gallup.com/poll/144869/americans-ratings-own-healthcare-quality-remain-high.aspx. November 22, 2010. Accessed July 28, 2011.

6 "However, in another 2010 ..." Mendes E. Americans' confidence in the medical system on the rebound. The Gallup Poll. gallup.com/poll/141815/americans-confidence-medical-system-rebound.aspx. August 9, 2010. Accessed July 28, 2011.

6 "Gallup conducted a worldwide poll ..." Deaton A. Income, health and wellbeing around the world: Evidence from the Gallup World Poll. *J Econ Perspect.* 2008;22(2):53-72.

6 "Paul Keckley ..." 2010 survey of health care consumers: Key findings, strategic implications. Deloitte Center for Health Solutions. deloitte.com/assets/Dcom-UnitedStates/Local%20Assets/Documents/US_CHS_2010SurveyofHealthCareConsumers_050310.pdf. 2010. Accessed July 28, 2011.

6 "A 2010 Employee Benefit Research Institute ..." 2010 health confidence survey: Health reform does not increase confidence in the health care system. Employee Benefit Research Institute Vol. 31, No. 9. September 2010.

7 "For example, a 2004 study found ..." Yusuf S, Hawken S, Ounpuu S, et al. Effect of potentially modifiable risk factors associated with myocardial infarction in 52 countries (the INTERHEART study): case-control study. *Lancet*. 2004;364(9438):937-952.

7 "Nearly 4 out of 10 U.S. deaths ..." Mokdad AH, Marks JS, Stroup DF, Gerberding JL. Actual causes of death in the United States, 2000. *JAMA*. 2004;291(10):1238-1245.

7 "Only half take medication ..." Parekh AK. Winning their trust. *N Engl J Med*. 2011; 364(24):e51.

7 "Declines in tobacco use ..." National Center for Health Statistics. *Health, United States, 2009: With special feature on medical technology*, Hyattsville MD. 2010.

Chapter 2. Health Reform

Page 15 "It is expected to reduce ..." Congressional Budget Office. Cost estimate for H.R. 4872, Reconciliation Act of 2010 (Final health care legislation): Table 4. 2010. goo.gl/S637o.

16 "With the exception ..." Morone JA. Presidents and health reform: From Franklin D. Roosevelt to Barack Obama. *Health Aff*. 2010;29(6):1096-1100.

18 "The Center for Public Integrity ..." Eaton J, Pell MB. Lobbyists swarm Capitol to influence health reform. The Center for Public Integrity website. iwatchnews.org/2010/02/24/2725/lobbyists-swarm-capitol-influence-health-reform. February 24, 2010. Accessed July 6, 2010.

18 "Ten key health-care groups ..." Vaida B. Doctors continued to spend big on lobbying in 2010. Kaiser Health News. kaiserhealthnews.org/Stories/2011/January/27/ama-lobbying.aspx. January 27, 2011. Accessed July 6, 2011.

19 "In a February 2010 ..." Brodie M, Altman D, Deane C, Buscho S, Hamel E. Liking the pieces, not the package: Contradictions in public opinion during health reform. *Health Aff*. 2010;29(6):1125-1130.

19 "The individual mandate ..." Grande D, Gollust SE, Asch DA. Polling analysis: Public support for health reform was broader than reported and depended on how proposals were framed. *Health Aff*. 2011;30(7):1242-1249.

19 "A January 2011 Kaiser/Harvard poll ..." Kaiser Family Foundation/Harvard School of Public Health. The Public's Health Care Agenda for the 112th Congress. kff.org/kaiserpolls/upload/8134-F.pdf. January 2011. Accessed July 7, 2011.

21 "A September 2010 ..." Alonso-Zaldivar R. Health insurance mandate began as a Republican idea. articles.boston.com/2010-03-28/news/29285190_1_individual-mandate-health-insurance-individual-requirement. March 28, 2010. Accessed July 6, 2011.

21 "In 1986, two-thirds ..." Brodie, op. cit.

22 "Republican pollster Frank Luntz ..." Kurtz H. How Fox News spun health-care debate. The Daily Beast. thedailybeast.com/articles/2010/12/09/how-fox-news-spun-the-health-care-debate.html. December 9, 2010. Accessed July 7, 2011.

22 "PolitiFact, the Pulitzer Prize-winning ..." Adair B, Holan AD. PolitiFact's Life of the Year: 'A government takeover of health care.' politifact.com/truth-o-meter/article/2010/dec/16/lie-year-government-takeover-health-care/. December 16, 2010. Accessed July 7, 2011.

22 "National Public Radio ..." Rovner J. Health law myths: Outside the realm of reality. NPR. npr.org/templates/story/story.php?storyId=129581493. September 3, 2010. Accessed July 6, 2011.

21 "As University of North Carolina ..." Oberlander J. Beyond repeal—the future of health care reform. *N Engl J Med*. 2010;363:2277-2279.

24 "According to one health blogger ..." Kuraitis V. Pilots, demonstrations & innovation in the

PPACA health care reform legislation. e-CareManagement.org blog. e-caremanagement.com/pilots-demonstrations-innovation-in-the-ppaca-healthcare-reform-legislation/. March 28, 2010. Accessed July 6, 2011.

24 "Wilbur Cohen ..." Kissick WL. *Medicine's Dilemma: Infinite Needs Versus Finite Resources.* New Haven: Yale University Press; 1994.

25 "These funding problems ..." Galewitz P. Some programs OK'd by health law lacking funding. Kaiser Health News. June 9, 2011. Accessed July 6, 2011.

26 "The CBO estimated ..." Effects of eliminating the individual mandate to obtain health insurance. Congressional Budget Office. cbo.gov/ftpdocs/113xx/doc11379/Eliminate_Individual_Mandate_06_16.pdf. June 16, 2010. Accessed July 11, 2011.

26 "According to an Urban Institute ..." Buettgens M, Garrett B, Holahan J. Why the individual mandate matters. Urban Institute. urban.org/publications/412280.html. December 2010. Accessed July 6, 2011.

26 "In 1996, it prohibited ..." Gruber J. Health care reform is a "three-legged stool". Center for American Progress. americanprogress.org/issues/2010/08/pdf/repealing_reform.pdf. August 2010. Accessed July 11, 2011.

26 "According to an Urban Institute computer simulation ..." Buettgens M, Dorn S, Carroll C. Consider savings as well as costs. Urban Institute. rwjf.org/files/research/72582qsonepage201107. pdf.July 2011. Accessed July 11, 2011; Dorn S, Buettgens M. Net effects of the Affordable Care Act on state budgets. Urban Institute. urban.org/UploadedPDF/1001480-Affordable-Care-Act.pdf. December 2010. Accessed July 6, 2011.

28 "Prior to the invasion of Iraq, Colin Powell ..." Woodward B. *Plan of Attack: The Definitive Account of the Decision to Invade Iraq.* New York: Simon & Schuster; 2004.

Chapter 3. Life Expectancy

Page 31 "Mathematician Benjamin Gompertz..." Gompertz B. On the nature of the function expressive of the law of human mortality. *Philos Trans R Soc Lond.* 1825.1:513-18.

31 "Life expectancy has been rising..." Christensen K, Doblhammer G, Rau R & Vaupel, JW. Ageing populations: The challenges ahead. *Lancet.* 2008;374:1196-1208.

31 "Life expectancy actually fell..." National Vital Statistics Reports. Vol. 59, No. 2. *Deaths: Preliminary Data for 2008.* Dec. 9, 2010.

32 "Of the 30-year increase..." Patel K, Rushefsky M. *The Politics of Public Health in the United States.* Armonk, NY: M.E. Sharpe; 2005.

32 "A 2002 *Health Affairs* journal article..." McGinnis JM, Williams-Russo, P, Knickman JR. The case for more active policy attention to health promotion. *Health Aff.* 2002; 21(2):78-93.

33 "Dr. David Heber..." Chilton FJ, Tucker L. Floyd Chilton, *The Gene Smart Diet: The Revolutionary Eating Plan that Will Rewrite Your Genetic Destiny—and Melt Away the Pounds.* New York, NY: Rodale; 2009.

34 "Patterns of death and disease have undergone several transitions..." Two excellent examinations of epidemiological transitions are: Gaziano JM. Fifth phase of the epidemiological transition: The age of obesity and inactivity. *JAMA.* 2010;303(3): 275-276, and Olshansky SJ, Ault AB. The fourth stage of the epidemiological transition: The age of delayed degenerative diseases. *The Milbank Quarterly* 1986; 64(1): 355-391.

34 "The probability of a 65-year-old..." Bell FC, Miller, ML. Life tables for the United States Social Security Area, 1900-2100. Baltimore, MD: Social Security Administration, Office of the Chief Actuary.

35 "In the early 1960s..." Flegal KM, Carroll MD, Kuczmarski RJ, Johnson CL. Overweight and obesity in the United States: prevalence and trends, 1960-1994. *Int J Obes.* 1998; 22(1):39-47.

35 "By 2008..." Flegal KM, Carroll MD, Ogden, CL, Curtin, LR. Prevalence and trends in obesity among US adults, 1999-2008. *JAMA.* 2010; 303(3):235-241.

35 "Obesity accounted for..." Finkelstein EA, Trogdon JG, Cohen JW, Dietz W. Annual medical spending attributable to obesity: payer- and service-specific estimates. *Health Aff.* 2009; 28(5):w822-w831.

35 "About 32 percent of school-age..." Ogden CL, Carroll MD, Curtin LR, Lamb MM, Flegal KM. Prevalence of high body mass index in US children and adolescents. 2007-2008. *JAMA.* 2010;303(3):242-249.

35 "Eighty percent of children..." Whitaker RC, Wright JA, Pepe MS, Seidel KD, Dietz WH. Predicting obesity in young adulthood from childhood and parental obesity. *N Engl J Med.* 1997;37(13):869–873.

35 "It has the potential..." Stewart ST, Cutler DM, Rose AB. Forecasting the effects of obesity and smoking on U.S. life expectancy. *N Engl J Med.* 2009;361(23):2252-2260.

35 "An estimated 25 percent of men..." Gaziano, op. cit.

36 "The four leading causes..." Goodarz D, Rimm EB, Oza S, Kulkarni SC, Murray CJ, Ezzati, M. The promise of prevention: The effects of four preventable risk factors on national life expectancy and life expectancy disparities by race and county in the United States. *PLoS Med.* 2010:7(3):e1000248.

36 "Ralph Keeney ..." Keeney RL. Personal decisions are the leading cause of death. *Oper Res.* 2008;56(6):1335-1347.

36 "Nearly one-quarter..." Nolte E, McKee CM. Measuring the health of nations: Updating an earlier analysis. *Health Aff.* 2008;27(1):58-71.

36 "In 1975, Americans who reached..." Michaud, P, Goldman D, Lakdawalla D, Gailey A, Zheng Y. International differences in longevity and health and their economic consequences. National Bureau of Economic Research. 2009;Working Paper No. 15235. nbe4r.org/papers/w15235. Accessed Dec. 23, 2010.

37 "A *Health Affairs* study ..." Muennig PA, Glied SA. What changes in survival rates tell us about U.S. health care. *Health Aff.* 2010;29(11):2105-2113.

38 "An often-cited 2003 study..." Lubitz J, Cai L, Kramarow E, Lentzner, H. Health, life expectancy, and health care spending among the elderly. *N Engl J Med.* 2003; 349(11):1048-55.

38 "The excess expense..." Sun W, Webb A, Zhivan, N. Center for Retirement Research at Boston College. Does staying healthy reduce your lifetime health care costs? May 2010; no. 10-8.

38 "According to the Employee Benefit Research Institute..." Fronstin P, Salisbury D, VanDerhei J. Employee Benefit Research Institute. Funding savings needed for health expenses for persons eligible for Medicare. December 2010;Issue Brief No. 351

38 "A 2008 Dutch study..." van Baal P, Polder JJ, de Wit GA, et al. Lifetime medical costs of obesity: Prevention to cure for increase health expenditure. *PLoS Medicine.* 2008;5(2):e29.

39 "The estimated medical cost..." Finkelstein EA, Trogdon JG, Cohen JW, Dietz, W. Annual medical spending attributable to obesity: Payer- and service-specific estimates. *Health Aff.* 2009;28(5):w822.

39 "The underweight..." Flega KM, Graubard BI, Williamson DF, Gail MH. Excess deaths associated with underweight, overweight, and obesity. *JAMA.* 2005;293(15):1861-1867.

39 "One study estimated..." Lakdawalla DN, Goldman DP, Shang B. The health and cost consequences of obesity among the future elderly. *Health Aff.* 2005;W5-R30.

39 "People over 50 ..." Neugarten BL, Havighurst RJ. *Extending the Human Life Span: Social Policy and Social Ethics.* Washington: National Science Foundation; 1977. Baltes MM. Environmental factors in dependency among nursing home residents: A social ecology analysis. In: Wills, TA, ed. *Basic Processes in Helping Relationships,* New York: Academic Press; 1982.

39 "It has been dubbed ..." Gruenberg EM. The failures of success. *Milbank Q.* 1977;55:3-24.

39 "It is also a failure. .." Fries, JF. Aging, natural death, and the compression of morbidity. *N Engl J Med.* 1980;303(3):130-135.

40 "For example, a 20-year-old today ..." Crimmins EM, Beltran-Sanchez, H. Mortality and morbidity trends: Is there compression of morbidity? *J Gerontol.* 2010

40 "Fries and his colleagues ..." Hubert HB, Bloch DA, Oehlert JW, Fries JF. Lifestyle habits and compression of morbidity. *J Gerontol.* 2002;57A(6):M347-M351.

40 "Plasticity of aging ..." Baltes, op. cit.

41 "Age-related decline ..." Fries, op. cit.

41 "Several studies show ..." Hubert, op. cit. Nusselder WJ, Looman CW, Mackenbach JP, et al. Smoking and compression of morbidity. *J Epidemiol Community Health.* 2000;54:566-74.

41 "The rate of disability ..." Fries, op. cit. and Molla MT, Madans JH. *Life expectancy free of chronic condition-induced activity limitations among white and black Americans, 2000–2006.* National Center for Health Statistics. Vital Health Stat. 2010;3(34).

41 "However, obesity may reverse ..." Sturm R, Ringel JS, Andreyeva T. Increasing obesity rates and disability trends. *Health Aff.* 2004;23(2):199-205.

41 "A 2009 study confidently ..." Christensen, op. cit.

41 "Another group of scientists ..." Oeppen J, Vaupel J. Broken limits to life expectancy. *Science.* 2002;296:1029-31.

41 "A more modest projection ..." Department of Economic and Social Affairs. World population to 2300. New York: United Nations, 2004.

41 "On the other hand ..." Olshansky SJ, Passaro DJ, Hershow RC et al. A potential decline in life expectancy in the United States in the 21st century. *N Engl J Med.* 2005;352(11):1138-1144.

41 "Researchers used a forecasting method ..." Reiter EN, Olshansky SJ, Yang Y. New forecasting methodology indicates more disease and earlier mortality ahead for today's younger Americans. *Health Aff.* 2011;30(8).

42 "If it is underestimated ..." Olshansky SJ, Goldman DJ, Zheng Y, Rowe JW. Aging in American in the twenty-first century: Demographic forecasts from the MacArthur Foundation Research Network on an aging society. *Milbank Q.* 2009;87(4):842-862.

42 "One trend is clear..." Kinsella K, He W. U.S. Census Bureau, International Population Reports, P95/09-1. An Aging World: 2008. Washington, D.C.: U.S. Government Printing Office.2009.

42 "Dr. Nortin Hadler..." Hadler, NM. *Worried Sick: A Prescription for Health in an Overtreated America.* Chapel Hill, NC: The University of North Carolina Press; 2008.

Chapter 4. Health Behavior

Page 43 "According to University of Pittsburgh researchers ..." Bambs C, Kip KE, Dinga A, Mulukutla SR, Aiyer AN, Reis SE. Low prevalence of "ideal cardiovascular health" in a community-based population. *Circulation.* 2011;123:850-857.

43 "But only 3 percent ..." Fine LJ, Philogene GS, Gramling R, Coups EJ, Sinha S. Prevalence of multiple chronic disease risk factors. 2001 National Health Interview Survey. *Am J Prev Med.*2004;27(2 Suppl):18-24.

43 "The opposite ..." Kvaavik E, Batty DG, Ursin G, Huxley R, Gale CR. Influence of individual and combined health behaviors on total and cause-specific mortality in men and women. *Arch Intern Med.*2009;170(8): 711-718.

43 "An English study found ..." Khaw KT, Wareham N, Bingham S, Welch A, Luben R, Day N. Combined impact of health behaviours and mortality in men and women: The EPIC-Norfolk Prospective Population Study. *PLoS Med.*2008;5(1):e12.

43 "In the United States ..." Woolf SH. The big answer: Rediscovering prevention at a time of crisis in health care. *Harv Health Policy Rev.* 2006;7:5-20.

43 "Nearly two-thirds ..." Thorpe KE. The rise in health care spending and what to do about it. *Health Aff.* 2005;24(6):1436-1445.

43 "It is the difference ..." Katz DL. Life and death, knowledge and power: Why knowing what matters is not what's the matter. *Arch Intern Med.*2009;169(15): 1362-1363.

43 "In a study of nearly ..." van Dam RM, Li T, Spiegelman D, Franco OH, Hu FB. Combined impact of lifestyle factors on mortality: Propsective cohort study in US women. *BMJ.*2008;337:a1440.

43 "Psychological factors also seem ..." Lachman ME, Agrigoroaei S. Promoting functional health in midlife and old age: Long-term protective effects of control beliefs, social support , and physical exercise. *PLoS One.*2010;5(10):e13297.

44 "As of mid-2009..." Koh HK. A 2020 vision for healthy people. *N Engl J Med.* 2010;368(18):1653-1656.

45 "One disturbing trend ..." King DE, Mainous AG, Carnemolla M, Everett CJ. Adherence to healthy lifestyle habits in US adults, 1988-2006. *Am J Med.* 2009;122(6):528-534.

46 "Those in this age group..." King DE, Mainous AG, Geesy ME. Turning back the clock: Adopting a healthy lifestyle in middle age. *Am J Med.* 2007;120:598-603.

46 "Despite large increases ..." Cutler DM, Glaeser EL, Rosen, AB. Is the US population behaving healthier? National Bureau of Economic Research: Cambridge, MA, April 2007. NBER Working Paper No. 13013.

46 "Doctors also do not think ..." Huang J, Yu H, Marin E, Brock S, Carden D, Davis T. Physicians' weight loss counseling in two public hospital primary care clinics. *Acad Med.* 2004;79(2):156-161.

46 "According to a survey ..." Foster GD, Wadden T, Makris, A et al. Primary care physicians' attitudes about obesity and its treatment. *Obes Res.* 2003;11(10):1168-1177.

46 "Physicians offer to help ..." Partnership for Prevention. Preventive care: A national profile on use, disparities and benefits. Washington, DC: Partnership for Prevention.; August 2007. rwjf.org/files/research/8-7-07%20-%20Partnership%20for%20Prevention%20Report%281%29.pdf. Accessed January 20, 2011.

46 "Barely 1 in 10 diabetics ..." Eliat-Adar S, Xu J, Zephier E, O'Leary V, Howard BV, Resnick, HE. Adherence to dietary recommendations for saturated fat, fiber, and sodium is low in American Indians and other US adults with diabetes. *J Nutr.* 2008;138(9):1699-1704.

46 "About 18 percent of heart disease ..." Soni, A. Personal health behaviors for heart disease prevention among the US adult civilian non-institutionalized population 2004. Rockville, MD: Agency for Healthcare Research and Quality; March 2007. MEPS statistical brief 165.

46 "Doctors advise only about one-third ..." Stafford RS, Farhat JH, Misra B, Shoenfeld DA. National patterns of physician activities related to obesity management. *Arch Fam Med.* 2000;9(7):156-161.

47 "In one study ..." Calfas KJ, Long BJ, Sallis JF, Wooten WJ, Pratt M, Patrick K. A controlled trial of physician counseling to promote the adoption of physical activity. *Prev Med.* 1996;25(3):225-233.

47 "The American Heart Association ..." Artinian NT, Fletcher GF, Mozaffarian D, et al. Interventions to promote physical activity and dietary lifestyle changes for cardiovascular risk factor reduction in adults. A scientific statement from the American Heart Association. *Circulation.* 2010;122:406-441.

47 "An extreme example is ..." Smokers refused operations. TVNZ. tvnz.co.nz/content/28552/425826.html. February 8, 2001. Accessed February 8, 2010.

47 "At least 40 percent of smokers ..." Ulene V. Why are unhealthy people so reluctant to change their lifestyles? *The Los Angeles Times.* May 23, 2011.

47 "In a group ..." Fadi TT, Krumholtz HM, Kosiborod M, et al. Predictdors of weight change in overweight patients with infarction. *Am Heart J.* 2007;154(4):711-717.

48 "In another study ..." Salisbury AC, Chan PS, Gosch KL, Buchanan DM, Spertus JA. Patterns and predictors of fast food consumption after acute myocardial infarction. *Am J Cardiol.* 2011;15:1105-1110.

48 "One out of 5 ..." Weaver KE, Rowland JH, Augustson E, Atienza AA. Smoking concordance in lung and colorectal cancer patient-caregiving dyads and quality of life. *Cancer Epidemiol Biomarkers Prevent.* 2011;20:239-248.

48 "A study of 9,000 cancer survivors ..." Blanchard CM, Courneya KS, Stein K. Cancer survivors' adherence to lifestyle behavior recommendations and associations with health-related quality of life: Results from the American Cancer Society's SCS-II. *J Clin Oncol.* 2008;26:2198-2204.

48 "However, their physicians ..." Sabatino SA, Coates RJ, Uhler RJ, Pollace LA, Alley LG, Zauderer LJ. Provider counseling about health behaviors among cancer survivors in the United States. *J Clin Oncol.* 2007;25:2100-2106.

48 "According to the Stanford ..." Bandura A. Self-efficacy: Toward a unifying theory of behavioral change. *Psychol Rev.* 1977;84:195-200.

48 "A World Health Organization report ..." World Health Organization. *Closing the gap in a generation: Health equity through action on the social determinants of health.* Geneva: WHO; 2008.

49 "A 2009 poll ..." GE Better Health 2010 study fact sheet: Patient-doctor disconnect on healthy living revealed. files.healthymagination.com/wp-content/uploads/2010/02/GE-Better-Health-Study-Fact-Sheet.pdf. Accessed January 21, 2011.

49 "The Vitality Group surveyed ..." The Vitality Group, 2008. My unhealthy lifestyle is your problem! findarticles.com/p/articles/mi_m0EIN/is_2008_July_23/ai_n27933814/. Accessed January 21, 2011.

50 "What cripples Americans' health ..." Weinstein ND. Unrealistic optimism about future life events. *J Pers Soc Psychol.*1980;39:306-320.

50 "A good example of optimism bias ..." College Board. Student descriptive questionnaire. Princeton, NJ: Educational Testing Service; 1976-1977.

50 "People with heart-attack symptoms ..." Johnson J, King K. Influence of expectations about symptoms on delay in seeking treatment during a myocardial infarction. *Am J Crit Care.* 1995;4:29-35.

51 "Likewise, a majority of patients ..." Meyer D, Leventhal H, Gutmann M. Common-sense models of illness: The example of hypertension. *Health Psychol.* 1985;4:115-135.

51 "Weinstein surveyed adults ..." Weinstein ND. Unrealistic optimism about susceptibility to health problems: Conclusions from a community-wide sample. *J Behav Med.* 1987;10(5):481-500; Weinstein ND 1980, op cit.

51 "Optimism bias is fairly immune ..." Helweg-Larsen M, Sheppard JA. Do moderators of the optimistic bias affect personal or target risk estimates? A review of the literature. *Personality and Social Psychology Review.* 2001;5(1):74-95.

51 "In international studies ..." Brownell KD. Personal responsibility and control over our bodies: When expectation exceeds reality. *Health Psychol.* 1991;10:303-310.

52 "The outlook reflects ..." Perloff LS, Fetzer BK. Self other judgments and perceived vulnerability to victimization. *J Pers Soc Psychol.* 1986; 50:502-510.

52 "A wealth of research shows ..." Harrison JA, Mullen PD, Green IW. A meta-analysis of studies of the health belief model with adults. *Health Education Review.* 1992;7:107-116.

52 "Indeed, a national survey ..." Niederdeppe J, Levy AG. Fatalistic beliefs about cancer prevention and three prevention behaviors. *Cancer Epidemiol Biomarkers Prevent.* 2007;16(5):998-1003.

Chapter 5. Nutrition

Page 53 "Animals, too, will pick food ..." Tordoff MG. Obesity by choice: The powerful influence of nutrient availability on nutrient intake. *Am J Physiol Integr Comp Physiol.* 2002;282(5):R1536-9.

53 "David Kessler, the former commissioner ..." Kessler D. *The End of Overeating: Taking Control of the Insatiable American Appetite.* New York: Rodale Books; 2009.

54 "Between 1990 and 2007 ..." Christian T, Rashad I. Trends in U.S. food prices, 1950-2007. *Econ and Human Biol.* 2009;7:113-20.

54 "One study claims ..." Powell, LM. Fast food costs and adolescent body mass index: Evidence from panel data. *J Health Econ.* 2009;28(5):963-970.

54 "In contrast, the cost ..." Auld MC, Powell LM. Economics of food energy density and adolescent body weight. *Economica.* 2009;76:719-740.

54 "The average American's daily calorie consumption ..." U.S. Department of Agriculture. Agriculture Fact Book 2001-2002. March 2003.

54 "The number of servings ..." Young L, Nestle M. The contribution of expanding portion sizes to the U.S. obesity epidemic. *Am J Public Health.* 2002;92:246-249; Bloom J. *American Wasteland: How America Throws Away Nearly Half of Its Food.* Philadelphia PA: Da Capo Press; 2010.

54 "Almost 90 percent ..." International Food Information Council. 2009 Food & Health Survey: Consumer attitudes toward food, nutrition and health. ific.org.

56 "Do not necessarily count ..." Adams KM, Kohlmeier M, Zeisel SH. Nutrition education in U.S. medical schools: Latest update of a national survey. *Acad Med.* 2010;85:1537-1542.

56 "The typical Western diet ..." Iqbal R, Anand S, Ounpuu S et al. Dietary patterns and the risk of acute myocardial infarction in 52 countries. *Circulation.* 2008;118:1929-1937.

56 "Diets rich in lean meat ..." Larson TM, Dalskov SM, van Baak M et al. Diets with high or low protein content and glycemic index for weight-loss maintenance. *N Engl J Med.* 2010;363(22):2102-13.

56 "An analysis of 21 studies ..." Sieri S, Krogh V, Berrino F. Dietary glycemic load and index and risk of coronary heart disease in a large Italian cohort: the EPICOR study. *Arch Inter Med.* 2010;170(7):640-7.

57 "Another study compared ..." Foster GD, Wyatt HR, Hill JO et al. Weight and metabolic outcomes after 2 years on a low-carbohydrate versus low-fat diet: A randomized trial. *Ann Intern Med.* 2010;153:147-157.

57 "A 2009 study was ..." Sacks FM, Bray GA, Carey VJ et al. Comparison of weight-loss diets with different compositions of fat, protein, and carbohydrates. *N Engl J Med.* 2009;360:859-873.

58 "According to a 2008 study ..." Miller TM, Abdel-Maksoud MF, Crane LA, Marcus AC, Byers TE. Effects of social approval bias on self-reported fruit and vegetable consumption: A randomized controlled trial. *Nutrition Journal.* 2008;7:118.

58 "A survey by Foodminds ..." Americans want Uncle Sam's help putting healthy foods on their dinner table. Foodminds. foodminds.com/index.php/news/food-temperance-survey-2010/. March 8, 2010. Accessed January 21, 2011.

59 "A GlaxoSmithKline Consumer Healthcare ..." Eight in 10 Americans say they're in control of their eating habits – but growing obesity crisis tells another story. GlaxoSmithKline Consumer Healthcare. us.gsk.com/html/media-news/pressreleases/2010/2010_us_pressrelease_10004.htm. January 13, 2010. Accessed January 21, 2011.

59 "Nearly 90 percent of Americans ..." Are we fooling ourselves? 90 percent of Americans say their diet is healthy, CR poll finds. Consumer Reports website. consumerreports.org/health/healthy-living/diet-nutrition/diets-dieting/healthy-diet/overview/index.htm January 2011. Accessed March 3, 2011.

60 "A September 2010 Harris Poll …" Large numbers of people claim to be changing their diets in ways that would improve their health. Harris Poll website. harrisinteractive.com/NewsRoom/HarrisPolls/tabid/447/ctl/ReadCustom%20Default/mid/1508/ArticleId/614/Default.aspx. November 9, 2010. Accessed February 11, 2011.

61 "Experts say the diet …" Konstantinidou V, Covas MI, Munoz-Aguayo D. In vivo nutrigenomic effects of virgin oil polyphenols within the frame of the Mediterranean diet: A randomized controlled trial. *The FASEB Journal.* 2010;24:2456-2557.

61 "The U.S. produces …" Putnam J, Allshouse J, Kanton LS. U.S. per capita food supply trends: More calories, refined carbohydrates, and fats. *Food Review.* Winter 2002(3). ers.usda.gov/publications/FoodReview/DEC2002/frvol25i3a.pdf. Accessed January 4, 2011.

61 "Yet 15 percent of the nation's households …" Robert Wood Johnson Foundation. Food Insecurity and Risk for Obesity Among Children and Families: Is There a Relationship? Princeton, NJ: April 2010.

61 "According to Jonathan Bloom …"Bloom J op cit.

61 "Tainted produce is …" Koro M, Anandan S, Quinlan JJ. Microbial quality of food available to populations of differing socioeconomic status. *Am J Prev Med.* 2010;38(5):478-481.

61 "About 85 percent of food-insecure …" Nord M. U.S. Department of Agriculture. Food insecurity in households with children. Washington, DC: EIB-56, U.S. Department of Agriculture, *Econ. Res. Serv;* 2009.

62 "People with more income …" Monsivais P, Drewnowski. Lower-energy-density diets are associated with higher monetary costs per kilocalorie and are consumed by women of higher socioeconomic status. *J Am Diet Assoc.* 2009;109(5):814-822.

62 "Another trick: …" Thomas M, Desai KK, Seenivasan S. How credit card payments increase unhealthy food purchases: Visceral regulation of vices. *Journal of Consumer Research.* 2010;38(5).

62 "People consume an average …" Bassett MT et al. Purchasing behavior and calorie information at fast-food chains in New York City, 2007. *Am J Prev Med.* 2008;98:1457-9.

62 "Super-sized portions …" Hurley J, Liebman B. Still supersized. Center for Science in the Public Interest. Nutrition Action Health Newsletter. September 2010. cspinet.org/nah/articles/supersized.html. Accessed Dec. 30, 2010.

62 "Beth Mansfield …" Bernstein S. "Eat less," U.S. says as fast-food chains super-size their offerings. *The Los Angeles Times.* February 2, 2011.

62 "A typical restaurant meal …" Hellmich N. Survey: Restaurants dishing out extra-large portions. USA Today. Oct 21, 2006. usatoday.com/news/health/2006-10-21-portions-restaurants_x.htm. Accessed January 5, 2010.

62 "Full-service and fast food meals …" Binkley J. Calorie and gram differences between meals at fast food and table service restaurants. *Review of Agricultural Economics.* 2008;30(4).

64 "People who live …" Mehta N, Chang V. Weight status and restaurant availability: A multilevel analysis. *Am J Prev Med .* 2008;34(2):127-133.

64 "Fast-food restaurants are up …" Powell L, Chaloupka F, Bao Y. The availability of fast-food and full-service restaurants in the United States: Associations with neighborhood characteristics. *Am J Prev Med.* 2007;33(4):S240-S245.

64 "Researchers found that adults …"Inagami S, Cohen D, Brown A, Asch S. Body mass index, neighborhood fast food and restaurant concentration, and car ownership. *J Urban Health.* 2009;86(5).

64 "The most frequently cited …" Rydell S, Harnack L, Oakes J, Story M, Jeffery R, French S. Why eat a fast-food restaurants: Reported reasons among frequent consumers. *J Am Diet Assoc.* 2008;108(12):2066-2070.

64 "More than half …" Boutelle K, Fulkerson J, Neumark-Sztainer D, Story M, French S. Fast food for family meals: Relationships with parent and adolescent food intake, home food availability and weight status. *Public Health Nutr.* 2007;10:16-23.

64 "An alarmed group ..." Ferenczi EA, Asaria P, Hughes AD, Chaturvedi N, Francis DP. Can a statin neutralize the cardiovascular risk of unhealthy dietary choices? *Am J Cardiol.* 2010;106(4):587.

65 "For example, a review of food sales..." Elbel B, Kersh R, Brescoll V, Dixon L. Calorie labeling and food choices: A first look at the effects of low-income people in New York City. *Health Aff.* 2009;28(6):w1110-1121.

65 "However, a separate New York City ..." Dumanovsky T, Huang CY, Nonas CA, Matte TD, Bassett MT, Silver LD. Changes in energy content of lunchtime purchases from fast food restaurants from introduction of calorie labelling: Cross sectional customer surveys. *BMJ.* 2011;343:d4464.

65 "About 200 diners ..." Burton S, Creyer EH, Kees J, Huggins K. Attacking the obesity epidemic: The potential health benefits of providing nutrition information in restaurants. *Am J Public Health.* 2006;96(9):1669-75.

65 "Researchers found that McDonald's ..." Chandon P, Wansik B. The biasing health halos of fast-food restaurant health claims: Lower calorie estimates and higher side-dish consumption intentions. *Journal of Consumer Research.* 2007;34(3).

66 "Jane Hurley ..." Bernstein, op. cit.

66 "The restaurant-labeling effort ..." Urban LE, Dallal GE, Robinson LM, Ausman LM, Saltzman E, Roberts SB. The accuracy of state energy contents of reduced-energy commercially prepared foods. *J Am Diet Assoc.* 2010;110(1):116-123.

66 "Less than one in 10 Americans ..." Kimmons J, Gillespie C, Seymour J, Serdula M, Blanck HM. Fruit and vegetable consumption intake among adolescents and adults in the United States: Percentage meeting individualized recommendations. *Medscape J Med.* 2009;11(1):26.

66 "The government and advocacy groups ..." U.S. Department of Agriculture. *Dietary assessment of major trends in U.S. food consumption.* Economic Research Service Report Summary, March, 2008.; U.S. Department of Agriculture, 2003 op. cit.

67 "The National Fruit and Vegetable Alliance ..." National Fruit & Vegetable Alliance. National action plan to promote health through increased fruit and vegetable consumption: 2010 report card. 2010.

67 "Orange juice is the top source ..." Kimmons J, op cit.

68 "A study of North Carolina young adults ..." Duffey KJ, Gordon-Larsen P, Shkany JM, Guilkey D, Jacobs Jr DR, Popkin BM. Food price and diet and health outcomes: 20 years of the CARDIA study. *Arch Intern Med.*2010;170(5):420-426.

68 "A U.S. Department of Agriculture analysis ..." Smith TA, Biing-Hwan L, Lee J. Taxing caloric sweetened beverages: Potential effects on beverage consumption, calorie intake, and obesity. ERR-100, U.S. Department of Agriculture, Economic Research Service, July 2010.

68 "Scientists tested the effectiveness ..." Epstein LH, Dearing KK, Roba LG, Finkelstein, E. The influence of taxes and subsidies on energy purchased in an experimental purchasing study. *Psychol Sci.* 2010;21(3):406-14.

Chapter 6. Physical Activity

Page 69 "Trips from home by automobile ..." Pucher J, Renne JL. Socioeconomics of urban travel: Evidence from 2001 NHTS. *Transportation Q.* 2003;57:49-77.

69 "Self-reported physical activity ..." U.S. Department of Health and Human Services. *Physical activity and health: A report of the Surgeon General.* Atlanta, GA: U.S. Department of Health and Human Services, Centers for Disease Control and Prevention, National Center for Chronic Disease Prevention and Health Promotion, 1996.

70 "A review of more than 40 studies ..." Alford L. What men should know about the impact of physical activity on their health. *Int J Clin Pract.* 2010;64(13):1731-1734.

70 "Eyes rolled ..." Lee I, Kjousse L, Sesso HD, Wang L, Buring JE. Physical activity and weight gain prevention. *JAMA* 2010;303(12):1173-1179.

70 "The study essentially reaffirmed ..."Institute of Medicine. *Dietary reference intakes for energy, carbohydrate, fiber, fat, fatty acids, cholesterol, protein, and amino acids.* Washington: National Academies Press; 2002.

70 "According to one ..." Farzaneh-Far R, Lin J, Epel E, Lapham K, Blackburn E, Whooley MA. Telomere length trajectory and its determinants in persons with coronary artery disease: Longitudinal findings from the heart and soul study. *PLoS One.* 2010; 5(1): e8612.

72 "The federal government released ..." U.S. Department of Health and Human Services. *2008 Physical activity guidelines for Americans.* Washington, DC: U.S. Department of Health and Human Services; 2008.

72 "In 2008 ..." Carlson SA, Fulton JE, Shoenborn CA, Loustalot F. Trend and prevalence based on the 2008 Physical Activity Guidelines for Americans. *Am J Prev Med.* 2010;39(4):305-313.

72 "Only about 5 percent ..." Tudor-Locke C, Johnson WD, Katzmarzyk PT. Frequently reported activities by intensity for U.S. adults. *Am J Prev Med.* 2010;39(4):e13-e20.

73 "However, even self-reported physical activity ..." Brownson RC, Boehmer TK, Luke DA. Declining rates of physical activity in the United States: What are the contributors? *Ann Rev Public Health.* 2005;26:421-443.

73 "The average U.S. adult ..." Bassett DR Jr., Wyatt HR, Thompson H, Peters JC, Hill JO. Pedometer-measured physical activity and health behaviors in U.S. adults. *Med Sci Sports Exerc.* 2010;42(10):1819-1825.

73 "Exercise may be the most popular..." Mendes E. Americans exercise less in 2009 than 2008. The Gallup Poll. gallup.com/poll/125102/americans-exercise-less-2009-2008.aspx. Accessed January 11, 2011.

73 "In fact, the most educated ..." Mullahy J, Robert SA. No time to lose? Time constraints and physical activity. NBER Working Paper No. 14513. November 2008.

73 "Dr. James Levine ..." Levine JA. *Move a Little, Lose a Lot: How N.E.A.T. Science Reveals How to Be Thinner, Happier, and Smarter.* New York: Crown Archetype; 2009.

74 "There is a direct correlation ..." Conroy D, Hyde A, Doerksen S, Ribeiro N. Implicit attitudes and explicit motivation prospectively predict physical activity. *Ann Behav Med.* 2010;39(2):112-118.

74 "Americans spend an average ..." Owen N, Bauman A, Brown W. Too much sitting: A novel and important predictor of chronic disease risk? *Br J Sports Med.* 2009;43(2):81-83.

74 "Men who spend more ..." Warren TY, Barry V, Hooker SP, Sui X, Church TS, Blair SN. Sedentary behaviors increase risk of cardiovascular disease mortality in men. *Med Sci Sports Exerc.* 2010;42(5):879-85.

74 "An Australian study ..." Dunstan DW, Barr ELM, Healy GN, et al. Television viewing time and mortality. *Circulation.* 2010;121:384-391.

75 "In one study..." Troiano RP, Berrigan D, Dodd KW, Masse LC, Tilert T, McDowell M. Physical activity in the United States measured by accelerometer. *Med Sci Sports Exerc.* 2008; 40(1):181-188.

75 "Only one-third of Americans ..." Bennett GG, Wolin KY, Puleo EM, Masse LC, Atienza AA. Awareness of national physical activity recommendations for health promotion among US adults. *Med Sci Sports Exerc.* 2009;41(10):1849-1855.

76 "About half of adults are dissatisfied ..." Garner DM. The 1997 body image survey results. *Psychology Today.* 1997;30:30-41.

76 "But, research shows exercising ..." Campbell A, Hausenblas HA. Effects of exercise interventions on body image. *Journal of Health Psychology.* 2009;14(6):780-793.

76 "Its index reflects ..." Mendes E. In U.S., nearly half exercise less than three days a week. The Gallup Poll. gallup.com/poll/118570/nearly-half-exercise-less-three-days-week.aspx. Accessed January 13, 2011.

76 "Duke University researchers ..." Blumenthal JA, Babyak MA, Doraiswamy PM et al. Exercise and pharmacotherapy in the treatment of major depressive disorder. *Psychosom Med.* 2007;69:587-596.

76 "People who walked ..." Nieman D. Exercise and immune function: Nutritional influences. ker.com/library/advances/320.pdf. Accessed January 13, 2011.

77 "People who take at least 5,000 steps ..." Sisson SB, Camhi SM, Church TS, Tudor-Locke C, Johnson WD, Katzmarzyk PT. Accelerometer-determined steps/day and metabolic syndrome. *Am J Prev Med.* 2010;38(6):682-3.

77 "Williams calculated that people ..." Williams PT. A cohort study of incident hypertension in relation to changes in vigorous physical activity in men and women. *J Hypertens.* 2008; 26(6):1085-1093.

77 "Weight training-related injuries ..." Kerr, ZY, Collins CL, Comstock RD. Epidemiology of weight training-related injuries presenting to United States emergency rooms, 1990 to 2007. *Am J Sports Med.* 2010;38(4):765-771.

78 "According to a 2000 study, ..." Muraven M, Baumeister RF. Self-regulation and depletion of limited resources: Does self-control resemble a muscle? *Psychol Bull.* 2000;126(2):247-259.

78 "Another dubious claim ..." Wang Z, Heshka S, Zhang K, Boozer CN, Heymsfield SB. Resting energy expenditure: Systematic organization and critique of prediction methods. *Obes Res.* 2001;9(5): 331.

78 "What exercise can do ..." NWCR Facts. nwcr.ws/Research/default.htm. Accessed February 1, 2011.

78 "British researchers examined ..." Shengxu L, Zhao JH, Luan J, et al. Physical activity attenuates the genetic predisposition to obesity in 20,000 men and women from EPIC-Norfolk prospective population study. *PLoS Medicine.* 2010;7(8):e1000332.

Chapter 7. Weight Control

Page 79 "Ten years ago ..." Sherry B, Blanck HM, Galuska DA, Dietz WH, Balluz L.Vital signs: State-specific obesity prevalence among adults—United States, 2009. *MMWR.* 2010;59(30):951-955.

79 "Obesity is the fastest-growing ..." Thorpe KE. The future of obesity: National and state estimates of the impact of obesity on direct health care expenses. fightchronicdisease.org/sites/default/files/docs/CostofObesityReport-FINAL.pdf. November 2009. Accessed July 31, 2011.

80 "The U.S. is the fattest ..." Organization for Economic Cooperation and Development. *Obesity and the economics of prevention: Fit, not fat.* OECD: Paris; 2010.

80 "America is adjusting ..." Nolin R. Overweight is the new normal. *The Sun Sentinel.* June 12, 2011.

80 "The statistics clearly indicate ..."Lee JM, Pilli S, Gebremariam A. Getting heavier, younger: Trajectories of obesity over the life course. *Int J Obes.* 2010;34(4):614-623.

80 "Men are more likely ..." Flegal KM, Carroll MD, Ogden CL. Prevalence and trends in obesity among US adults, 1999-2008. *JAMA.* 2010;303(3):235-241.

81 "The 'personal responsibility' argument ..." Brownell KD, Kersh R, Ludwig DS, et al. Personal responsibility and obesity: A contstructive approach to a controversial issue. *Health Aff.* 2010;29(3):379-387.

82 "American public opinion ..." Center for Consumer Freedom (home page). Washington DC: Center for Consumer Freedom. consumerfreedom.com. Accessed February 2, 2011.

82 "Many believe obese ..." Puhl RM, Heuer CA. Obesity stigma: Important considerations for public health. *Am J Public Health.* 2010;100(6):1019-1028.

82 "There is a misguided belief ..." Puhl RM, Brownell KD. Confronting and coping with weight stigma: An investigation of overweight and obese adults. *Obesity.* 2006;(14)10:1802-1815.

82 "Examples of weight bias do not get..." Pomeranz JL. A historical analysis of public health, the law, and stigmatized social groups: The need for both obesity and weight bias legislation. *Obesity.* 2008;16:S93-S102.

82 "Remarkably, discrimination against excess weight ..." Puhl R, Brownell KD. Bias, discrimination, and obesity. Obes Res. 2001;9(12):788-805; Puhl R, Brownell KD. Weight bias: A review and update. *Obesity.* 2009;17(5):941-964.

82 "A Fort Lauderdale (FL) Sun-Sentinel ..." Lamendola B. Some ob-gyns in South Florida turn away overweight women. *The Sun Sentinel.* May 17, 2011.

83 "Emory University professor ..." Thorpe KE. The future costs of obesity: National and state estimates of the impact of obesity on direct health care expenses. nccor.org/downloads/CostofObesityReport-FINAL.pdf. November 2009. Accessed August 2, 2011.

84 "More than two-thirds..." Puhl *Obesity,* op. cit.

84 "Many overweight people ..." Saguy AC, Riley KW. Weighing both sides: Morality, mortality, and framing contests over obesity. *J Health Polit Policy Law.* 2005;30(5):869-923.

84 "One of the reasons ..." Silk AW, McTigue KM. Reexamining the physical examination for obese patients. *JAMA.* 2011;305(2):193-194.

84 "People yearn to be thin ..." The Harris Poll. Would Americans rather be younger, thinner, richer or smarter? August 26, 2010. harrisinteractive.com/NewsRoom/HarrisPolls/tabid/447/mid/1508/articleId/555/ctl/ReadCustom%20Default/Default.aspx. Accessed January 25, 2011.

85 "A survey by the Rudd Center ..." Puhl RM, Heuer CA. Public opinion about laws to prohibit weight discrimination in the United States. *Obesity.* 2011;19(1):74-82.

85 "One theory is that ..." Kolata G. *Rethinking Thin: The New Science of Weight Loss—and the Myths and Realities of Dieting.* New York: Picador; 2007.

85 "If one parent is obese ..." Obesity in children and teens. American Academy of Child & Adolescent Psychiatry website. aacap.org/cs/root/facts_for_families/obesity_in_children_and_teensUpdated May 2008. Accessed February 4, 2011.

86 "An August 2010 Harris Interactive ..." Overweight? Obese? Or normal weight? Americans have hard time gauging their weight. Harris Interactive website. harrisinteractive.com/NewsRoom/HarrisPolls/tabid/447/mid/1508/articleId/558/ctl/ReadCustom%20Default/Default.aspx. September 2, 2010. Accessed February 11, 2011.

86 "A group of Dallas researchers ..." Powell TM, de Lemos JA, Banks K. Body size misperception: A novel determinant in the obesity epidemic. *Arch Intern Med.* 2010;170(18): 1695-1696

87 "The 'health belief model' ..." Behavior change: A summary of four major theories. Family Health International website. fhi.org/nr/rdonlyres/ei26vbslpsidmahhxc332vwo3g233xsqw22er3vofqvrfjvubwyzclvqjcbdgexyzl3msu4mn6xv5j/bccsummaryfourmajortheories.pdf. November 2004. Accessed February 11, 2011.

87 "Overweight men are more likely ..." Gregory CO, Blanck HM, Gillespie C, Maynard LM, Serdula, MK. Perceived health risk of excess body weight among overweight and obese men and women: Differences by sex. *Prev Med.* 2008;47(1): 46-52.

88 "In a study of more than 300 black women ..." Moore SE, Harris C, Wimberly Y. Perception of weight and threat to health. *J Natl Med Assoc.* 2010;102:119-124.

88 "According to a Dutch study ..." Luttikhuis HG, Stolk RP, Sauer PJ. How do parents of 4- to 5-year-old children perceive the weight of their children? *Acta Paediatr.* 2010;99(2):263-267.

89 "For example, the Pima Indians ..." Obesity and Diabetes. National Institutes of Health website. diabetes.niddk.nih.gov/dm/pubs/pima/obesity/obesity.htm. Accessed February 4, 2011.

89 "An Australian researcher declared ..." Swinburn B. Increased energy intake along virtually explains all the increase in body weight in the United States from the 1970s to the 2000s. 2009 European Congress on Obesity; May 6-9, 2009; Amsterdam, the Netherlands. Abstract T1:RS3.3.

89 "A Canadian researcher, however, blamed ..." Juneau C, Potvin L. Trends in leisure-, transport-, and work-related physical activity in Canada 1994-2005. *Prev Med.* 2010;51(5): 384-386.

89 "In 1960, about 50 percent ..." Church TS, Thomas DM, Tudor-Locke C, et al. Trends over 5 decades in U.S. occupation-related physical activity and their associations with obesity. *PLoS One.* 2011;6(5):e19657.

89 "Nearly 80 percent ..." Must A, Spandano J, Coakley EH, Field AE, Colditz G, Dietz WH. The disease burden associated with overweight and obesity. *JAMA.* 1999;282:1523-1529.

90 "Some researchers have concluded ..." Jia H, Lubetkin EI. Trends in quality-adjusted life-years lost contributed by smoking and obesity. Am J Prev Med. 2010;38(2):138-144; Jia H, Lubetkin EI. Obesity-related quality-adjusted life years lost in the U.S. from 1993 to 2008. *Am J Prev Med.* 2010;39(3):220-227.

90 "Others say that ..." Stewart ST, Cutler DM, Rosen AB. Forecasting the effects of obesity and smoking on US life expectancy. *N Engl J Med.*2009;361:2252-2260.

90 "North Carolina economists analyzed ..." Finkelstein EA, Brown DS, Wrage LA, Allaire BT, Hoerger TJ. Individual and aggregate years-of-life-lost associated with overweight and obesity. *Obesity.* 2010;18(2):333-339.

90 "Another study involving ..." deGonzalez A, Hartge P, Cerhan JR, et al. Body-mass index and mortality among 1.46 million white adults. *N Engl J Med.*2010;363:2211-2219.

90 "But once a heart ailment is acquired ..." Lavie CJ, Milani RV, Ventura HO. Obesity and cardiovascular disease: Risk factor, paradox, and impactc of weight loss. *J Am Coll Cardiol.* 2009;53:1925-1932.

91 "One in 3 obese people ..." Wildman RP, Muntner P, Reynolds K, et al. The obese without cardiometabolic risk factor clustering and the normal weight with cardiometabolic risk factor clustering. *Arch Intern Med.* 2008;168(15):1617-1624.

91 "A study that tracked ..." Sui S, LaMonte MJ, Laditka JN. Cardiorespiratory fitness and adiposity as mortality predictors in older adults. *JAMA.*2007;298(21):2507-2516.

91 "Only about one in 6 ..."Kraschnewski JL, Boan J, Esposito J, et al. Long-term weight loss maintenance in the United States. *Intl J Obes.* 2010;34:1644-1654.

91 "A review of 31 long-term ..." Mann T, Tomiyama AJ, Westling E, Lew A, Samuels B, Chatman J. Medicare's search for effective obesity treatments: Diets are not the answer. *Am Psychol.* 2007;62(3):220-223.

91 "The scientific community believes diets ..." Puhl RM, *Am J Public Health,* op. cit.

92 "Bacon tracked 78 obese women ..." Bacon L, Stern JS, Van Loan MD, Keim, NL. Size acceptance and intuitive eating improve health for obese, female chronic dieters. *J Am Diet Assoc.* 2005;105(6):929-936.

Chapter 8. Tobacco and Alcohol

Page 93 "If the trend continues ..." Schroeder S, Warner KE. Don't forget tobacco. *N Eng J Med.* 20101;363(3):201-204.

93 "Nevertheless, the rate essentially ..." Dube SR, McClave A, James C, Caraballo R, Kaufmann R. Vital signs: Current cigarette smoking among adults aged 18 or over—United States, 2009. *MMWR.* 2010;59(35):1135-1140.

93 "The U.S. government ..." Dube SR, Asman K, Malarcher A, Carabollo R. Cigarette smoking among adults and trends in smoking cessation—United States, 2008. *MMWR.* 2010;58(44):1227-1232.

93 "The percentage of people ..." Pierce JP, Messer K, White MM, Cowling DW, Thomas DP. Prevalence of heavy smoking in California and the United States, 1965-2007. *JAMA.* 2001; 305(11):1106-1112.

94 "University of Wisconsin researchers boldly ..." Fiore MC, Baker TB. Stealing a march in the 21st century: Accelerating progress in the 100-year war against tobacco addiction in the United States. *Am J Public Health*. 2009;99(7):1170-1175.

94 "On the other hand ..." Selected facts and figures from The Tobacco Atlas, third edition. World Lung Foundation and American Cancer Society website. tobaccoatlas.org/downloads/TA3-ChineseFactSheet.pdf. Accessed January 26, 2011.

94 "Nearly 3 out of 4 ..." Leistikow BN, Kabir Z, Connolly GN, Clancy L, Alpert HR. Male tobacco smoke load and non-lung cancer mortality associations in Massachusetts. *BMC Cancer*. 2008;8:341.

94 "Half of all smokers ..."Peto R, Lopez AD, Borcham J, Health TM. *Mortality from smoking in developed counties 1950-2000: Indirect estimation from national vital statistics.* Oxford: Oxford University Press; 1994.

95 "About half of the 50 states ..." Tynan M, Babb S, MacNeil A, Griffin M. State smoke-free laws for worksites, restaurants, and bars – United States, 2000-2010. *MMWR*. 2011;60(15): 472-475.

95 " Dr. Tim McAfee ..." Cammeron B. A smoke-free nation? CDC predicts nationwide ban by 2020. *The New York Daily News*. April 22, 2011.

96 "A 2009 Gallup poll ..." Jones JM. Majority disapproves of new law regulating tobacco. Gallup website. gallup.com/poll/121079/majority-disapproves-of-new-law-regulating-tobacco.aspx. June 22. 2009. Accessed January 26, 2011.

97 "The surgeon general's office ..." Office of the Surgeon General . *How tobacco smoke causes disease: The biology and behavioral basis for smoking-attributable disease.* Rockville, MD: U.S Department of Health and Human Services; 2010.

97 "Cigarettes alter a smoker's DNA ..." Zhong Y, Carmelia SG, Upadhyaya P, et al. Immediate consequences of cigarette smoking: Rapid formation of polycyclic aromatic hydrocarbon diol epoxides. *Chem Res Toxicol*. 2011;24(2):246-252.

97 "Smokers' arteries stiffen ..." Tomiyama H, Hashimoto H, Tanaka H, et al. Continuous smoking and progression of arterial stiffening. *J Am Coll Cardiol*. 2010;55:1979-1987.

97 "A 55-year-old smoker ..." Woloshin S, Schwartz LM, Welch HG. The risk of death by age, sex, and smoking status in the United States: Putting health risks in context. J *Natl Cancer Inst*. 2008;100:845-853.

97 "The number of cigarettes ..." Strandberg AY; Strandberg TE, Pitkala K, Salomaa VV, Tilvis RS, Miettinen TA. The effect of smoking in midlife on health-related quality of life in old age: A 26-year prospective study. *Arch Inter Med*. 2008;168(18):1968-1974.

97 "Pipe and cigars ..." Rodriguez J, Jiang R, Johnson WC, MacKenzie BA, Smith LJ, Barr RG. The association of pipe and cigar use with cotinine levels, lung function, and airflow obstruction: A cross-sectional study. *Ann Intern Med*. 2010;152:201-210.

97 "For every $1 spent ..." Rumberger JS, Hollenbeak CS, Kline D. Potential costs and benefits of smoking cessation: An overview of the approach to state-specific analysis. American Lung Association website. lungusa.org/stop-smoking/tobacco-control-advocacy/reports-resources/cessation-economic-benefits/reports/SmokingCessationTheEconomicBenefits.pdf. April 30, 2010. Accessed January 26, 2011.

97 "According to a Vanderbilt economist ..." Viscusi K. How to value a life. *PLoS Med*. 2008;5(2):e29.

97 "A 2008 Dutch study ..."van Baal PHM, Polder JJ, de Wit GA, et al. Lifetime medical costs of obesity: Prevention no cure for increasing health expenditure. *PLoS Med*. 2008;5(2):e29.

98 "Four proven strategies ..." Schroeder S., op. cit.

98 "Tobacco has long been ..." Ali MK, Koplan JP. Promoting health through tobacco taxation. *JAMA*. 2010;303(4):357-358.

98 "For example, more than 40 percent ..." Ong MK, Zhou Q, Sung H. Sensitivity to cigarette prices among individuals with alcohol, drug, or mental disorders. *Am J Public Health.* 2010;100: 1243-1245.

100 "Cigarette tax increases would be ..." Tobacco taxes: A win-win for cash-strapped states. Campaign for Tobacco-Free Kids website. tobaccofreekids.org/reports/state_tax_report/ downloads/Tax_Report_Complete.pdf. February 10, 2010. Accessed January 26, 2011.

100 "In 2009, tobacco companies spent ..." Ribisl KM, Patrick R, Eidson S, Tynan M, Francis J. State cigarette minimum price laws—United States, 2009. *MMWR.* 2010;59(13):389-392.

100 "Nearly two-thirds of Americans..." Schroeder S., op. cit.

100 "At one time..." Babb S, Tynan M, MacNeil A. State Pre-emption of local smoke-free laws in government work sites, private work sites, and restaurants—United States, 2005-2009. *MMWR.* 2010;59(4):105-108.

100 "Fatal heart attacks ..." Dove MS, Dockery DW, Mittleman MA, et al. The impact of Massachusetts' smoke-free workplace laws on acute myocardial infarction deaths. *Am J Public Health.* 2010;100(11):2206-2212.

100 "Studies in other states ..." Callinan J, et al. Legislative smoking bans for reducing secondhand smoke exposure, smoking prevalence and tobacco consumption. *Cochrane Database of Syst Rev.* 2010; issue 6.

100 "However, research has consistently ..." Engelen M, Farrelly M. The health and economic impact of New York's Clean Indoor Air Act. Albany: New York State Department of Health; July 2006; Klein E, Forster JL, Erickson DJ, Lytle LA, Schillo B. Economic effects of clean indoor air policies on bars and restaurant employment in Minneapolis and St. Paul, Minnesota. *J Public Health Manag Pract.* 2010;16:285-293.

101 "An Oklahoma study found ..." Tobacco smoke pollution in Oklahoma workplaces. Oklahoma Tobacco Research Center. University of Oklahoma Health Sciences Center website. February 2010. ouhsc.edu/otrc/research/documents/PreliminaryIAQreport.pdf. Accessed January 26, 2011.

101 "Second-hand smoke annually ..." Oberg M, Jaakkola, Woodward A, Peruga A, Pruss-Ustun A. Worldwide burden of disease from exposure to second-hand smoke: A retrospective analysis of data from 192 countries. *The Lancet.* November 26, 2010. who.int/quantifying_ehimpacts/publications/smoking.pdf. Accessed January 26, 2011.

101 "Smokers are at additional risk ..." Piccardo MT, Stella A, Valerio F. Is the smokers exposure to environmental tobacco smoke negligible? *Environmental Health.* 2010;9(5).

101 "The residue from ..." Winickoff JP, Friebely J, Tanski SE, et al. Beliefs about the health effects of "thirdhand" smoke and home smoking bans. *Pediatrics.* 2009;123:e74-e79.

101 "It is not surprising..." Kaufmann RB, Babb S, O'Halloran A, et al. Vital signs: Nonsmokers' exposure to secondhand smoke—United States, 1999-2008. *MMWR.* 2010;59(35):1141-1146.

101 "States spent $517 million ..." A broken promise to our children: The 1998 state tobacco settlement 12 years later. Campaign for Tobacco-Free Kids website. tobaccofreekids.org/ reports/settlements/FY2011/StateSettlementReport_FY2011_web.pdf. November 2010. Accessed January 26, 2011.

101 "Countries that have completely ..." Blecher E. The impact of tobacco advertising bans on consumption in developing countries. *Journal of Health Economics.* 2008;27(4):930-942.

102 "Americans are drinking ..." Newport, F. U.S. drinking rate edges up slightly to 25-year high. Gallup Website. July 30, 2010. gallup.com/poll/141656/drinking-rate-edges-slightly-year-high.aspx. Accessed January 21, 2011.

102 "Two out of 3 ..." Caetano R, Baruah J, Ramisetty-Mikler S, Ebama MS. Sociodemographic predictors of pattern and volume of alcohol consumption across Hispanics,

blacks, and whites: 10-year trend (1992-2002). *Alcohol Clin Exp Res.* 2010;34(10):1-11; National Institute on Alcohol Abuse and Alcoholism. *Rethinking drinking: Alcohol and your health.* Washington, DC: U.S. Department of Health and Human Services; September 2009.

102 "A national survey ..." National Institute on Alcohol Abuse and Alcoholism. National Epidemiologic Survey on Alcohol and Related Conditions: Selected findings. *Alcohol Research & Health.* 2006;29(2):71-155.

102 "Even people ages 45 to 64 ..." King DE, Mainous AG, Geesey ME. Adopting moderate alcohol consumption in middle age: Subsequent cardiovascular events. *Am J Med.* 2008;121(9):e9.

102 "But it could be ..." Hansel B, Thomas F, Pannier B, et al. Relationship between alcohol intake, health and social status and cardiovascular risk factors in the urban Paris-Ile-De-France Cohort: is the cardioprotective action of alcohol a myth? *Eur J Clin Nutr.* 2010;64:361-368.

103 "It is a leading preventable ..." Naimi TS, Nelson DE, Brewer RD. The intensity of binge alcohol consumption among US adults. Am J Prev Med. 2010;38(2):201-207; Sociodemographic differences in binge drinking among adults—14 states, 2004. *MMWR.* 2009;58(12):301-304.

103 "But it also leads ..." National Institute on Alcohol Abuse and Alcoholism, op cit.

103 "The economic impact ..." Lee MH, Mello MJ, Reinert S. Emergency department charges for evaluating minimally injured alcohol-impaired drivers. *Annals of Emergency Medicine.* 2009;54(4):593-599.

103 "Almost 1 out of 8 ..." Naimi TS, Nelson DE, Brewer RD. Driving after binge drinking. *Am J Prev Med.* 2009;37(4):314-320.

103 "Professional sporting events ..." Erickson DJ, Toomey TL, Lenk KM, Kilian GR, Fabian EA. Can we assess blood alcohol levels of attendees leaving professional sporting events? *Alcohol Clin Exp Res.* 2011;35(4).

103 "A study of social networks ..." Rosenquist JN, Murabit J, Fowler JH, Christakis NA. The spread of alcohol consumption behavior in a large social network. *Ann Intern Med.* 2010;152: 426-433.

104 "University of Florida researchers ..." Wagenaar AC, Salois MJ, Komro KA. Effects of beverage alcohol price and tax levels on drinking: A meta-analysis of 1003 estimates from 112 studies. *Addiction.* 2009;104:2.

104 "Doubling alcohol taxes ..." Wagenaar AC, Tobler AL, Komro KA. Effects of alcohol tax and price policies on morbidity and mortality: A systematic review. *Am J Public Health.* 2010;100(11):2270-2278.

104 "But alcohol prices are ..." Elder RW, Lawrence B, Ferguson A, et al. The effectiveness of tax policy interventions for reducing excessive alcohol consumption and related harms. *Am J Prev Med.* 2010;38(2):217-229.

Chapter 9. Personalized Medicine

Page 105 "Swedish scientists followed ..." Wilhelmsen L, Svardsudd K, Eriksson H, et al. Factors associated with reaching 90 years of age: A study of men born in 1913 in Gothenburg, Sweden. *J Intern Med.* December 22, 2010. onlinelibrary.wiley.com/doi/10.1111/j.1365-2796. 2010.02331.x/full. Accessed March 15, 2011.

105 "However, another important study ..." Sebastiani P, Solovieff N, Puca A. Genetic signatures of exceptional longevity in humans. *Science.* July 1, 2010.sciencemag.org/cgi/ gca?gca=science.1190532v1&sendit.x=0&sendit.y=0. Accessed March 15, 2011.

107 "The harsh reality is ..." Spear BB, Heath-Chiozzi M, Huff J. Clinical application of pharmacogenetics. *Trends Mol Med.* 2001;7(5):201-204.

108 "According to a February 2008 study ..." Mallal S, Phillips E, Carosi G, et al. HLA-B*5701 screening for hypersensitivity to abacavir. *N Engl J Med.* 2008;358:568-579.

108 "Paradoxically, sales increased ..." Frueh FW. Considerations for a business model for the

effective integration of novel biomarkers into drug development. *Personalized Medicine*. 2008; 5(6):641-649.

108 "The market for targeted therapeutics ..." The new science of personalized medicine: Translating the promise into practice. Pricewaterhouse Coopers website. pwc.com/us/en/health-industries/topics/personalized-medicine.jhtml. 2009. Accessed March 12, 2011.

108 "However, the price of DNA sequencing ... " Wade, N. A decade later, genetic map yields few new cures. *The New York Times*. June 12, 2010.

108 "According to one estimate ..."Personalized medicines are shaping the way R&D is done, according to Tufts Center for the Study of Drug Development. CSDD website. csdd.tufts.edu/news/complete_story/pr_ir_nov-dec_2010. November 16, 2010. Accessed March 13, 2011; Pollack A. Drug companies purse personalized medicine approach. *The New York Times*. November 16, 2010.

109 "A Government Accountability Office ..." *Direct-to-consumer genetic tests: Misleading test results are further complicated by deceptive marketing and other questionable practices*. Government Accountability Office website. gao.gov/products/GAO-10-847T. July 22, 2010. Accessed March 11, 2011.

109 "A 2006 report argued ..." Watson K, Cook ED, Litt D, Helzlsour K. Direct-to-consumer online genetic testing and four principles: An analysis of the ethical issues. *Ethics Med*. 2006; 22(2):83-91.

109 "A Federal Trade Commission ..." At-home genetic tests: A healthy dose of skepticism may be the best prescription. Federal Trade Commission website. ftc.gov/bcp/edu/pubs/consumer/health/hea02.shtm. July 2006. Accessed March 15, 2011.

110 "Australian journalist Ray Moynihan ..." Moynihan R. Beware the fortune tellers peddling genetic tests. *BMJ*. 2011;342:c7233.

110 "In a poll taken ..." Sandroff R. Direct-to-consumer genetic tests and the right to know. *Hastings Cent Rep*. 2010;40(5):24-25.

110 "People appear willing to pay ..." Neumann PJ, Cohen JT, Hammitt JK. Willingness-to-pay for predictive tests with no immediate treatment implications: A survey of US residents. *Health Economics*. onlinelibrary.wiley.com/doi/10.1002/hec.1704/full. December 28, 2010. Accessed March 15, 2011.

110 "Four of 5 Americans ..." Kaufman D, Murphy J, Scott J, Hudson K. Subjects matter: A survey of public opinions about a large genetic cohort study. *Genetics in Medicine*. 2008;10(11): 831-839.

111 "Younger adults are especially ..." O'Neill SC, McBride CM, Hensley S, Kaphiingst KA. Preferences for genetic and behavioral health information: The impact of risk factors and disease attributions. *Ann Behav Med*. 2010;40(2):127-137.

112 "A study in the New England Journal of Medicine ..." Bloss CS, Schork NJ, Topol EJ. Effect of direct-to-consumer genomewide profiling to assess disease risk. *N Engl J Med*. 2011; 264(6):524-534.

112 "A separate study ..." Bernhardt BA, Gollust S, Griffin G, et al. "It's not like judgment day": Public understanding of and reactions to personalized genomic risk. American Society of Human Genetics 60th annual meeting. Washington, D.C. Nov. 2-6, 2010.

112 "With genetic tests ..." Shim M; Cappella JN; Lerman C. Familial risk cues in direct-to-consumer prescription drug advertisements: Impacts on intentions to adopt healthy lifestyles and pharmaceutical choices. *Journal of Applied Communication Research*. 2010;38(3):230-247.

112 "A Cleveland Clinic researcher ..." Eng, C. American Society of Human Genetics 60th annual meeting. Washington, D.C. Nov. 2-6, 2010.

113 "Likewise, researchers collected ..." Paynter NP, Chasman DI, Pare G, et al. Association between a literature-based genetic risk score and cardiovascular events in women. *JAMA*.2010; 303(7):631-637.

113 "Family members often take ..." Quillin JM, Bodurtha JN, Siminoff LA, Smith TJ. Exploring hereditary cancer among dying cancer patients—a cross-sectional study of hereditary risk and perceived awareness of DNA testing and banking. *J Genet Couns*. 2010;19(5): 497-525.

113 "An international research consortium ..." Winslow R. Gene sites tied to obesity identified in new research. *The Wall Street Journal*. October 11, 2010.

114 "Dr. Robert Marion ..." Gardner, A. Medicine's future could lie in each patient's genome. *Bloomberg Businessweek*. March 11, 2010.

114 "Congress passed ..." PricewaterhouseCoopers op. cit.

115 "However, according to a survey ..." Stanek EJ, Sanders CL. National pharacogenomics physician survey: Who are the physicians adoping pharmacogenomics and how does knowledge impact adoption? American Society of Human Genetics 59th annual meeting. Honolulu, HI. Oct. 20-24, 2009.

115 "A Baylor College of Medicine ..." Plon SE, Cooper HP, Parks B. Genetic testing and cancer risk management recommendations by physicians for at-risk relatives. *Genetics in Medicine*. 2001;13(2):148-154.

115 "Hank Greely ..." Stein, R. Company plans to sell genetic testing kit at drugstores. *The Washington Post*. May 11, 2010.

116 "BusinessWeek chief economist Michael Mandel... " Mandel, M. The great stagnation and evidence-based medicine. innovationandgrowth.wordpress.com/2011/02/05/the-great-stagnation-and-evidence-based-medicine/. February 5, 2011. Accessed March 16, 2011; Lee DH, Vielemeyer O. Analysis of overall level of evidence behind Infectious Diseases Society of America practice guidelines. 2011;171(1):18-22.

Chapter 10. Health Care Disparities

Page 118 "Columbia University researchers ..." Galea S, Tracy M, Hoggatt KJ, DiMaggio C, Adam Karpati. Estimated deaths attributable to social factors in the United States. *Am J Public Health*. 2011;e1-e10. ajph.aphapublications.org/cgi/content/abstract/AJPH.2010.300086v1. June 16, 2011. Accessed July 28, 2011.

119 "Many Americans are unaware ..." Booske BC, Robert SA, Rohan AM. Awareness of racial and socioeconomic health disparities in the United States: The National Opinion Survey on Health and Health Disparities. *Preventing Chronic Disease*. cdc.gov/pcd/issues/2011/jul/10_0166.htm. July 2011. Accessed July 27, 2011.

119 "Low-SES Americans have levels of illness ..." Williams DR, Jackson PB. Social sources of racial disparities. *Health Aff*. 2005;24(2):325-334.

122 "Researchers in the MacArthur Study of Successful Aging ..." Allostatic load network. MacArthur Foundation website. macses.ucsf.edu/research/allostatic/allostatic.php August 2009. Accessed June 9, 2011.

122 "This is reflected ..." Isaacs SL, Schroeder SA. Class—The ignored determinant of health. *N Engl J Med*. 2004;351(11):1137-1142.

123 "Government is more likely... " Mechanic D, Tanner J. Vulnerable people, groups, and populations: Societal view. *Health Aff*. 2007;26(5):1220-1230.

123 "University of Oxford researchers ..." Stuckler D, Basu S, McKee M. Budget crises, health, and social welfare programmes. *BMJ*. 2010;340:c3311.

123 "However, a 1998 study examined ..." Lantz PM, House JS, Lepkowski JM, Williams DR, Mero RP, Chen J. Socioeconomic factors, health behaviors, and mortality. *JAMA*. 1998;279(21):1703-1708.

124 "This medicalization of social reform ..." Lantz PM, Lichtenstein RL, Pollack HA. Health policy approaches to population health: The limits of medicalization. *Health Aff*. 2007;26(5): 1253-1257.

124 "Canadian researchers wanted ..." Alter DA, Stukel T, Chong A, Henry D. Lesson from Canada's universal care: Socially disadvantaged patients use more health services, still have poorer health. *Health Aff.* 2011;30(2):274-283.

124 "Likewise, SES health disparities ..." Adler NE, Newman K. Socioeconomic disparities in health: Pathways and policies. *Health Aff.* 2002;21(2):60-76.

124 "On the other hand ..." Mechanic D. Policy challenges in addressing racial disparities and improving population health. *Health Aff.* 2005;24(2):335-342.

125 "A group of 89 retired generals ..." Ready, willing and unable to serve. missionreadiness.org/PAEE0609.pdf. 2009. Accessed June 12, 2011.

125 "A 2011 study reached ..." Reynolds AJ, Temple JA, Ou S, White BA. School-based early childhood education and age-28 well-being: Effects by timing, dosage, and subgroups. *Science.* sciencemag.org/content/early/2011/06/08/science.1203618. June 9, 2011. Accessed June 11, 2011.

126 "There is some debate ..." Deaton A. Policy implications of the gradient of health and wealth. *Health Aff.* 2002;21(2):13-30.

126 "According to one analysis ..." Woolf SH. Public health implications of government spending reductions. *JAMA.* 2011;305(18):1902-1903.

126 "A Review of Economic Studies journal article ..." Lleras-Muney A. The relationship between education and adult mortality in the United States. *The Review of Economic Studies.* 2005;72(1):189-221.

126 "In developed nations ..." Deaton, op. cit.

126 "If adults who had not completed ..." Overcoming obstacles to health. Robert Wood Johnson Foundation website. rwjf.org/files/research/obstaclestohealth.pdf February 2008. Accessed June 8, 2011.

126 "The life-course model ..." Forrest CB, Riley AW. Childhood origins of adult health: A basis for life-course health policy. *Health Aff.* 2004;23(5):155-163.

128 "Less than 3 percent ..." Kaplan G. The poor pay more—poverty's high cost to health. deepblue.lib.umich.edu/bitstream/2027.42/64129/1/The%20Poor%20Pay%20More-Povertys%20High%20Cost%20to%20Health_2009.pdf September 2009. Accessed June 8, 2011.

128 "Smoking rates were similar ..." Pamuk E, Makus D, Heck K, Reuben C, Lochner K. *Socioeconomic Status and Health Chartbook. Health, United States, 1998.* Hyattsville MD: National Center for Health Statistics; Vital signs: Current cigarette smoking among adults age 18 or older—United States, 2009. *MMWR.* 2010;59(35):1135-1140.

128 "Each additional year ..." Loucks EB, Abrahamowicz M, Xiao Y, Lynch JW. Associations of education with 30 year life course blood pressure trajectories: Framingham Offspring Study. *BMC Public Health.* 2011;11:139.

128 "Education's health benefits ..." Cutler DM, Lleras-Muney A, Vogl T. Socioeconomic status and health dimensions and mechanisms. National Bureau of Economic Research Working Paper 14333. September 2008.

128 "About 30 percent ..." Education matters for health. Robert Wood Johnson Foundation website. rwjf.org/files/research/sdohseries2011education.pdf April 2011. Accessed June 8, 2011.

129 "Income affects health ..." Marmot M. The influence of income on health: Views of an epidemiologist. *Health Aff.* 2002;21(2):31-46.

129 "A 25-year-old man ..." Kaplan, op. cit.

129 "The U.S. poverty rate ..." Poverty. U.S. Census Bureau website. census.gov/hhes/www/poverty/about/overview/index.html. Accessed June 11, 2011.

129 "A task force of the Center for American Progress ..." Greenberg M, Dutta-Gupta I, Minoff E. From Poverty to Prosperity: A National Strategy to Cut Poverty in Half. Washington DC: Center for American Progress; 2007.

129 "Survey data show ..." Schlesinger M. Reprivatizing the public household? Medical care in the context of American values. *J Health Polit Policy Law*. 2007;29(4-5):969-1004.

130 "The U.S. elderly poverty rate ..." Kaplan G, op. cit.

130 "People who unfavorably compare ..." Brunner E, Marmot MG. Social organization, stress, and health. In: Marmot MG, Wilkinson RG, eds. *Social Determinants of Health*. 2nd ed. Oxford: Oxford University Press; 2006.

130 "Some attempt to cope ..." Kawachi I, Kennedy BP. *The Health of Nations: Why Inequality Is Harmful to Your Health*. New York: New Press; 2002.

130 "Perhaps because of the nation's history ..." Isaacs SL, op. cit.

131 "One comprehensive review ..." Williams DR, Collins C. U.S. socioeconomic and racial differences in health: Patterns and explanations. *Annu Rev Sociol*. 1995;21:349-386.

131 "For example, the U.S. Census Bureau ..." The 2011 U.S. Census Bureau statistical abstract. census.gov/compendia/statab/cats/births_deaths_marriages_divorces/life_expectancy. html. Accessed June 11, 2011.

131 "Great Britain tracks ..." Issacs SL, op. cit.

132 "Social status itself ..." Redelmeier DA, Singh SM. Survival in Academy Award-winning acts and actresses. *Ann Intern Med*. 2001;134:955-962.

132 "Racial health disparities ..." Kawachi I, Daniels N, Robinson DE. Health disparities by race and class: Why both matter. *Health Aff*. 2005;24(2):343-352.

132 "More starkly ..." Sen AK. Mortality as an indicator of economic success and failure. *Economic Journal*. 1998;108:1-25.

132 "U.S. income inequality ..." Who saw the most income growth? (A breakdown of income group, 1979-2007). Economic Policy Institute website. epi.org/economic_snapshots/entry/top_incomes_grow_while_bottom_incomes_stagnate/September 8, 2010. Accessed June 8, 2011.

132 "The combined net worth ..." Inequality by the numbers. The Program on Inequality and the Public Good website. October 2008.

133 "Between 1978 and 2005 ..." Economic mobility: Is the American dream alive and well? Economic Mobility Project website. economicmobility.org/assets/pdfs/EMP%20American%20 Dream%20Report.pdf. Accessed June 8, 2011.

133 "The racial and ethnic wealth gap ..." Kochlar R, Fry R, Taylor P. Wealth gaps rise to record highs between whites, blacks, Hispanics. Pew Research Center. pewsocialtrends.org/ 2011/07/26/wealth-gaps-rise-to-record-highs-between-whites-blacks-hispanics/. July 26, 2011. Accessed July 28, 2011.

133 "The American Dream seems ..." Isaacs JB. International comparisons of economic mobility. The Brookings Institution. economicmobility.org/assets/pdfs/EMP_International Comparisons_ChapterIII.pdf. Accessed June 8, 2011.

133 "Less than one-third ..." Economic Mobility Project, op. cit.

133 "Environmental risk factors ..." Pruss-Ustun A, Carvalan. How much disease burden can be prevented by environmental interventions? *Epidemiology*. 2007;18(1):167-178.

134 "More than 80,000 new synthetic ..." Landrigan PL, Goldman LR. Children's vulnerability to toxic chemicals: A challenge and opportunity to strengthen health and environmental policy. *Health Aff*. 2011;30(5):842-850.

134 "However, numerous studies..." deFur PL, Evans GW, Hubal EA, Kyle AD, Morello-Frosch RF, Williams DR. Vulnerability as a function of individual and group resources in cumulative risk assessment. *Environ Health Perspect*. 2007;115:817-524.

134 "Nearly one-fifth ..." Where we live matters to our health: Neighborhoods and health. Robert Wood Johnson Foundation website. rwjf.org/files/research/commissionneighborhood 102008.pdf. September 2008. Accessed June 8, 2011.

134 "Substandard housing also ..." Jacobs DE. Environmental health disparities in house. Am J Public Health. 2011. ajph.aphapublications.org/cgi/content/abstract/AJPH.2010.300058v1 May 6. Accessed June 8, 2011.

134 "However, the National Center for Healthy Housing ..." National Center for Healthy Housing (NCHH). State of health housing, 2009. nchh.org/Policy/State-of-Healthy-Housing.aspx. Accessed June 8, 2011

135 "In addition to residential environmental ..." Gochfield M, Burger J. Disproportionate exposures in environmental justice and other populations: The importance of outliers. *Am J Public Health*. 2011; e1-e11.

135 "Children have ..." Landrigan PL, op. cit.

135 "A study of Michigan public schools ..." Mohai P, Kweon B, Lee S, Ard K. Air pollution around schools is linked to poorer student health and academic performance. *Health Aff*. 2011;30(5):852-862.

Chapter 11. Prevention

Page 137 "The CBO cited a lack ..." Congressional Budget Office. Letter to Sen. Kent Conrad, chairman, U.S. Senate Committee on Budget. budget.senate.gov/democratic/documents/2009/CBO%20Letter%20HealthReformAndFederalBudget_061609.pdf. June 16, 2009. Accessed February 9, 2011.

138 "Nearly 3 out of 4 ..." Poll finds Americans think disease prevention central to health reform. Robert Wood Johnson Foundation website. rwjf.org/healthpolicy/product.jsp?id=51652. November 13, 2009. Accessed February 9, 2011.

138 "Advocates correctly point out ..." Goetzel RZ. Do prevention or treatment services save money? The wrong debate. *Health Aff*. 2010;28(1):37-41.

139 "Steven Woolf, a physician..." Woolf SH, Husten CG, Lewin LS, Marks JS, Fielding JE, Sanchez EJ. The economic argument for disease prevention: Distinguishing between value and savings. Partnership for Prevention website. prevent.org/data/files/initiatives/economicargumentfordiseaseprevention.pdf. February 2009. Accessed February 9, 2011.

140 "The rule of thumb..." Woolf SH. A closer look at the economic argument for disease prevention. *JAMA*. 2009;301(5):536-538.

140 "Placing an economic value ..." Appelbaum B. As U.S. agencies put more value on a life, businesses fret. *The New York Times*. February 16, 2011.

141 "Of the 30-year increase..." Patel K, Rushefsky M. *The Politics of Public Health in the United States*. Armonk, NY: M.E. Sharpe; 2005.

141 "Public-health measures..." Centers for Disease Control and Prevention. Ten great public health achievements—United States, 1900-1999. *MMWR*. 1999;48(12):241-243.

142 "Research has repeatedly shown..." Blueprint for a healthier America: Modernizing the federal health system to focus on prevention and preparedness. Trust for America's Health website. healthyamericans.org/report/55/blueprint-for-healthier-america. October 2008. Accessed February 16, 2011.

142 "Despite widespread support..." Sensening A. Estimates of public health spending as measured in the National Health Expenditures Accounts: The U.S. experience. *Journal of Public Health Management and Practice*. 2007;13(2):103-114.

142 "Trust for America's Health..." Prevention for a healthier America: Investments in disease prevention yield significant savings, stronger communities. Trust for America's Health website. healthyamericans.org/reports/prevention08/Prevention08.pdf. February 2009. Accessed February 16, 2011.

142 "The top 20 percent of communities..." Mays GP, Smith SA. Geographic variation in public health spending: Correlates and consequences. *Health Ser Res*. 2009;44(5, Part 2):1807-1808.

142 "More spending translates…" Mays G, McHugh M, Shim K, et al. Getting what you pay for: Public health spending and the performance of essential public health services. *Journal of Public Health Management and Practice*. 2004;10(5):435-443.

142 "A 2011 *Health Affairs* journal study …" Mays GP, Smith SA. Evidence links increases in public health spending to declines in preventable deaths. *Health Aff*. 2011;30(8).

143 "The average state budget's …" Lav I, McNichol E. State budget troubles worsen. Center on Budget and Policy Priorities website. cbpp.org/cms/index.cfm?fa=archivePage&id=9-8-08sfp.htm Updated November 12, 2008. Accessed February 16, 2011.

143 "About 55 percent of local health departments…" Meyer J, Weiselberg L. County and city health departments: The need for sustainable funding through health reform. Naples, FL: Healthcare Management Associates; 2009.

143 "The $35 billion spent…" Levy J, St. Laurent R, Segal L, Vinter S. Shortchanging America's health: A state-by-state look at how public health dollars are spent. Trust for America's Health website. healthyamericans.org/report/74/federal-spending-2010. March 2010. Accessed February 16, 2011.

143 "Only 28 percent of smokers…" Preventive care: A national profile on use, disparities, and health benefits. Robert Wood Johnson Foundation website. rwjf.org/files/research/8-7-07%20-%20Partnership%20for%20Prevention%20Report%281%29.pdf. August 7, 2007. Accessed February 16, 2011.

143 "A New York City health department…" Farley TA, Dalal MA, Mostashari F, Frieden TR. Deaths preventable in the U.S. by improvements in use of clinical preventive services. *Am J Prev Med*. 2010;38(6):600-609.

144 "If 90 percent of Americans …" Maciosek MV, Coffield AB, Flottemesch TJ, Edwards NM, Solberg LI. Greater use of preventive services in U.S. health care could save lives at little or no cost. *Health Aff*. 2010;29(9):1656-1660.

144 "For example, the National Commission …" Bernstein J, Chollet D, Peterson GG. Encouraging appropriate use of preventive health services. Mathematica Policy Research website. mathematica-mpr.com/publications/PDFs/Health/reformhealthcare_IB2.pdf. May 2010. Accessed February 9, 2011.

144 "TFAH argues …" Trust for America's Health, 2009, op cit.

144 "A 5 percent reduction …" Ormond BA, Spillman BC, Waldmann TA, Caswell KJ, Tereshchenko. Potential national and state medical savings from primary disease prevention. *Am J Pub Health*. 2011; 101(1):157-164.

145 "A 2008 study estimated …" Kahn R, Robertson RM, Smith R, Eddy D. The impact of prevention on reducing the burden of cardiovascular disease. *Circulation*. 2008;118:576-585.

145 "A 2007 study illustrated …" Russell LB. Prevention's potential for slowing the growth of medical spending. Institute for Health, Health Care Policy and Aging Research website. ihhcpar.rutgers.edu/downloads/nchc_report.pdf. October 2007. Accessed February 10, 2011.

145 "One out of 4 Americans …" National Center for Healthcare Statistics. *Health, United States 2010: With special feature on death and dying*. Washington, DC: Centers for Disease Control; 2011.

145 "Researchers had Australian doctors …" Brown D. In the balance: Some candidates disagree, but studies show it's often cheaper to let people get sick. *The Washington Post*. April 8, 2008.

146 "Researchers reviewed hundreds …" Cohen JT, Neumann PJ, Weinstein MC. Does preventive care save money? Health economics and the presidential candidates. *N Engl J Med*. 2008;358(7):661-663.

146 "For example, screening 35-year-olds …" Hoerger TJ, Harris R, Hicks KA, Donahue K, Sorensen S, Engelgau M. Screening for Type 2 diabetes Mellitus: A Cost-Effectiveness Analysis. *Ann Intern Med*. 2004;140(9):689-699.

146 "Russell illustrated the effect …" Russell LB, op cit.

146 "Consumer Reports ..." 44 percent of health adults getting unneeded heart screenings. Consumer Reports website. pressroom.consumerreports.org/pressroom/2011/02/my-entry.html. February 3, 2011. Accessed February 9, 2011.

147 "One in 5 people ..." Radolf JD, Park IU, Chow JM, et al. Discordant results from reverse sequence syphilis screening—five laboratories, United States, 2006-2010. *MMWR.* 2011; 60(5):133-137.

147 "In a national survey ..." Schwartz LM, Woloshin S, Fowler FJ, Welch HG. Enthusiasm for cancer screening in the United States. *JAMA.* 2004;291:71-78.

147 "But a comprehensive review ... " Welch HG, Schwartz LM, Woloshin S. Are increasing 5-year survival rates evidence of success against cancer? *JAMA.* 2000;283(22):2975-2978.

147 "Cancer screening finds lots ..." Welch, HG. *Should I Be Tested for Cancer? Maybe Not and Here's Why.* Berkley, CA: University of California Press; 2006.

147 "Dr. Laura Esserman ..." Esserman L, Shieh Y, Thompson I. Rethinking screening for breast cancer and prostate cancer. *JAMA.* 2009;302(15):1685-1692.

148 "Welch calculated ..." Welch HG. Overdiagnosis and mammography screening. *BMJ.* 2009;339:b1425.

149 "In another example ..." National Lung Screening Trial (NLST) Initial Results: Fast Facts. National Cancer Institute website. cancer.gov/newscenter/pressreleases/NLSTFastFacts. November 4, 2010. Accessed February 17, 2011.

149 "News reports hailed the results ..." Harris G. CT scans cut cancer deaths, study finds. *The New York Times.* November 4, 2010. Accessed February 17, 2011.

149 "An earlier study showed ..." Croswell JM, Baker SG, Marcus PM, Clapp JD, Kramer BS. Cumulative incidence of false-positive test results in lung cancer screening: A randomized trial. *Ann Intern Med.* 2010;152(8):505-512.

149 "Americans use preventive services ..." McGlynn EA, Asch SM, Adams J, et al. The quality of health care delivered to adults in the United Stataes. *N Engl J Med.* 2008;348(26):2635-2645.

149 "If everyone received ..." Yarnall KS, Pollak KI, Ostbye T, Krause KM, Michener JL. Primary care: Is there enough time for prevention? *Am J Public Health.* 2003;93(4):635-641.

149 "A survey by the Midwest Business Group on Health ..." Japsen B. Emphasis on preventive care no guarantee that employees use benefits. *The Chicago Tribune.* August 18, 2010.

149 "The CDC named vaccination ..." Ten great public health achievements—United States, 1990-1999. *MMWR.* 1999; 48:241-243.

150 "As a result, adults represent ..." Tan, L. Improving adult immunization rates of today and preventing the pandemic of tomorrow; Novick L. Living today for a better tomorrow: Helping adults understand the value of immunization to long-term health. Partnership for Prevention website. prevent.org/data/files/initiatives/tan5-8-09slides.pdf Congressional briefing May 8, 2009. Accessed February 10, 2011.

150 "A National Foundation for Infectious Diseases poll ..." National survey on adult vaccination reports low consumer awareness of vaccines and the risks of vaccine-preventable diseases. nfid.org/pdf/pressconfs/adultimm08/nfidsurvey.pdf. 2008. Accessed June 12, 2011.

150 "For example, nearly half of Americans ..." Vaccine-autism link: Sound science or fraud? HealthDay website. healthday.com/press/healthday-harris-vaccine-autism.html. January 20, 2011. Accessed February 9, 2011.

150 "The original research ..." Godlee F, Smith S, Marcovitch H. Wakefield's article linking MMR vaccine and autism was fraudulent. *BMJ.* 2011;342:c7452.

Chapter 12. Workplace Wellness

Page 151 "Nearly 60 percent of an average company's ..." Milani RV, Lavie CJ. Impact of worksite wellness intervention on cardiac risk factors and one-year health care costs. *Am J Cardiol.* 2009;104(10):1389-1392.

151 "Starbucks, for example ..." Kowitt B. Starbucks CEO: "We spend more on health care than coffee". CNN website. money.cnn.com/2010/06/07/news/companies/starbucks_schultz_healthcare.fortune/index.htm. June 7, 2010. Accessed May 1, 2011.

152 "Dee Edington ..." Edington, DW. *Zero Trends: Health as a Serious Economic Strategy.* Ann Arbor: Health Management Research Center; 2009.

153 "According to a 2010 international survey ..." Working well: A global survey of health promotion and workplace wellness strategies. Buck Consultants. vielife.com/downloads/research/gw/Global_Wellness_2009_ExecSumm_English.pdf. 2009. Accessed March 4, 2011.

153 "In most of the world ..." Working well: A global survey of health promotion and workplace wellness strategies. Buck Consultants. bucksurveys.com/bucksurveys/product/tabid/139/p-51-working-well-a-global-survey-of-health-promotion-and-workplace-wellness-strategies.aspx. Accessed March 4, 2011.

153 "Large employers consider wellness programs ..." What employers want from health insurers—now. PricewaterhouseCoopers Research Institute. pwchealth.com/cgi-local/hregister.cgi?link=reg/what_employers_want.pdf. 2008. Accessed March 4, 2011.

154 "Workplaces suffered ..." Work matters for health. Robert Wood Johnson Foundation website. commissiononhealth.org/PDF/0e8ca13d-6fb8-451d-bac8-7d15343aacff/Issue%20Brief%204%20Dec%2008%20-%20Work%20and%20Health.pdf. December 2008. Accessed March 4, 2011.

154 "About 2 out of 3 employers ..." Purchasing value in health care: Selected findings from the 15th annual National Business Group on Health/Towers Watson Survey Report—2010. Towers Watson website. towerswatson.com/assets/pdf/1258/WT-2010-15571.pdf. Accessed March 4, 2011.

155 "According to a survey ..." Roberts, S. Employers prepare to expand wellness efforts: Survey. Business Insurance website. businessinsurance.com/article/20100523/ISSUE01/305239981. May 24, 2010. Accessed March 4, 2011.

155 "Anything less than a robust wellness program ..." Tu H, Mayrell, RC. Employer wellness initiatives grow, but effectiveness varies widely. National Institute for Health Care Reform research brief. nihcr.org/Employer-Wellness-Initiatives.html. July 2010. Accessed March 4, 2011.

155 "A Kaiser Family Foundation survey ..." Employer health benefits 2010 annual survey. Kaiser Family Foundation website. ehbs.kff.org/pdf/2010/8085.pdf. 2010. Accessed March 4, 2011.

156 "An Integrated Benefits Institute survey ..." More than health promotion: How employers manage health and productivity. Integrated Benefits Institute website. ibiweb.org/do/viewdocument/DocumentList?linkId=37837&aId=F7DF5BD5F9A54439EF1C80F3DEAC2516. January 2010. Accessed March 4, 2011.

156 "The tip of the spear ..." Baicker K, Cutler D, Song Z. Workplace wellness programs can generate savings. *Health Aff.* 2010;29(2): 1-8.

156 "They are more likely ..." Health risk appraisals: How sharp is this tool in shaping employee behavior? Changes in Health Care Financing & Organization. academyhealth.org/files/publications/HCFOBriefDecember2009.pdf. December 2009. Accessed March 4, 2011.

156 "Participation in wellness programs ..." MetLife 8th annual study of employee benefit trends. MetLife website. metlife.com/assets/institutional/services/insights-and-tools/ebts/Employee-Benefits-Trends-Study.pdf. April 2010. Accessed March 4, 2011.

156 "Clinics were common ..." Tu HT, Boukus ER, Cohen GR. Workplace clinics: A sign of growing employer interest in wellness. Center for Studying Health System Change Research Brief No. 17. hschange.com/CONTENT/1166/. December 2010. Accessed March 4, 2011.

157 "Many companies that have taken ..." Workplace health programs and cost containment. Health Care Financing & Organization website. hcfo.org/publications/workplace-health-programs-and-cost-containment. December 2009. Accessed March 4, 2011.

157 "One of the most comprehensive studies ..." Baicker K, op. cit.

157 "A *Harvard Business Review* study ..." Berry LL, Mirabito AM, Baun WB. What's the hard return on employee wellness programs? Harvard Business Review website. hbr.org/2010/12/whats-the-hard-return-on-employee-wellness-programs/ar/1 December 2010. Accessed March 4, 2011.

157 "Wellness programs are relatively inexpensive ..." New study finds most employers spend nearly 2% of health care claims budget on wellness programs. National Business Group on Health website. businessgrouphealth.org/pressrelease.cfm?ID=149. January 25, 2010. Accessed March 4, 2011.

158 "The payback rises ..." Aldana SG. Financial impact of health promotion programs: A comprehensive review of the literature. *American Journal of Health Promotion.* 2001:15(5):296-320.

158 "The most consistent performers ..." Employers raising the bar on financial incentives to improve worker health, National Business Group on Health/Towers Watson survey finds. National Business Group on Health website. businessgrouphealth.org/pressrelease.cfm?ID=153. March 11, 2010. Accessed May 1, 2011.

158 "They spend about $10,000 ..." More workers seeking health information from employers, health plans, National Business Group on Health survey finds. businessgrouphealth.org/pressrelease.cfm?ID=168. February 1, 2011. Accessed March 4, 2011.

158 "For example ..." Interview with wellness director Leia Spoor, January 20, 2011.

159 "According to Edington ..." Edington, op cit.

159 "A Midwest Business Group on Health survey ..." Japsen B. Emphasis on preventive care no guarantee that employees use benefits. The Chicago Tribune. articles.chicagotribune.com/2010-08-18/health/ct-biz-0819-notebook-health-20100818_1_preventive-care-larry-boress-insurers-and-employers. August 18, 2010. Accessed March 4, 2011.

159 "The presence of insurance ..." Hughes MC, Hannon PA, Harris JR, Patrick DL. Health behaviors of employed and insured adults in the United States, 2004-2005. *American Journal of Health Promotion.* 2010;24(5):315.

159 "In focus groups ..." New research finds employers need to rethink their approach to engaging employees and dependents in managing their health. Midwest Business Group on Health. prnewswire.com/news-releases/new-research-finds-employers-need-to-rethink-their-approach-to-engaging-employees-and-dependents-in-managing-their-health-92990054.html. Accessed March 4, 2011.

160 " ... despite the fact that 86 percent ..." Smith TW, Kim J. Paid sick days: Attitudes and experiences. Public Welfare Foundation website. publicwelfare.org/resources/DocFiles/psd2010 final.pdf. June 2010. Accessed March 4, 2011.

160 "More than 8 out of 10 ..." Paid sick days improve our public health. National Partnership for Women & Families fact sheet. July 2011. Accessed July 28, 2011.

160 "According to a University of Pennsylvania survey ..." Long JA, Helweg-Larsen M, Volpp KG. Patient opinions regarding "pay for performance for patients." *J Gen Intern Med.* 2008; 23(10):1647-1652.

161 "An Integrated Benefits Institute survey ..." Jinnett K, Parry T, Molmen W. Employer incentives for workforce health and productivity. Integrated Benefits Institute. ibiweb.org/do/PublicAccess?documentId=955. October 2008. Accessed March 4, 2011.

161 "However, according to a Towers Watson survey ..." Changes ahead: Health care reform in a challenging economy. Towers Watson website. towerswatson.com/assets/pdf/2884/Towers Watson-HC-Changes-Flash-5-NA-2010-17151.pdf. September 2010. Accessed May 1, 2011.

161 "The average per-employee incentive ..." Annual wellness study finds significant jump in incentive dollars as employers report improved employee participation. Fidelity website. fidelity.com/inside-fidelity/employer-services/2011-wellness-survey. February 8, 2011. Accessed March 4, 2011.

162 "Harvard researchers calculated ..." Schmidt H, Voigt K, Wikler D. Carrots, sticks and health care reform—problems with wellness incentives. *N Engl J Med*. 2010;362(2):e3.

162 "A 2005 *Wall Street Journal* and Harris Interactive poll ..." Kicking a bad habit could pay off. *The Wall Street Journal*, January 6, 2006.

Chapter 13. Patient Engagement

Page 163 "How many do this? ..." Snapshot of people's engagement in their health care. Center for Advancing Health. cfah.org/activities/snapshot.cfm. May 20, 2010. Accessed May 2, 2011.

164 "What do engaged patients do? ..." Hibbard JH, Stockard J, Mahoney ER, Tusler, M. Development of the Patient Activation Measure (PAM): Conceptualizing and measuring activation in patients and consumers. *Health Serv Res*. 2004;39(4 Pt 1):1005-1026.

164 "Consider that physicians spend ..." Choice in medical care: When should the consumer decide? Academy Health website. academyhealth.org/files/issues/ConsumerDecide.pdf. October 2007. Accessed May 4, 2011.

164 "They forget 40-80 percent ..." Kessels, RP. Patients' memory for medical information. *J R Soc Med*. 2003;96(5):219-222.

165 "Six out of 10 ..." Jammed access: Widening the front door to healthcare. PricewaterhouseCoopers website. pwc.com/us/en/healthcare/publications/jammed-access-widening-the-front-door-to-healthcare.jhtml. July 2009. Accessed May 2, 2011.

165 "Researcher Judith Hibbard ..." Hibbard J. Engaging consumers to improve health and reduce costs. Presentation, Alliance for Health Reform. March 5, 2010.

166 "The typical health consumer ..." Center for Advancing Health, op. cit.

166 "In his book *Tracking Medicine* ..." Wenner JE. *Tracking Medicine: A Researcher's Quest to Understand Health Care*. New York: Oxford; 2010.

168 "The average physician visit ..." Mauksch LB. Relationship, communication, and efficiency in the medical encounter. *Ann Intern Med*. 2008;168(13):1387-1395.

168 "The average patient ..." Marvel MK. Soliciting the patient's agenda: Have we improved? *JAMA*. 1999;281(3):283-287.

168 "In a University of Michigan study ..." Zulman DM, Kerr EA, Hofer TP, Heisler M, Zikmund-Fisher BJ . Patient-provider concordance in the prioritization of health conditions among hypertensive diabetes patients. *J Gen Intern Med*. 2010; 25(5):408-414.

169 "Seven out of 10 ..." Newport F. Most Americans take doctor's advice without second opinion. Gallup website. gallup.com/poll/145025/americans-doctor-advice-without-second-opinion.aspx. December 2, 2010. Accessed May 2, 2011.

170 "A 2-year-old is diagnosed ..." Institute of Medicine. *Health Literacy: A Prescription to End Confusion*. Washington, D.C.: The National Academies Press; 2004.

170 "As preposterous as this true story seems ..." Parker RM, Ratzan SC, Lurie N. Health literacy: A policy challenge for advancing high-quality health care. *Health Aff*. 2003;22(4): 147-153.

171 "One hospital study found ..." Williams, M, Parker R, Baker D, et al. Inadequate functional health literacy among patients at two public hospitals. *JAMA*.1995;274(21):1677-1682.

171 "Almost half of the U.S. population ..." Kirsch I, Jungeblut A, Jenkins L, Kolstad A. *Adult Literacy in America: A First Look at the Results of the National Adult Literacy Survey*. Washington, D.C.: U.S. Department of Education, National Center for Education Statistics, 1993; 1993.

171 "One out of 4 patients ..." Lipkus IM, Samsa G, Rimer BK. General performance on a numeracy scale among high education samples. *Med Decis Making*. 2001;21(1):37-44.

171 "Educational attainment certainly is important ..." Institute of Medicine, op. cit.

171 "For example, 16 percent of highly educated people ..." Lipkus IM, op. cit.

171 "A classic example: ..." Schmitz M. Rudy Giuliani's battle with prostate cancer. About.com

website. prostatecancer.about.com/od/patientandfamilysupport/a/rudygiulianiprostatecancer.htm. December 30, 2009. Accessed May 2, 2011.

171 "Unfortunately, patients often either hide ..." Institute of Medicine, op. cit.

171 "In a study at a women's clinic ..." Lindau S, Tomori C, Lyons T, Langseth I, Bennett C, Garcia P. The association of health literacy with cervical cancer prevention knowledge and health behaviors in a multiethnic cohort of women. *Am J Obster Gynecol*. 2002;186:938-943.

171 "Literacy skills predict health status ..." Wilson J. The crucial link between literacy and health. *Ann Intern Med*. 2003;139(10):875-878.

171 "A review of 96 studies ..." Berkman ND, Sheridan SL, Donahue KE, Halpern DJ, Crotty K. Low health literacy and health outcomes: An updated systematic review. *Ann Intern Med*. 2011;155(2):97-107.

172 "More than 300 studies ..." Institute of Medicine, op. cit.

172 "An analysis of Medicaid applications ..." Susmita P, Kavanagh J, Song L, et al. Literacy level of Medicaid applications and child Medicaid retention rates: Comparison across 50 states. Presentation, American Academy of Pediatrics annual meeting, Vancouver, B.C., May 1, 2010.

172 "The National Work Group on Literacy and Health ..." Wilson J, op. cit.

173 "The American Medical Association ..." Kon, AA. The shared decision-making continuum. *JAMA*. 2010;304(8):903-904.

173 "Patients make a large number ..." Wennberg D, Barbeau B, Gerry E. Power to the Patient: The importance of shared decision-making. Health Dialog website. resources. healthdialog.com/Power-to-the-Patient-Research.html. June 2009. Accessed May 2, 2011.

173 "One study found a 20 to 30 percent reduction ..." O'Connor A, Stacey D, Entwistle V, et al. Decision aids for people facing health treatment or screening decisions. *Cochrane Database Syst Rev*. 2003;(2):CD001431.

174 "There are other benefits ..." Crawford M, Rutter D, Manley C, et al. Systematic review of involving patients in the planning and development of health care. *BMJ*. 2002;325:1263-1266.

174 "Wennberg and several colleagues ..." Wennberg JE, op. cit.

174 "In another study of treatment ..." Barry MJ, Fowler FJ, Mulley AG, Henderson JV, Wennberg JE. Patient reactions to a program designed to facilitate patient participation in treatment decisions for benign prostatic hyperplasia. *Medical Care*. 1995;33(8):771-782.

174 "A study of nine common medical decisions ..." Zikmund-Fisher, Couper MP, Singer E, et al. The DECISIONS Study: A nationwide survey of United States adults regarding 9 common medical decisions. *Med Decis Making*. 2010:30(5 suppl.): 20S-34S.

175 "Use of decision aids ..." O'Connor AM, Bennett CL, Stacey D, et al. Decision aids for people facing health treatment or screening decisions. *Cochrane Database of Systematic Reviews*. 2009; (3):CD001431.

175 "In one study ..." Wennberg JE, op. cit.

175 "In theory, physicians are in favor of decision aids ..." Wennberg D, op. cit.

176 "One out of 2 patients ..." Health reform—prospering in a post-reform world. PricewaterhouseCoopers website. pwc.com/us/en/health-industries/publications/prospering-in-a-post-reform-world.jhtml. May, 2010. Accessed May 2, 2011; The customization of diagnosis, care and cure. pwc.com/us/en/healthcast/index.jhtml?wt.ac=healthindustries_healthcast. May 2010. Accessed May 11, 2011

176 "In fact, seeking health information ..." Fox, S. 80% of Internet users look for health information online. Pew Research Center website. pewinternet.org/Reports/2011/HealthTopics.aspx. February 1, 2011. Accessed May 2, 2011.

176 "The avid users ..." "Cyberchondriacs" on the rise? Harris Interactive website. harrisinteractive.com/NewsRoom/HarrisPolls/tabid/447/mid/1508/articleId/448/ctl/ReadCustom%20Default/Default.aspx. August 4, 2010. Accessed May 2, 2011.

176 "The most frequent reasons ..." McDaid D, Park A. Online health: Untangling the Web. Bupa website. bupa.com/jahia/webdav/site/bupacom/shared/Documents/PDFs/media-centre/Health%20Pulse%20-%20HW/Online%20Health%20-%20Untangling%20the%20Web.pdf. January 4, 2011. Accessed May 2, 2011.

176 "More than half who sought ..." Tu HT, Cohen GR. Striking jump in consumers seeking health care information. Center for Studying Health System Change. hschange.org/CONTENT/1006/. August 2008. Accessed May 2, 2011.

176 "Researchers reviewed 343 website pages ..." Bernstam EV, Walji MF, Sagaram S, et al. Commonly cited website quality criteria are not effective at identifying inaccurate online information about breast cancer. *Cancer.* 2008;112(6):1206-1213.

177 "A large 1979 California study ..."Berkman LF, Syme SI. Social networks: Host resistance and mortality: A nine-year follow-up study of Alameda County residents. *Am J Epidemiol.* 1979;109:186-204.

177 "People trust information ..." 2008 Edelman trust barometer. Edelman website. edelman.com/trust/2008/trustbarometer08_Final.pdf. Accessed May 2, 2011.

177 "A 2009 poll found ..." Kaiser Health tracking poll: 2009. kff.org/kaiserpolls/upload/7944.pdf. Accessed May 11, 2011.

177 "Dr. Michael Fisch ..." Parker-Pope T. You're sick. Now what? Knowledge is power. *The New York Times,* September 30, 2008.

178 "Most U.S. adults still trust ..." Fox, S. Mobile Health 2010. PewResearchCenter website. pewinternet.org/Reports/2010/Mobile-Health-2010.aspx. October 19, 2010. Accessed May 2, 2011.

Chapter 14. Chronic Disease

Page 179 "Of every Medicare dollar ..." 2009 almanac of chronic disease: The impact of chronic disease on U.S. health and prosperity. Partnership to Fight Chronic Disease. fightchronicdisease.org/pdfs/2009_PFCDAlmanac.pdf. 2009. Accessed March 5, 2011.

179 "Chronic conditions account for about three-quarters ..." Coordinating chronic care management through health information exchanges. Deloitte Center for Health Solutions. deloitte.com/assets/Dcom-UnitedStates/Local%20Assets/Documents/us_chs_ChronicCare ManagementHIEs_w.pdf. 2007. Accessed March 5, 2011.

179 "Now more than 1 in 4 Americans ..." Cassil, A. Rising rates of chronic health conditions: What can be done? Center for Studying Health System Change Research Brief 125. hschange.com/CONTENT/1027/November 2008. Accessed March 5, 2011.

180 "Mental illness and chronic disease ..." The power of prevention: Chronic disease ... the public health challenge of the 21st century. Centers for Disease Control. cdc.gov/chronicdisease/pdf/2009-Power-of-Prevention.pdf. 2009. Accessed March 5, 2011.

180 "Chronic disease is increasing ..." Chronic care: A call to action for health reform. AARP Public Policy Institute. assets.aarp.org/rgcenter/health/beyond_50_hcr.pdf. March 2009. Accessed March 5, 2011.

181 "A person who turns 65 years old ..." AARP Public Policy Institute, op. cit.

181 "Regardless, more than two-thirds ..." CDC, op. cit.

182 "World federations representing ..." Mbanya JC, Squire SB, Cazop E, Puska P. Mobilising the world for chronic NCDs. *The Lancet.* 2010;377(9765):536-537.

182 "As a result, nearly one in 6 ..." AARP Public Policy Institute, op. cit.

183 "About 81 million people ..." Brody J. Tackling care as chronic ailments pile up. *The New York Times.* February 21, 2011.

183 "The National Cancer Institute ..." Mariotto AB, Yabroff KR, SHao Y, Feuer EJ, Brown ML. Projections of the cost of cancer care in the United States: 2010-2020. *J Natl Cancer Inst.* 2011;103:1-12,

183 "The cost of treating ..." Heidenreich PA, Trogdon JG, Khavjou OA. Forecasting the future of cardiovascular disease in the United States. *Circulation.* 2011;123(8):933-944.

183 "More than 50 percent ..." The United States of diabetes: Challenges and opportunities in the decade ahead. UnitedHealth Group's Center for Health Reform & Modernization. united healthgroup.com/hrm/UNH_WorkingPaper5.pdf. November 2010. Accessed August 2, 2011.

184 "More than half of people..." Re-Forming health care: Americans speak out about chronic conditions and the pursuit of healthier lives. National Council on Aging fact sheet. ncoa.org/ assets/files/pdf/FINAL_Survey_Fact_Sheet_DC.pdf March 2009. Accessed March 4, 2011.

184 "According to one estimate ..." Ostbye T, Yarnall KS, Krause KM, Pollak KI, Gradison M, Michener JL. Is there time for management of patients with chronic diseases in primary care? *Ann Fam Med.* 2005;3:209-214.

185 "A 2005 review of studies ..." Heisler M. Health system strategies to improve chronic disease management and outcomes: What works? Center for Studying Health System Change website. hschange.com/CONTENT/1002/Heisler.pdf. July 31, 2008. Accessed March 22, 2011.

185 "In a 2001 survey ..." Anderson, G. Chronic care: Making the case for ongoing care. Robert Wood Johnson Foundation. rwjf.org/pr/product.jsp?id=50968. February 2010. Accessed March 5, 2011.

186 "Less than a third of U.S. physician practices ..." Carrier E, Reschavsky J. Expectations outpace reality: Physicians' use of care management tools for patients with chronic conditions. Center for Studying Helth System Change Research Brief No. 129. hschange.com/CONTENT/1101/. December 2009. Accessed March 5, 2011.

186 "Chronic disease hits people ..." Cassil, op. cit.

186 "Thirteen out of 15 Medicare ..." Peikes D, Chen A, Schore A, Brown R. Effects of care coordination on hospitalization, quality of care, and health care expenditures among Medicare beneficiaries: 15 randomized trials. *JAMA.*2009;301(6):603-608.

187 "A 2008 *Health Affairs* survey ..." Schoen C, Osborn R, How S, Doty MM, Peugh J. In chronic condition: Experiences of patients with complex health care needs, in eight countries, 2008. *Health Aff.* 2009;28(1):w1-w16.

188 "According to research ..." Bernstein J, Chollet D, Peterson GG. Disease management: Does it work? Mathematica Policy Research. mathematica-mpr.com/publications/PDFs/health/ reformhealthcare_IB4.pdf. May 2010. Accessed March 5, 2011.

188 "Other factors that contribute to success ..." Brandt, S, Hartmann S, Hehner S. How to design a successful disease-management program. McKinsey Quarterly. mckinseyquarterly.com/ How_to_design_a_successful_disease-management_program_2685. October 2010. Accessed March 5, 2011.

188 "The gold standard in disease management ..." Wagner EH, Austin BT, Davis C, Hindmarsh, Schaefer J, Bonomi A. Improving chronic illness care: Translating evidence into action. *Health Aff.* 2001;20(6):64-78.

189 "Chronic-disease management nationally increased ..." Shortell S, Gillies R, Siddque J, et al. Improving chronic illness care: A longitudinal cohort analysis of large physician organizations. *Med Care.* 2009;47(9):932-939.

189 "Chronic disease is an unquestionable financial drain ..." AARP Public Policy Institute, op. cit.

190 "How much a person ..." Joyce GF, Keeler EB, Shang B, Goldman DP. The lifetime burden of chronic disease among the elderly. *Health Aff.* 2005;W5-R18-R29.

190 "Chronic-disease sufferers often ..." Cunningham PJ. Chronic burdens: The persistently high out-of-pocket health care expenses faced by many Americans with chronic conditions. The Commonwealth Fund. commonwealthfund.org/Content/Publications/Issue-Briefs/2009/Jul/ Chronic-Burdens-The-Persistently-High-Out-of-Pocket-Health-Care-Expenses-Faced-by-Many-Americans.aspx July 2009. Accessed March 5, 2011.

190 "Therefore it is not surprising ..." National Council on Aging fact sheet, op. cit.

190 "The uninsured often simply suffer ..." Wilper AP. A national study of chronic disease prevalence and access to care in uninsured U.S. adults. *Ann Intern Med.* 2008:149(3):170-176

190 "If they make it to age 65 ..." McWilliams J, Meara E, Zaslavsky A, Ayanian JZ. Health of previously uninsured adults after acquiring Medicare coverage. *JAMA.* 2007;298(24):2886-2894.

190 "The Milken Institute calculated ..." The economic burden of chronic disease on the United States. The Milken Institute. chronicdiseaseimpact.com/. October 2007. Accessed March 5, 2011.

191 "Two decades ago ..." Thorpe KE, Ogden TL, Galactionova K. Chronic conditions account for rise in Medicare spending from 1987 to 2006. *Health Aff.* 2010;29(4): 718-724.

191 "A patient's engagement ..." AARP Public Policy Institute, op. cit.

192 "Research has confirmed ..." Sarasohn-Kahn, J. Participatory health: Online and mobile tools help chronically ill manage their care. California HealthCare Foundation. chcf.org/publications/2009/09/participatory-health-online-and-mobile-tools-help-chronically-ill-manage-their-care September 2009. Accessed March 5, 2011.

192 "An AARP survey ..." Barrett LL. Healthy @ home. AARP website. assets.aarp.org/rgcenter/il/healthy_home.pdf. March 2008. Accessed April 5, 2011.

192 "However, once they go online ..." Fox, S. E-patients with a disability or chronic disease. Pew Internet & American Life Project. pewinternet.org/Reports/2007/Epatients-With-a-Disability-or-Chronic-Disease.aspx October 8, 2007. Accessed March 5, 2011.

192 "Those with chronic diseases also ..." Fox S, Purcell K. Chronic disease and the Internet. Pew Internet & American Life Project. pewinternet.org/Reports/2010/Chronic-Disease.aspx March 24, 2010. Accessed March 5, 2011.

Chapter 15. National Health Costs

Page 195 "Health care costs grew ..." Martin A, Lassman D Whittle L, Catlin A. Recession contributes to slowest annual rate of increase in health spending in five decades. *Health Aff.* 2011;30(1):11-22.

195 "Health costs reached another ..." Consumer price index—April 2011. U.S. Bureau of Labor Statistics website. bls.gov/news.release/archives/cpi_08132010.pdf. August 13, 2010. Accessed May 24, 2011.

195 "Employer health costs were expected ..." PricewaterhouseCoopers. Behind the numbers: Medical cost trends for 2012. pwc.com/us/en/health-industries/publications/behind-the-numbers-medical-cost-trends-2012.jhtml. May 2011. Accessed May 24, 2011.

195 "Health spending is rising faster ..." Health care spending in the United States and selected OECD countries, April 2011. Kaiser Family Foundation website. kff.org/insurance/snapshot/OECD042111.cfm. April 2011. Accessed May 24, 2011.

196 "The U.S. is expected to spend ..." Keehan SP, Sisko AM, Truffer CJ, et al. National health spending projections through 2020: Economic recovery and reform drive faster spending growth. *Health Aff.* 2011;30(8); OECD Health Data 2010: Statistics and Indicators. oecd.org/document/30/0,3746,en_2649_37407_12968734_1_1_1_37407,00.html. Accessed May 24, 2011.

196 "Peter Orszag, former director ..." Congressional testimony, Committee on the Budget, U.S. Senate. June 21, 2007.

196 "The current trend ..." Dentzer S. Rolling the rock up the mountain. *Health Aff.* 2009; 28(5):1250-1252.

196 "Federal Reserve Chairman ..." Irwin N, Montgomery L. Federal Reserve Chairman Ben Bernanke sounds a warning on growing deficit. *The Washington Post.* April 8, 2010.

196 "Americans clearly do not ..." Murray M. NBC/WSJ poll: Voters deficit-worried but wary of cuts. msnbc.msn.com/id/41876558/ns/politics/. March 2, 2011. Accessed May 24, 2011;

McClatchy-Marist poll. maristpoll.marist.edu/418-mcclatchy-marist-poll/ April 18, 2011. Accessed June 6, 2011.

196 "About half believe neither program ..." AP-GfK poll: Medicare doesn't have to be cut. abcnews.go.com/Politics/wireStory?id=13662567. May 23, 2011. Accessed May 24, 2011.

196 "From late 2007 to February 2011 ..." Health sector economic indicators. Altarum Institute website. altarum.org/files/imce/CSHS-Labor-Brief_May%202011_051711.pdf. May 17, 2011. Accessed May 24, 2011.

197 "McKinsey Global Institute ..." Accounting for the cost of U.S. health care: A new look at why Americans spend more. McKinsey Global Institute. mckinsey.com/mgi/publications/US_healthcare/Executive_Summary.asp. December 2008. Accessed May 24, 2011.

198 "In a classic *Health Affairs* study ..." Anderson GF, Reinhardt UE, Hussey PS, Petrosyan V. It's the prices, stupid: Why the United States is so different from other countries. *Health Aff.* 2003;22(3):89-103.

198 "For example, the U.S. consumes ..." McKinsey, op. cit.

198 "It also has the lowest ..." Vladeck BC, Rice T. Market failure and the failure of discourse: Facing up to the power of sellers. *Health Aff.* 2009;28(5):1305-1315.

199 "Mike Leavitt ..." Leavitt: Gov't should stay out of drug pricing. MSNBC website. msnbc.msn.com/id/15703562/ns/politics/t/leavitt-govt-should-stay-out-drug-pricing/ November 13, 2006. Accessed June 6, 2011.

200 "Other nations do not have ..." Fuchs, VR. Government payment for health care—causes and consequences. *N Engl J Med.* 2010;363(23):2181-2183.

200 "The International Federation of Health Plans ..." IFHP survey of medical costs by unit shows price differences of more than 300 percent between countries. International Federation of Health Plans website. ifhp.com/documents/IFHP_news_release_FINAL_000.pdf. November 22, 2010. Accessed May 24, 2011.

200 "Even though U.S. physicians ..." Bodenheimer T. High and rising health care costs. Part 3: The role of health care providers. *Ann Intern Med.* 2005;142:996-1002.

202 "The U.S. spends about six times ..." Goodell S, Ginsburg PB. High and rising health care costs: Demystifying U.S. health care spending. Robert Wood Johnson Foundation website. rwjf.org/files/research/101508.policysynthesis.costdrivers.brief.pdf. October 2008. Accessed May 24, 2011.

203 "The comparative lack of productivity gains ..." Goodell , op. cit.

203 "Increased productivity requires ..." Vladeck, op. cit.

204 "The National Center for Health Statistics ..." National Center for Health Statistics. *Health, United States, 2009: With special feature on medical technology.* Hyattsville, MD: U.S. Department of Health and Human Services.

204 "Health-care providers have aggressively ..." McKinsey op cit.

206 "An average of 2,200 U.S. physicians ..." Behind the numbers: Medical cost trends for 2012. PricewaterhouseCoopers website. pwc.com/us/en/health-industries/publications/behind-the-numbers-medical-cost-trends-2012.jhtml. May 2011. Accessed June 1, 2011.

206 "The Center for Studying Health System Change ..." Felland LE, Grossman JM, Tu HT. Key findings from HSC's 2010 site visits: Health care markets weather economic downturn, brace for health reform. Center for Studying Health System Change. hschange.org/CONTENT/1209/. May 2011. Accessed June 1, 2011.

207 "However, Massachusetts Inspector ..." McConville C. IG seeks power to rein in rising health-care cost. *The Boston Herald.* June 28, 2011.

207 "After a wave of hospital mergers ..." Vogt WB, Town R. How has hospital consolidation affected the price and quality of hospital care? Robert Wood Johnson Foundation Research Synthesis Report No. 9. Robert Wood Johnson Foundation website. rwjf.org/files/research/no9researchreport.pdf. February 2006. Accessed April 18, 2011.

207 "According to an investigation …" Investigation of health care cost trends and cost drivers. Office of the Massachusetts. Attorney General Martha Coakley. mass.gov/Cago/docs/healthcare/Investigation_HCCT&CD.pdf. January 29, 2010. Accessed April 20, 2011.

207 "In 2009, Medicare and Medicaid paid hospitals …" TrendWatch Chartbook 2011. American Hospital Association website. aha.org/aha/research-and-trends/chartbook/index.html. Accessed June 1, 2010.

208 "On average, commercial-insurance rate …" Berenson RA, Ginsburg PB, Kemper N. Unchecked provider clout in California foreshadows challenges to health reform. *Health Aff.* 2010;29(4):699-705.

208 "For example, some California …" Berenson RA, Ginsburg PB, Kemper N. Unchecked provider clout in California foreshadows challenges to health reform. *Health Aff.* 2010;29: 699-705.

208 "In a HealthDay/Harris Interactive poll …" Goodwin J. Poll finds Americans blame insurers, drug companies for rising health costs. HealthDay. March 24, 2010.

208 "A 2009 analysis of hospital finances …" Fox M. U.S. hospital profits fall to zero: Thomson Reuters. reuters.com/article/2009/03/02/us-hospitals-usa-idUSTRE5216G320090302. March 2, 2009. Accessed June 1, 2011.

209 "According to a 2007 Congressional Budget Office …" Congressional Budget Office. Financing projected spending in the long-run. cbo.gov/ftpdocs/82xx/doc8295/07-09-Financing_Spending.pdf. July 9, 2007. Accessed June 1, 2011.

210 "Steven Schroeder, distinguished professor …" Schroeder SA. Personal reflections on the high cost of American medical care. *Arch Intern Med.* 2011;171(8):722-727.

Chapter 16. Consumer Health Costs

Page 211 "In less than a decade …" 2011 Milliman Medical Index: Health care costs for American families double in less than nine years. publications.milliman.com/periodicals/mmi/pdfs/milliman-medical-index-2011.pdf May 2011. Accessed May 23, 2011.

211 "Most people have only a vague notion …" Congressional Budget Office. The long-term budget outlook: Federal debt held by the public under two budget scenarios. cbo.gov/ftpdocs/115xx/doc11579/06-30-LTBO.pdf June 2010 (revised August 2010). Accessed May 23, 2011; Estimated state median income, by family size and by state for FY 2009. August 2010). Accessed May 23, 2011; Estimated state median income, by family size and by state for FY 2009. cec.sped.org/Content/NavigationMenu/SpecialEdCareers/ESTIMATED_STATE_MEDIAN_INCOME.pdf. Accessed May 26, 2011.

212 "Before the introduction of Medicare …" Baicker K, Goldman D. Patient cost-sharing and healthcare spending growth. Journal of Economic Perspectives. 2011;25(2):47-68; Accounting for the cost of U.S. health care: A new look at why Americans spend more. McKinsey Global Institute. mckinsey.com/mgi/publications/US_healthcare/Executive_Summary.asp. December 2008. Accessed May 24, 2011.

212 "A Deloitte study estimates …" The hidden costs of U.S. health care for consumers: A comprehensive analysis. Deloitte website. deloitte.com/assets/Dcom-UnitedStates/Local%20Assets/Documents/US_CHS_HiddenCostsofUSHealthCareforConsumers_032111.pdf. March 2011. Accessed May 23, 2011.

212 "The inability to pay medical bills …" Medical bills still top consumer woe, CR poll finds. Consumer Reports website. news.consumerreports.org/health/2011/03/medical-bill-still-top-consumer-woe-cr-poll-finds.html. March 22, 2011. Accessed May 23, 2011.

212 "About 40 percent of Americans …" Herman PM, Rissi JJ, Walsh ME. Health insurance status, medical debt, and their impact on access to care in Arizona. *Am J Public Health.* 2011;101(8):1437-1443.

212 "Even more disturbing ..." Kaiser Health tracking poll. kff.org/kaiserpolls/8058.cfm. March 2010. Accessed May 23, 2011.

212 "Nearly 6 out of 10 say ..." Stremikis K, Schoen C, Fryer A. A call for change: The 2011 Commonwealth Fund survey of public views of the U.S. health system. The Commonwealth Fund. commonwealthfund.org/~/media/Files/Publications/Issue%20Brief/2011/Apr/1492_Stremikis_public_views_2011_survey_ib.pdf. April 2011. Accessed May 23, 2011.

214 "According to an ongoing ..." Cunningham PJ, Felland LE. Falling behind: Americans' access to medical care deteriorates, 2003-2007. Center for Studying Health System Change. hschange.org/CONTENT/993/. June 2008. Accessed May 23, 2011.

214 "Even two-thirds ..." Stremikis K, op cit.

214 "Women experience greater ..." Rustgi SD, Doty MM, Collins SR. Women at risk: Why many women are forgoing needed health care. The Commonwealth Fund. commonwealthfund.org/~/media/Files/Publications/Issue%20Brief/2009/May/Women%20at%20Risk/PDF_1262_Rustgi_women_at_risk_issue_brief_Final.pdfMay 2009. Accessed May 23, 2011.

214 " For the 40 percent ..." Collins SR, Doty MM, Robertson R, Garber T. Help on the horizon: How the recession has left millions of workers without health insurance, and how health reform will bring relief. The Commonwealth Fund. commonwealthfund.org/~/media/Files/Publications/Fund%20Report/2011/Mar/1486_Collins_help_on_the_horizon_2010_biennial_survey_report_FINAL_v2.pdf. March 2011. Accessed May 23, 2011.

215 "More than 25 percent of Americans ..." Lusardi A, Schneider DJ, Tufano P. The economic crisis and medical care usage. National Bureau of Economic Research. nber.org/papers/w15843. March 2010. Accessed May 23, 2011.

215 "About 70 percent of U.S. hospitals ..." Hospitals continue to feel lingering effects of the economic recession, June 2010. American Hospital Association website. aha.org/aha/research-and-trends/index.html. Accessed May 28, 2011.

216 "Health plans have reported record profits ..." Pear R. Insurers told to justify rate increases over 10 percent. *The New York Times*. May 19, 2011.

216 "A February 2010 Moody's Investor Service ..." Moody's says benefits changes help curb care use. Associated Press. finance.yahoo.com/news/Moodys-says-benefits-changes-apf-1503081562.html?x=0&.v=1. February 16, 2011. Accessed May 18, 2011.

216 "However, according to a forecast ..." PricewaterhouseCoopers. Behind the numbers: Medical cost trends for 2012. pwc.com/us/en/health-industries/publications/behind-the-numbers-medical-cost-trends-2012.jhtml. May 2011. Accessed May 24, 2011.

217 "An American Psychological Association survey ..." 2010 stress in America report. American Psychological Association website. apa.org/news/press/releases/stress/national-report.pdf. November 9, 2010. Accessed June 2, 2011.

217 "About 40 percent of employees ..." Darling H. The recession's toll on employees' health: Results of a new National Business Group on Health survey. National Business Group on Health website. wbgh.org/pdfs/PRESS%20CONFERENCE-%20RECESSION%20IMPACT%20ON%20EMPLOYEES%20052009.pdf. May 27, 2009. Accessed May 26, 2011.

218 "The risk of heart attack ..." Gallo W, Teng H, Falba T, Kasl S Krumholz H, Bradley E. The impact of late career job loss on myocardial infarction and stroke: A 10 year follow up using the Health and Retirement survey. *Occup Environ Med*. 2006;10:683-687.

218 "A 2006 study ..." Strully K. Job loss and health in the U.S. labor market. *Demography*. 2009;46(2):221-246.

218 "The death rate of high-seniority male employees ..." Sullivan D, Von Wachter T. Mortality mass layoffs, and career outcomes: An analysis using administrative data. Nation Bureau of Economic Research Working Paper No. 13626. nber.org/papers/w13626 November 2007. Accessed May 28, 2011.

218 "A University of North Carolina economics professor ..." Ruhm C. Are recessions good for your health? *Quarterly Journal of Economics.* 2000;115(2):617-650.

218 "He also discovered ..." Ruhm C. Health living in hard times. *Journal of Health Economics.* 2005;24:341-363.

218 "Other health behaviors ..." Biddle J, Hamermes D. Sleep and the allocation of time. *Journal of Political Economics.* 1990;98:922-943; Granados T. Increasing mortality during the expansions of the U.S. economy, 1900-1996. Int J Epidemiol. 2005;34(6):1194-1202.

218 "Low-income workers ..." Edwards R. Who is hurt by procyclical economy? *Soc Sci Med.* 2008;67(12):2051-2058.

218 "Difficult economic times ..." Catalon R. Health, medical care, and economic crisis. *N Engl J Med.* 2009;360(8):749-751.

218 "In 2010, employers and health plans ..." PricewaterhouseCoopers. Behind the numbers: Medical cost trends for 2012. pwc.com/us/en/health-industries/publications/behind-the-numbers-medical-cost-trends-2012.jhtml. May 2011. Accessed May 24, 2011.

219 "A recession even affects ..." Guttmacher Institute. A real-time look at the impact of the recession on women's family planning and pregnancy decisions. guttmacher.org/pubs/RecessionFP.pdfSeptember 2009. Accessed May 26, 2011.

220 "The uninsured are especially disadvantaged ..." Shortchanged by medical debt fact sheet. Families USA. familiesusa.org/assets/pdfs/medical-debt-fact-sheet.pdf November 2009. Accessed May 23, 2011.

220 "Only 1 out of 8 ..." Chappel A. *The value of health insurance: Few of the uninsured have adequate resources to pay potential hospital bills.* ASPE Research Brief; May 2011.

220 "Medical expenses contributed ..." Himmelstein DJ, Thorne D, Warren E, Woolhandler S. Medical bankruptcy in the United States, 2007: Results of a national study. *Am J Med.* 2009; 122(8):741-746; Medical bills underlie 60 percent of U.S. bankruptcies: study. Reuters website. reuters.com/article/2009/06/04/us-healthcare-bankruptcy-idUSTRE5530Y020090604. June 4, 2009. Accessed May 26, 2011.

221 "Besides having a better medical safety nets ..." Oberlander J, White J. Public attitudes toward health care spending aren't the problem; prices are. *Health Aff.* 2009;28(5):1285-1293.

221 "Himmelstein also examined ..." Himmelstein DJ, Thorne D, Woolhandler S. Medical bankruptcy in Massachusetts: Has health reform made a difference? *Am J Med.* 2011;124(3): 224-228.

221 "Other researchers say ..." Dranove D, Millenson ML. Medical bankruptcy: Myth versus fact. *Health Aff.* 2006;25:w74-w83.

221 "A study of medical financial burden ..." Robertson CT, Egelhof R, Hoke M. Get sick, get out: The medical causes of home mortgage foreclosures. *Health Matrix: Journal of Law-Medicine.* 2008;18(65).

222 "A study focusing on the elderly ..." Pottow JA. The rise in elder bankruptcy filings and failure of U.S. bankruptcy law. Public Law and Legal Theory Working Paper Series. University of Michigan Law School. papers.ssrn.com/sol3/papers.cfm?abstract_id=1669298 . August 2010. Accessed May 23, 2011.

222 "Seniors spend about 10 percent ..." Desmond KA, Rice T, Cubanski J, Neuman P. The burden of out-of-pocket health spending among older versus younger adults: Analysis from the consumer expenditure survey, 1998-2003. Kaiser Family Foundation website. kff.org/medicare/upload/7686.pdf. September 2007. Accessed May 23, 2011.

222 "According to Fidelity Investments ..." Fidelity Investments estimates couples retiring in 2010 will need $250,000 to pay medical expenses during retirement. fidelity.com/inside-fidelity/employer-services/fidelity-estimates-couple-retiring-in-2010-will-need-250000-to-cover-healthcare-costs. March 25, 2010. Accessed May 26, 2011.

222 "The Center for Retirement Research ..." Webb A, Zhivan N. What is the distribution of lifetime health care costs from age 65? Center for Retirement Research at Boston College website. prudential.com/media/managed/Distri_of_Lifetime_Health_Costs_from_age65.pdf March 2010. Accessed May 26, 2011.

222 "Retirees spend about 10 percent ..." Johnson RW, Mommaerts C. Will health care costs bankrupt aging boomers? Urban Institute. urban.org/uploadedpdf/412026_health_care_costs.pdf. February 2010. Accessed May 23, 2010.

223 "Three out of 4 baby boomers ..." New MainStay investments survey finds that 76 percent of pre-retirees are willing to work longer and save more today to live more comfortably tomorrow. nylim.com/portal/site/nylim/menuitem.f550dba0610de3f1d629658ada48c1ca/?vgnextoid=d6bc855d9be3a210VgnVCM100000ac841cacRCRD&vgnextchannel=a185195231e64210VgnVCM100000ac841cacRCRD. August 5, 2010. Accessed May 23, 2011.

223 "The number of workers enrolled ..." The Kaiser Family Foundation and Health Research & Educational Trust. Employer Health Benefits 2010 Annual Survey. ehbs.kff.org/pdf/2010/8085.pdf. Accessed May 18, 2011.

223 "The average deductible ..." Health benefit cost growth accelerates to 6.9% in 2010. Mercer website. mercer.com/press-releases/1400235. November 17, 2010. Accessed May 18, 2011.

224 "Companies with at least 50 percent ..." Purchasing value in health care. Towers Watson website. towerswatson.com/assets/pdf/1258/WT-2010-15571.pdf. 2010. Accessed May 18, 2011.

224 "Nearly 25 percent ..." Kullgren JT, Galbraith AA, Hinrichsen VL, et al. Health care use and decision making among lower-income families in high-deductible health plans. *Arch Intern Med.* 2010;170(21):1918-1925.

224 "Nearly two-thirds ..." Majority of large employers revising health benefit programs for 2011, National Business Group on Health survey finds. businessgrouphealth.org/pressrelease.cfm?ID=162. August 18, 2010. Accessed May 26, 2011.

224 "The typical CDHP member ..." Fronstin P. Health savings accounts and health reimbursement arrangements: Assets, account balances, and rollovers, 2006-2009. Employee Research Benefit Institute issue brief. June (343):1-30

225 "The average household income ..." Health Savings Accounts: Participation increased and was more common among individuals with higher incomes. gao.gov/new.items/d08474r.pdf. Government Accounting Office website. April 1, 2008. Accessed May 18, 2011.

225 "They are less likely ..." Findings from the 2010 EBRI/MGA consumer engagement in health care survey. Employee Benefit Research Institute website. ebri.org/pdf/briefspdf/EBRI_IB_12-2010_No352_CEHCS.pdfDecember 2010. Accessed May 18, 2011.

225 "RAND Corp. conducted groundbreaking ..." Manning WG, Newhouse JP, Keeler EB, Leibowitz A, Marquis MS. Health insurance and the demand for medical care: Evidence from a randomized experiment. *American Economic Review.* 1987;77(3):251-277.

226 "Another recent RAND study ..." Haviland AM, Sood N, McDevitt R, Marquis MS. How do consumer-directed health plans affect vulnerable populations? *Forum for Health Economics & Policy.* 2011;14(2).

226 "One study of health plans ..." Trivedi AN, Moloo H, Mor V. Increased ambulatory care copayments and hospitalizations among the elderly. *N Engl J Med.* 2010;362(4):320-328.

226 "For example, Pitney Bowes ..." Mahoney JJ. Value-based benefit design: Using a predictive modeling approach to improve compliance. *Journal of Managed Care Pharmacy.* 2008;14(6 Suppl. B):3-8.

226 "A 2007 study concluded ..." Goldman DP, Joyce G, Zheng. Varying pharmacy benefits with clinical status: The case of cholesterol-lowering therapy. *JAMA.* 2007;298(1):61-69.

227 "What is puzzling is that HDHPs ..." Buntin MB, Haviland AM, McDevitt R, Sood N.

Healthcare spending and preventive care in high-deductible and consumer-directed health plans. *Am J Manag Care*. 2011;17(3):222-230.

227 "For example, high cost-sharing ..." Solomon MD, Goldman DP, Joyce GF, Escarce JJ. Cost sharing and the initiation of drug therapy for the chronically ill. *Arch Intern Med*. 2009;169(8):740-748.

227 "The healthiest 50 percent ..." Blumberg LJ. High-risk pools—merely a stopgap reform. *N Engl J Med*. 2011;364:e39.

227 "The harsh reality ..." An unequal burden: The true cost of high-deductible health plans for communities of color. FamiliesUSA website. familiesusa.org/assets/pdfs/unequal-burden.pdf. September 2008. Accessed May 18, 2011.

228 "A 2008 consumer survey ..." Cordina J, Singhai S. What consumers want in health care. The McKinsey Quarterly. mckinseyquarterly.com/What_consumers_want_in_health_care_2145. June 2008. Accessed May 18, 2011.

228 "UCLA Medical Center included ..." Weaver C. Want to know what a hospital charges? Good luck. Kaiser Health News. kaiserhealthnews.org/Stories/2010/June/29/Hospital-Prices.aspx. June 29, 2010. Accessed May 18, 2011.

228 "More than 30 states ..." Sinaiko AD, Rosenthal MB. Increased price transparency in health care—challenges and potential effect. *N Engl J Med*. 2011;364(10):891-894.

229 "Consumers do not even shop ..." Tu HT, May JH. Self-pay markets in health care: Consumer nirvana or caveat emptor. *Health Aff*. 2007;26(2):w217-w226.

Chapter 17. Waste and Overtreatment

Page 231 "A 2005 report ..." National Academy of Sciences, National Academy of Engineering and Institute of Medicine. *Rising Above the Storm, Revisited*. Washington, D.C.: The National Academies Press; 2005.

232 "It is difficult to fathom ..." McGlynn EA, Asch SM, Adams J, et al. The quality of health care delivered to adults in the United States. *N Engl J Med*. 2003;348(26):2635-2645.

232 "However, delivering all of the ..." Bodenheimer T, Pham HH. Primary care: Current problems and proposed solutions. *Health Aff*. 2010;29(5):799-805.

232 "Dr. Jack Wennberg ..." State of the nation's health. Dartmouth Medicine website. dartmed.dartmouth.edu/spring07/pdf/atlas.pdf. Spring 2007. Accessed June 5, 2011.

232 "The Congressional Budget Office ..." Congressional Budget Office. Opportunities to increase efficiency in health care. Statement of director Peter R. Orszag at the Health Reform Summit, June 16, 2008.

232 "PricewaterhouseCoopers' (PwC) Health Research Institute ..." The price of excess. PricewaterhouseCoopers website. pwc.com/us/en/healthcare/publications/the-price-of-excess. jhtml. 2010. Accessed June 5, 2011.

232 "A Thomson Reuters analysis ..." Kelley B, Fabius R. A path to eliminating $3.6 trillion in wasteful health-care spending. Thomson Reuters website. thomsonreuters.com/content/healthcare/pdf/white_papers/path_eliminating_36_trillion. 2010. Accessed May 25, 2011.

232 "A 2008 RAND Corp. study ..." Bentley TG, Effros RM, Palar K, Keeler EB. Waste in the U.S. health care system: A conceptual framework. *Milbank Q*. 2008;86(4):629-659.

233 "In 2002, 180 patients ...´Moseley JB, O'Malley K, Petersen NJ, et al. A controlled trial of arthroscopic surgery for osteoarthritis of the knee. *N Engl J Med*. 2002;347(2):137-139.

233 "A second set of researchers ..." Kirkley A, Birmingham TB, Litchfield RB, et al. A randomized trial of arthroscopic surgery for osteoarthritis of the knee. *N Engl J Med*. 2008; 359: 1097-1107.

233 "Two recent randomized trials ..." Kallmes DF, Comstock BA, Heagerty PJ, et al. A randomized controlled trial of vertebroplasty for osteoporotic spine fractures. *N Engl J Med*.

2009;361(6):569-579; Buchbinder R, Osborne RH, Ebeling PR, et al. A randomized trial of vertebroplast for painful osteoporatic vertebral fractures. *N Engl J Med.* 2009;361(6):557-568.

234 "Brookings Institution economist Henry Aaron ..." Aaron HJ. The costs of health care administration in the United States and Canada—questionable answers to a questionable question. *N Eng J Med.* 2003;349:801-803.

234 "For example, Johns Hopkins Health System ..." PricewaterhouseCoopers, op. cit.

234 "Billing and insurance-related functions ..." Kahn JG, Kronick R, Kreger M, Gans DN. The cost of health insurance administration in California: Estimates for insurers, physicians and hospitals. *Health Aff.* 2005;24:1629-1639.

234 "Health-care clerical workers ..." Cutler DM. Where are the health care entrepreneurs? The failure of organizational innovation in health care. National Bureau of Economic Research Working Paper 16030. nber.org/papers/w16030. May 2010. Accessed May 25, 2011.

234 "The U.S. spends about three times ..." Davis K, Schoen C, Guterman S, Shih T, Schoebaum SC, Weinbaum I. Slowing the growth U.S. health care expenditures: What are the options? Commonwealth Fund website. commonwealthfund.org/usr_doc/Davis_slowinggrowth UShltcareexpenditureswhatareoptions_989.pdf. January 2007. Accessed June 5, 2011.

234 "Brookings economist Aaron ..." Aaron, op. cit.

235 "In an essay ..." Brody H. Medicine's ethical responsibility for health care reform—the top five list. *N Engl J Med.* 2010;362(4):283-285.

235 "Brody told Newsweek magazine ..." Begley S. This won't hurt a bit. Newsweek. newsweek.com/2010/03/04/this-won-t-hurt-a-bit.html March 5, 2010. Accessed June 5, 2011.

236 "Only 40 percent ..." Straus SE, Tetroe JM, Graham ID. Knowledge translation is the use of knowledge in heath care decision making. *J Clin Epidemiol.* 2011;64:6-10.

236 "The U.S. Department of Health and Human Services ..." Guidelines by top. Agency for Healthcare Research and Quality website. guideline.gov/browse/by-topic.aspx. Accessed June 5, 2011.

236 "For example, a 2011 study ..." Lee DH, Vielemeyer O. Analysis of overall level of evidence behind Infectious Diseases Society of America practice guidelines. *Arch Intern Med.* 2011;171(1):18-22.

236 "Another 2011 study ..." Mendelson TB, Meltzer M, Campbell EG, Caplan AL, Kirkpatrick JN. Conflicts of interest in cardiovascular clinical practice guidelines. *Arch Intern Med.* 2011;171(6):577-585.

237 "The National Cancer Institute estimates ..." Prostate cancer. National Cancer Institute website. cancer.gov/cancertopics/types/prostate. Accessed June 7, 2011; Learn about cancer. American Cancer Society website. cancer.org/cancer/cancerbasics/cancer-prevalence. Accessed June 7, 2011.

237 "Of the 150 patients treated ..." Bell L. The magic bullet for prostate cancer. *Men's Health* website. menshealth.com/health/prostate-cancer-proton-therapy. February 1, 2011. Accessed June 7, 2011.

238 "A course of PRT can cost ..." Goozner M. The proton beam debate: Are facilities outstripping the evidence? *J Natl Cancer Inst.* 2010;102(7):450-453.

238 "Anthony Zietman is a radiation oncologist ..." Pollack A. Cancer fight goes nuclear, with heavy price tag. *The New York Times.* December 26, 2007.

238 "The latest U.S. research ..." Hensley S. Surgery no better than waiting for most men with prostate cancer. National Public Radio. May 17, 2011.

238 "Zietman and colleagues explained ..." Zietman A, Goitein M, Tepper JE. Technology evolution: Is it survival of the fittest? *J Clin Oncol.* 2010;28:4275-4279.

239 "One study found ..." Woolf SH, Johnson RE. The break-even point: When medical advances are less important than improving the fidelity with which they are delivered. *Ann Fam Med.* 2005;3:545-552.

239 "Older men diagnosed with low-risk ..." Hayes JH, Ollendorf DA, Pearson SD, et al. Active surveillance compared with initial treatment for men with low-risk prostate cancer: A decision analysis. *JAMA*. 2010;304(12):2373-2380.

239 "Recovery from small heart attacks ..." Di Nisio M, Middeldorp S, Buller R. Direct thrombin inhibitors. *N Engl J Med*. 2005;353:1028-1040.

239 "Similarly, 22 percent of elderly Americans ..." Tu J, Pashos CL, Naylor CD et al. Use of cardiac procedures and outcomes in elderly patients with myocardial infarction in the United States and Canada. *N Engl J Med*. 1997;336(21):1500-1505.

239 "One out of 5 heart defibrillators ..." Al-Katib SM, Hellkamp A, Curtis J, et al. Non-evidence-based ICD implanations in the United States. *JAMA*. 2001;305(1):43-49.

239 "Americans spent nearly $86 billion ..." Martin BI, Deyo RA, Mirza SK, et al. Expenditures and health status among adults with back and neck problems. *JAMA*. 2008; 299(6):656-664.

239 "Medical imaging ..." Kolata, G. Good or useless, medical scans cost the same. *The New York Times*. March 1, 2009.

240 "Patients of doctors ..." Schreibati JB, Baker LC. The relationship between low back MRI, surgery, and spending: Impact of physician self-referral status. *Health Serv Res*. 2011. onlinelibrary. wiley.com/doi/10.1111/j.1475-6773.2011.01265.x/abstract. April 21, 2011. Accessed May 25, 2011; Hendee WR, Becker GJ, Borgstede JP, et al. Addressing overutilization in medical imaging. *Radiology*. radiology.rsna.org/content/early/2010/08/05/radiol.10100063.abstract. August 24, 2010. Accessed May 25, 2011.

240 "In a 2006 essay ..." Leff B, Finucane TE. Gizmo idolatry. *JAMA*.2008;299(15):1830-1832.

242 "The thresholds for disease ..." Kaplan RM. *Disease, Diagnoses, and Dollars: Facing the Ever-Expanding Market for Medical Care*. New York: Copernicus Books; 2009.

242 "However, there are physicians ..." Fuchs VR, Milstein A. The $640 billion question—why does cost-effective care diffuse so slowly? *N Engl J Med*. 2011;364:1985-1987.

243 "Most Americans have two perspectives ..." Health care in America 2006 survey. Kaiser Family Foundation website. kff.org/kaiserpolls/upload/7572.pdf. October 2006. Accessed May 25, 2011.

243 "A 2000 World Health Organization report ranked ..." The world health report 2000—health systems: improving performance. Geneva: World Health Organization; 2000; Murray CJ, Frank J. A framework for assessing the performance of health systems. *Bull World Health Organ*. 2000;78:717-713.

243 "The Commonwealth Fund ranked ..." Davis K, Schoen C, Stremikis K. Mirror, mirror on the wall: How the performance of the U.S. health care system compares internationally. Commonwealth Fund website. commonwealthfund.org/~/media/Files/Publications/Fund %20Report/2010/Jun/1400_Davis_Mirror_Mirror_on_the_wall_2010.pdf. June 2010. Accessed May 25, 2011.

244 "Gov. Mitch Daniels ..." Top Republicans headline today's CPAC. C-SPAN.org. cspan.org/Events/Top-Republicans-Headline-Todays-CPAC/10737419537-2/. February 11, 2011. Accessed July 28, 2011.

244 "The FBI estimates ..." Lind KD. Attacking waste, fraud, and abuse in health reform. AARP Public Policy Institute. assets.aarp.org/rgcenter/ppi/health-care/fs186-fraud.pdf. May 2010. Accessed May 25, 2011.

244 "By comparison, credit-card fraud ..." Combating health care fraud in a post-reform world: Seven guiding principles for policymakers. The National Health Care Anti-Fraud Association website. sas.com/resources/asset/health-insurance-third-party-white-paper-nhcaa.pdf. October 6, 2010. Accessed May 25, 2011.

244 "Health reform augmented efforts ..." Health care fraud prevention and enforcement efforts recover record $4 billion; new Affordable Care Act tools will help fight fraud. U.S.

Department of Health & Human Services website. hhs.gov/news/press/2011pres/01/20110124a. html. January 24, 2011. Accessed May 25, 2011.

244 "According to the Government Accounting Office ..." Fraud detection systems. gao.gov/ new.items/d11822t.pdf. July 12, 2011. Accessed July 28, 2011.

Chapter 18. Employer and Individual Insurance

Page 245 "Employers were unimpressed ..." Health care reform: Looming fears mask unprecedented employer opportunities to mitigate costs, risks and reset total rewards. Towers Watson website. towerswatson.com/assets/pdf/1935/Post-HCR_Flash_survey_bulletin_5_25_ 10%281%29.pdf. May 2010. Accessed May 18, 2011.

245 "The people most affected ..." Employer and employee reactions to health reform: Findings from the 2010 EBRI/MGA Consumer Engagement in Health Care Survey and the 2010 SHRM organization's response to health care reform poll. Employee Benefit Research Institute Notes. 2011;32(1): 2.

245 "That exemption will cost ..." Joint Committee on Taxation. Background information on tax expenditure analysis and historical survey of tax expenditure estimates. Scheduled for a public hearing before the Senate Committee on Finance. 67.192.62.149/publications.html?func= startdown&id=3739 . February 28, 2011. Accessed May 18, 2011.

246 "About 52 percent of employees ..." Fronstin P. The impact of the 2007-2009 recession on workers' health coverage. Employee Benefit Research Institute. ebri.org/pdf/briefspdf/EBRI_IB_ 04-2011_No356_Rccsn-HlthCvg.pdf. April 2011; Gould E. Health insurance eroding for working families: Employer-provided coverage declines for fifth consecutive year. Economic Policy Institute. epi.org/publications/entry/bp175/. September27, 2006. Accessed May 18, 2011.

246 "According to the U.S. Census Bureau ..." Income, poverty, and health insurance coverage in the United States: 2009. U.S. Census Bureau website. census.gov/prod/2010pubs/p60-238.pdf. September 2010. Accessed May 26, 2011.

246 "The percentage paid ..." Changes ahead: Health care reform in a challenging economy. Towers Watson website. towerswatson.com/assets/pdf/2884/TowersWatson-HC-Changes-Flash-5-NA-2010-17151.pdf. September 2010. Accessed May 18, 2011.

246 "The current recession illustrates ..." Fronstin P. The impact of the recession on employment-based health coverage. Employee Benefit Research Institute. ebri.org/publications/ ib/index.cfm?fa=ibDisp&content_id=4539May 2010. Accessed May 18, 2011.

247 "Another one: ..." Medicaid, SCHIP and economic downturn: Policy challenges and policy responses. Kaiser Family Foundation. kff.org/medicaid/upload/7770.pdf. April 2008. Accessed May 19, 2011.

248 "In fact, small businesses ..." Gabel J, McDevitt R, Gandolfo L, et al. Generosity and adjusted premiums in job-based insurance: Hawaii is up, Wyoming is down. *Health Aff.* 2006;25(3):832-843.

248 "Three-quarters of small businesses ..." Holve E, Brodie M, Levitt L. Small business executives and health insurance: Findings from a national survey of very 248 small firms. *Managed Care Interface.* 2003;16(9):19-24.

248 "More than a quarter ..." Gardiner T. Small Business Majority presentation for Alliance for Health Reform, Washington, D.C. September 8, 2010. Accessed May 18, 2011.

248 "Small business owners were ready ..." McInturff WD, Weigel L. Deja vu all over again: The similarities between political debates regarding health care in the early 1990s and today. *Health Aff.* 2008;27(3):699-704.

248 "Nearly 70 percent ..." Doty MM, Collins SR, Rustgi SD, Nicholson JL. Out of options: Why so many workers in small businesses lack affordable health insurance, and how health care

reform can help. Commonwealth Fund. commonwealthfund.org/Content/Publications/Issue-Briefs/2009/Sep/Out-of-Options.aspx September 2009. Accessed May 19, 2011.

248 "In 2007, more than half ..." Collins SR, Davis K, Nicholson JL, Stremikis K. Realizing health reform's potential: Small businesses and the Affordable Care Act of 2010. Commonwealth Fund. commonwealthfund.org/Content/Publications/Issue-Briefs/2010/Sep/Small-Businesses.aspx. September 2, 2011. Accessed May 18, 2011.

250 "The Congressional Budget Office predicts ..." Congressional Budget Office. An analysis of health insurance premiums under the Patient Protection and Affordable Care Act. cbo.gov/ftpdocs/107xx/doc10781/11-30-Premiums.pdf. November 30, 2009. Accessed May 18, 2011.

250 "However, more than half ..." Collins SR, op cit.

251 "Analysts have differed widely ..." Small business tax credits. Health Affairs health policy brief. healthaffairs.org/healthpolicybriefs/brief.php?brief_id=38. January 14, 2011. Accessed May 18, 2011.

253 "A May 2010 survey ..." Mercer's 2010 survey on health reform – sizing up the challenge. mercer.com/press-releases/1380755. May 2010. Accessed May 18, 2011.

253 "A Towers Watson analysis ..." Cadillace health plan tax to penalize majority of employers by 2018. Towers Watson website. towerswatson.com/press/1895. May 19, 2010. Accessed May 20, 2011.

254 "A survey of small California businesses ..." Levey NN. California small businesses still unclear on provisions of healthcare reform law, poll finds. *The Los Angeles Times.* March 20, 2011.

254 "The CBO estimated ..." Congressional Budget Office, op cit.

254 "The RAND Corporation ..." Eibner C, Hussey PS, Girosi F. The effects of the Affordable Care Act on workers' health insurance coverage. *N Engl J Med.* 2010;363(15):1393-1395.

254 "A 2008 survey found ..." The 2008 health confidence survey: Rising costs continue to change the way Americans use the health care system. Employee Benefit Research Institute. ebri.org/pdf/notespdf/EBRI_Notes_10-2008.pdf. October 2008. Accessed May 26, 2011.

254 "The average out-of-pocket maximums ..." Whitmore H, Gabel JR, Pickreign J, McDevitt R. The individual insurance market before reform: Low premiums and low benefits. *Med Res Rev.* April 17, 2011. mcr.sagepub.com/content/early/2011/01/29/1077558711399767.abstract. Accessed May 19, 2011.

255 "Viewed from another angle ..." McDevitt R, Gabel J, Lore R, Pickreign J, Whitemore H, Brust T. Group insurance: A better deal for most people than individual plans. *Health Aff.* 2010;29(1):156-164.

255 "These are often stopgap policies ..." Nearly 11 million Americans have individual health insurance policies, but some only for a short time. Agency for Healthcare Research and Quality website. ahrq.gov/news/nn/nn010709.htm. January 7, 2009. Accessed May 18, 2011.

255 "Buying individual insurance ..." New report: 129 million Americans with a pre-existing condition could be denied coverage without new health reform law. U.S. Department of Health & Human Services website. hhs.gov/news/press/2011pres/01/20110118a.html. January 18, 2011. Accessed May 19, 2011.

255 "One in 7 who applied for individual insurance ..." Adamy J. Insurers denied coverage to 1 in 7. *The Wall Street Journal.* October 13, 2010.

255 "Suffice to say that ..." Dorn S. Uninsured and dying because of it: Updating the Institute of Medicine analysis on the impact of uninsurance on mortality. urban.org/publications/411588.html January 8, 2008. Accessed May 20, 2011.

255 "That is a direct result ..." Wilper AP, Wollhandler S, Lasser KE, McCormick D, Bor DH, Himmelstein DU. A national study of chronic disease prevalence and access to care in uninsured U.S. adults. *Ann Intern Med.* 2008;149:170-176.

Chapter 19. Government Insurance

Page 257 "According to federal actuaries ..." Truffer CJ, Keehan S, Smith S, et al. Health spending projections through 2019: The recession's impact continues. Health Aff. 2010;29(3).

257 "They currently make up ..." Congressional Budget Office Director's blog. The long-term budget outlook. cboblog.cbo.gov/?p=328. July 16, 2009. Accessed June 28, 2011.

258 "Barely half of Americans ..." Kaiser Family Foundation tracking poll. kff.org/kaiserpolls/upload/8190-F.pdf. May 2011. Accessed June 28, 2011.

258 "Commentators had a field day ..." Rucker P. Sen. DeMint of S.C. is voice of opposition to health-care reform. *The Washington Post.* July 28, 2009.

258 "However, nearly 4 out of 10 Medicare ..." Mettler S. Reconstituting the submerged state: The challenges of social policy reform in the Obama era. *Perspectives on Politics.* 2010;8(3):803-824.

258 "About half of Americans ..." Newport F. U.S. still split on whether gov't should ensure health care. Gallup Poll website. gallup.com/poll/144839/split-whether-gov-ensure-healthcare.aspx. November 18, 2010. Accessed June 28, 2011.

260 "Medicaid covers about 60 million ..." Kaiser Family Foundation. Medicare at a glance. kff.org/medicare/1066.cfmSeptember 2010. Accessed June 28, 2011.

260 "When Medicaid expanded ..." Currie J, Gruber J. Health insurance eligibility, utilization of medical care, and child health. *The Quarterly Journal of Economics.* 1996.111(2):431-466.

260 "A 2011 study of 10,000 people ..." Finkelstein A, Taubman S, Wright B, et al. The Oregon health insurance experiment: Evidence from the first year. National Bureau of Economic Research Working Paper No. 17190. nber.org/papers/w17190.pdf. July 2011. Accessed July 8, 2011.

260 "This group of nearly nine million ..." The Kaiser Family Foundation Program on Medicare Policy. The role of Medicare for the people dually eligible for Medicare and Medicaid. kff.org/medicare/upload/8138.pdf. January 2011. Accessed June 28, 2011.

261 "On average, about 17 percent ..." Kaiser Commission on Medicaid and the Uninsured. The role of Medicaid in state economies: A look at the research executive summary. kff.org/medicaid/upload/7075_02_ES.pdf January 2009. Accessed June 28, 2011.

262 "Medicaid enrollment rose ..." Iglehart JK. After midterm elections, changes are in store. *Health Aff.* 2011;30(1):8-10.

262 "Every state added enrollment ..." Kaiser Commission on Medicaid and the Uninsured. Hoping for economic recovery, preparing for health reform: A look at Medicaid spending, coverage and policy trends. kff.org/medicaid/8105.cfm September 2010. Accessed June 28, 2011.

262 "According to the Kaiser Family Foundation ..." Holahan J, Garrett AB. Rising unemployment, Medicaid and the uninsured. Kaiser Commission on Medicaid and the Uninsured. kff.org/uninsured/upload/7850.pdf. January 2009. Accessed June 28, 2011.

262 "Oregon's Medicaid program ..." Wright BJ, Carlson MJ, Allen H, Holmgren AL, Rustvold DL. Raising premiums and other costs for Oregon health plan enrollees drove many to drop out. *Health Aff.* 2010;29(12):2311-2316.

263 "In an attempt ..." Adamy J. Arizona proposes Medicaid fat fee. *The Wall Street Journal.* April 1, 2011.

264 "For example, every out-of-state ..." Jacob S. Why the dump-Medicaid idea makes no sense. *The Dallas Morning News.* November 30, 2010.

264 "In the 21 states ..." Ku L. Ready, set plan, implement: Executing the expansion of Medicaid. *Health Aff.* 2010;29(6):1173-1177.

264 "The CBO estimated ..." Congressional Budget Office, "Long-Term Analysis of a Budget Proposal by Chairman Ryan." cbo.gov/ftpdocs/121xx/doc12128/04-05-Ryan_Letter.pdf. April 5, 2011. Accessed June 28, 2011.

265 "About 40 percent ..." Sommers BD, Epstein AM. Medicaid expansion—the soft underbelly of health care reform? *N Engl J Med.* 2010;363(22):2085-2087.

265 "According to a *Health Affairs* ..." Kenney GM, Lynch V, Cook A, Phong S. Who and where are the children yet to enroll in Medicaid and the Children's Health Insurance Program? *Health Aff.* 2010;29(10):1920-1929.

266 "For example, Medicaid ..." Yoo, B, Berry A, Kasajima M, Szilagyi, PG. Association between Medicaid reimbursement and child influenza vaccination rates. *Pediatrics.* 2010;126(5): e998-e1010.; Preidt R. Doctors lose money giving flu shots to kids on Medicaid. *USA Today.* October 19, 2010.

266 "Researchers posed as the parent ..." Bisgaier J, Rhodes KV. Auditing access to specialty care. *N Engl J Med.* 2011;(364(24):2324-2333.

266 "Prior to Medicare's enactment ..." Kaiser Family Foundation. Medicare: A Primer. 2010. kff.org/medicare/7615.cfm. Accessed June 29, 2011.

267 "Nearly half of those on Medicare ..." Kaiser Family Foundation. Medicare spending and financing fact sheet. kff.org/medicare/upload/7305-05.pdf. August 2010. June 28, 2011.

267 "A Wayne State University ..." Jankowski TB, Booza JC, Leach CA. Invisible poverty: New measure unveils financial hardship in Michigan's older adult population. Seniors Count! Working Paper Series. freep.com/assets/freep/pdf/C4177040720.PDF. July 20, 2011. Accessed July 27, 2011.

267 "Medicare Advantage costs ..." Health Affairs policy brief. Medicare Advantage Plans. healthaffairs.org/healthpolicybriefs/brief.php?brief_id=48 June 15, 2011. Accessed June 28, 2011.

268 "Annual Medicare expenditures ..." Kaiser Family Foundation fact sheet. Medicare spending and financing. kff.org/medicare/upload/7305-05.pdf. August 2010. Accessed June 29, 2011.

268 "About 25 percent account ..." Reschovsky JD, Hadley J, Saiontz-Martinez CB, Boukus ER. Following the money: Factors associated with the cost of treating high-cost Medicare beneficiaries. *Health Ser Res.* hschange.com/CONTENT/1185/1185.pdf. January 11, 2011. Accessed June 28, 2011.

268 "One study calculated ..." Berenson RA, Hammons T, Gans DN, et al. A house is not a home: Keeping patients at the center of practice redesign. *Health Aff.* 2008;27(5):1219-1230.

268 "Medicare spending historically has grown ..." Congressional Budget Office. The long-term outlook for health care spending. cbo.gov/ftpdocs/87xx/doc8758/11-13-LT-Health.pdf. November 2007. Accessed June 29, 2011.

268 "The typical couple ..." Steuerle CE, Rennane S. Social Security and Medicare taxes and benefits over a lifetime. Urban Institute. urban.org/UploadedPDF/social-security-medicare-benefits-over-lifetime.pdf. January 2011. Accessed June 28, 2011.

268 "Median out-of-pocket spending ..." Kaiser Family Foundation fact sheet, op. cit.

269 "Yet a majority of Americans ..." Seib GF. In battle over Medicare, new prescription needed. *The Wall Street Journal.* June 21, 2011.

269 "Medicare trustees estimated ..." Shatto JD, Clemens MK. Projected Medicare expenditures under an illustrative scenario with alternative payment updates to Medicare providers. Centers for Medicare & Medicaid Services. cms.gov/ReportsTrustFunds/Downloads/2011TRAlternativeScenario.pdf. May 13, 2011. Accessed June 28, 2011.

270 "According to the CBO, " Congressional Budget Office, April 5, 2010, op. cit.

271 "According to a Kaiser Family Foundation ..." Neuman T, Cubanski J, Waldo D, Eppig F, Mays J. Raising the age of Medicare eligibility: A fresh look following implementation of health reform. Kaiser Family Foundation website. kff.org/medicare/upload/8169.pdf. March 2011. Accessed June 29, 2011.

271 "In a March 2010 report ..." Government Accountability Office. Medicare and

Medicaid fraud, waste, and abuse. gao.gov/new.items/d11409t.pdf. March 9, 2011. Accessed June 28, 2011.

271 "The Office of Management and Budget tracks ..." High-error programs. Payment Accuracy. paymentaccuracy.gov/high-priority-programs. Accessed July 28, 2011.

272 "The Dartmouth Atlas Project ..." Fisher ES, Bynum JP, Skinner JS. Slowing the growth of health care costs—lessons from regional variation. *N Engl J Med.* 2009;360(9):849-852.

272 "In a June 2011 report ..." Medicare Payment Advisory Commission. Report to the Congress: Medicare and the Health Care Delivery System. medpac.gov/documents/Jun11_EntireReport.pdf June 2011. Accessed June 30, 2011.

Chapter 20. The Doctor

Page 275 "Their income essentially has stayed ..." Cunningham P, Hadley J. Effects of changes in incomes and practice circumstances on physicians' decisions to treat charity and Medicaid patients. *Milbank Q.* 2008;86(1):91-123.

275 "Their workdays are brutal ..." Baron RJ. What's keeping us so busy in primary care? A snapshot from one practice. *N Engl J Med.* 2010;362(17):1632-1636.

275 "Many patients do not get ..." Bodenheimer T, Pham HH. Primary care: Current problems and proposed solutions. *Health Aff.* 2010;29(5):799-805.

276 "Primary-care physicians' share ..." Berenson RA, Hammons T, Gans DN, et al. A house is not a home: Keeping patients at the center of practice redesign. *Health Aff.* 2008;27(5): 1219-1230.

276 "If payers cut reimbursement ..." Aaron HJ, Ginsburg PB. Is health spending excessive? If so, what can we do about it. *Health Aff.* 2008;28(5):1260-1275.

276 "However, they control 80 cents ..." Health reform and the decline of physician private practice. The Physicians Foundation website. physiciansfoundation.org/uploadedFiles/ Health%20Reform%20and%20the%20Decline%20of%20Physician%20Private%20Practice.pdf. October 2010. Accessed May 11, 2011.

276 "In a 2006 survey ..." Merritt J, Hawkins J, Miller PD. *Will the Last Physician in America Please Turn Off the Lights?* Independence MO: Practice Support Resources Inc.; 2004.

276 "Medical liability system costs ..." Mello MM, Chandra A, Gawande AA, Studdert DM. National costs of the medical liability system. *Health Aff.* 2010;29(9):1569-1577.

276 "However, physician concerns ..." Carrier ER, Reschovsky JD, Mello MM, Mayrell RC, Katz D. Physicians' fears of malpractice lawsuits are not assuaged by tort reforms. *Health Aff.* 2010;29(9):1585-1592.

278 "The average work week ..." Staiger DO, Auerbach DI, Buerhaus PI. Trends in the work hours of physicians in the United States. *JAMA.* 2010;303(8):747-753.

278 "Only 1 out of 4 say..." Physician Foundation op cit.

278 "The recession has prompted ..." Commins J. Healthcare workers delaying retirement. Media Health Leaders website. healthleadersmedia.com/page-1/TEC-266573/Healthcare-Workers-Delaying-Retirement. May 25, 2011. Accessed July 28, 2011.

278 "Qliance, a Seattle-based primary-care practice ..." Presentation, Disruptive Innovation in Healthcare Services Workshop, Southwest Healthcare Transactions Conference, Dallas, April 27, 2011.

280 "For example, many economic sectors ..." Blanchfield BB, Heffernan JL, Osgood B, Sheehan RR, Meyer GS. Saving billions of dollars—and physicians' times—by streamlining billing practices. *Health Aff.* 2010;29(6):1248-1254.

280 "Physicians have to hustle ..." Beck M. The doctor will see you eventually. *The Wall Street Journal.* October 18, 2010.

280 "The average physician ..." Casalino LP, Nicholson S, Gans DN, et al. What does it cost physician practices to interact with health insurance plans? *Health Aff.* 2009;28(4):w533-w543.

281 "The Congressional Budget Office ..." Congressional Budget Office. *Key issues in analyzing major health insurance proposals.* Washington, D.C.: CBO; 2008.

281 "For example, two-thirds of Texas physicians ..." TMA survey: Physicians confused, anxious; believe health system is broken. Texas Medical Association website. texmed.org/template.aspx?id=20613. February 11, 2011. Accessed May 11, 2011.

282 "About 1 in 3 Medicare beneficiaries ..." Reforming the delivery system. Medicare Payment Advisory Commission website. medpac.gov/documents/jun08_entirereport.pdf. June 2008. Accessed May 11, 2011.

282 "The problem is that ..." Hillman BJ, Goldsmith J. Imaging: The self-referral boom and the ongoing search for effective policies to contain it. *Health Aff.* 2010;29(12):2231-2236.

282 "An analysis of ..." Hughes DR, Bhargavan M, Sunshine J. Imaging self-referral associated with higher costs and limited impact on duration of illness. *Health Aff.* 2010;29(12): 2244-2251.

282 "So much for good intentions ..." Sunshine J, Bhargavan M. The practice of imaging self-referral doesn't produce much one-stop service. *Health Aff.* 2010;29(12):2237-2243.

283 "The U.S. has the about the same number ..." Bodenheimer T, Chen E, Bennett HD. Confronting the growing burden of chronic disease: Can the U.S. health care workforce do the job? *Health Aff.* 2009;28(1):64-74.

283 "A study of 11 industrialized nations ..." Schoen C, Osborn R, Squires D, Doty MM, Pierson R, Applebaum S. How health insurance design affects access to care and costs, by income, in eleven countries. Health Aff. 2010;29(12):2323-2334.

283 "Massachusetts reformed its state health system ..." 2011 patient access to health care study: A survey of Massachusetts Physicians' Offices. Massachusetts Medical Society website. massmed.org/AM/Template.cfm?Section=Research_Reports_and_Studies2&CONTENTID=54336&TEMPLATE=/CM/ContentDisplay.cfm. 2011. Accessed May 17, 2011.

284 "The U.S. trains ..." Pardes H. The coming doctor shortage. *The Wall Street Journal.* January 19, 2011.

284 "This was an intentional shortage ..." Merritt J, op cit.

284 "About 80 percent of new physicians ..." Goodman DC. Twenty-year trends in regional variations in the U.S. physician workforce. *Health Aff.* 2004;w90-w97.

285 "Only 1 out of 14 ..." Bodenheimer, op cit.

285 "Primary-care physicians earn ..." Vaughn BT, DeVrieze SR, Reed SD, Schulman KA. Can we close the income and wealth gap between specialists and primary care physicians? *Health Aff.* 2010;29(5):933-940.

285 "In a 2010 interview ..." Health care reform, doctor shortage, and the importance of market forces. Modern Medicine website. modernmedicine.com/modernmedicine/Family+Medicine/Health-Care-Reform-Doctor-Shortage-and-the-Importa/ArticleStandard/Article/detail/662139. March 25, 2010. Accessed May 11, 2011.

286 "A Mayo Clinic pilot study ..." Adamson SC, Bachman JW. Pilot study of providing online care in a primary care setting. *Mayo Clin Proc.* 2010;85(8):704-710.

283 "A 2010 Health Affairs article ..." Margolius D, Bodenheimer T. Transforming primary care: From past practice to the practice of the future. *Health Aff.* 2010;29(5):779-784.

287 "An estimated 40,000 ..." Associated Press. "Medical home" health care model, focusing on prevention, shows results and cuts costs. *The Washington Post.* July 20, 2011.

287 "Seattle-based Group Health ..." Presentation, Disruptive Innovation in Healthcare Services Workshop, Southwest Healthcare Transactions Conference, Dallas, April 27, 2011.

287 "In a survey at its Bellevue clinic ..." Meyer H. Group Health's move to the medical home: For doctors, it's often a hard journey. *Health Aff.* 2010;29(5):844-851.

287 "In an Internet survey ..." Chen P. Fueling the anger of doctors. The New York Times. April 29, 2010.

288 "Seattle's GH invested ..." Meyer, opt cit.

Chapter 21. The Hospital

Page 289 "Charges can run ..." Friedman B, Henke RM, Wier LM. *Most expensive hospitalizations, 2008.* Agency for Healthcare Research and Quality Statistical Brief #97. hcup-us.ahrq.gov/reports/statbriefs/sb97.pdf. October 2010. Accessed April 16, 2011.

289 "Days spent in the hospital ..." Hall MJ, DeFrances CJ, Williams SN, Golosinskly A, Schwartzman A. *National hospital discharge survey: 2007 survey.* National Health Statistics Reports No. 29. October 26, 2010. Accessed April 16, 2011.

289 "Hospital care's portion of health-care costs ..." The cost of caring: Drivers of spending on hospital care. American Hospital Association website. aha.org/aha/trendwatch/2011/11mar-tw-costofcaring.pdf. March 2011. Accessed April 20, 2011.

289 "Nonetheless, the hospitals are tied ..." Oil, pharmaceutical, health insurance, and tobacco top the list of industries that people think should be more regulated. Harris Interactive website. harrisinteractive.com/NewsRoom/HarrisPolls/tabid/447/mid/1508/articleId/648/ctl/ReadCustom%20Default/Default.aspx. December 2, 2010. Accessed April 16, 2011.

290 "About 3 out of 4 ..." Hospitals continue to feel lingering effects of the economic recession. American Hospital Association website. aha.org/aha/content/2010/pdf/10june-econimpact.pdf. June 23, 2010. Accessed April 16, 2011.

290 "According to an American Hospital Association (AHA) survey ..." Report on the Capital Crisis: Impact on Hospitals. aha.org/aha/content/2009/pdf/090122capitalcrisisreport.pdf. January 22, 2009. Accessed April 18, 2011.

290 "Hospitals employ more than five million ..." Hospital facts to know. AHA website. aha.org/aha/content/2008/pdf/08-issue-facts-to-know-.pdf. Accessed April 18, 2011.

293 "However, the Medicare's Office ..." Testimony of Richard Foster, chief Medicare actuary. The estimated effect of the Affordable Care Act on Medicare and Medicaid outlays and total national health care expenditures. Committee on Energy and Commerce Subcommittee on Health, U.S. House of Representatives, May 16, 2011.

293 "Richard Foster ..." Daly R. Risk to hospital profitability highlighted. *Modern Healthcare.* July 13, 2011.

294 "Consultant Steven Lieberman ..." Proposed CMS regulation kills ACOs softly. Health Affairs blog. April 6, 2011. healthaffairs.org/blog/2011/04/06/proposed-cms-regulation-kills-acos-softly/

294 "The Medicare Physician Group Practice ..." Inglehart J. The ACO regulations—some answers, more questions. *N Engl J Med.* April 13, 2011. nejm.org/doi/full/10.1056/NEJM p1103603

296 "Outpatient surgeries accounted ..." Cullen KA, Hall MJ, Golosinskiy. *Ambulatory surgery in the United States, 2006.* National Health Statistics Reports No. 11. Hyattsville, MD: National Center for Health Statistics; 2009.

298 "Physician alignment..." Thompson J. Considering key factors for hospital-physician alignment. Healthcare Finance News website. healthcarefinancenews.com/news/considering-key-factors-hospital-physician-alignment. July 16, 2010. Accessed April 20, 2011.

298 "A 2011 study found ..." Goodall AH. Physician-leaders and hospital performance: Is there an association? Soc Sci Med. sciencedirect.com/science/article/pii/S0277953611003819. July 6, 2011. Accessed July 28, 2011.

298 "According to a 2010 PricewaterhouseCooper's (PwC) survey ..." From courtship to

marriage. Part I: Why health reform is driving physicians and hospitals closer together. PricewaterhouseCoopers website. pwc.com/us/en/health-industries/publications/from-courtship-to-marriage.jhtml. December 2010. Accessed April 20, 2011.

299 "Physicians are ready ..." Mathews AW. When the doctor has a new boss. *The Wall Street Journal.* November 8, 2010.

299 "The percentage of physicians ..." Isaacs SL, Jellinek PS, Ray WL. The independent physician—going, going ... *N Engl J Med.* 2009;360(7):655-657.

299 "According to a 2010 HealthLeaders ..." Cantlupe J. Physician alignment in an era of change. HealthLeaders Media website. content.hcpro.com/pdf/content/256536.pdf. September 2010. Accessed April 20, 2011.

300 "In 1999, the Institute of Medicine ..." To err is human: Building a safer health system. Institute of Medicine website. iom.edu/Reports/1999/To-Err-is-Human-Building-A-Safer-Health-System.aspx. November 1, 1999. Accessed April 16, 2011; Landrigan CP, Parry GJ, Bones CB, Hackbarth AD, Goldman DA, Sharek PJ. Temporal trends in rates of patient harm resulting from medical care. *N Engl J Med.* 2010;363:2124-2134.

300 "Even more disturbing ..." Classen DC, Resar R, Frances G, et al. "Global Trigger Tool" shows that adverse events in hospitals may be ten times greater than previously mention. *Health Aff.* 2011;30(4):581-589.

301 "A 2009 *Journal of the American Medical Association* ..." Pronovost PJ, Colantuoni E. Measuring preventable hard: Helping science keep pace with policy. *JAMA.* 2099;301(102): 1273-1275.

301 "The disregard for patient safety ..." McGuckin M, Waterman R, Govednik J. Hand hygiene compliance rates in the United States—a one-year multicenter collaboration using product/volume usage measurement and feedback. *Am J Med* Qual. 2009;24(3):205-213; Korniewicz DM, El-Masri M. Exploring the factors associated with hand hygiene compliance of nurses during routine clinical practice. *Applied Nursing Research.* 2010;23(2):86-90; Millenson ML. NYC train station bathroom yields cleaner hands than hospitals. The Health Care Blog. thehealthcareblog.com/blog/2010/09/16/nyc-train-station-bathroom-yields-cleaner-hands-than-hospitals/. September 16, 2010. Accessed April 16, 2011.

301 "Consequently, it is no surprise ..." U.S. Department of Health and Human Services. *National Healthcare Quality Report 2009.* Rockville, MD: Agency for Healthcare Research and Quality. March 2010.

301 "An association of medical professionals ..." Preventable bloodstream infections still a problem in hospitals, infection prevention group finds. Association for Professionals in Infection Control and Epidemiology website. apic.org/AM/Template.cfm?Section=Featured_News_and_Events&CONTENTID=15870&TEMPLATE=/CM/ContentDisplay.cfm. July 12, 2010. Accessed April 18, 2011.

301 "Among the hospitals who have conducted ADEs studies ..." Agency for Healthcare Research and Quality. *Reducing and preventing adverse drug events to decrease hospital costs.* Research in Action, Issue 1. AHRQ website. March 2001. Accessed April 18, 2011.

302 "According to a 2009 study ..." Jha AK, DesRoches CM, Campbell EG, et al. Use of electronic health records in US hospitals. *N Engl J Med.* 2009;360:1628-1638.

302 "A 2007 Institute of Medicine ..." Aspden P, Wolcot JA, Bootman JL, Cronenwett, ed. *Preventing Medication Errors.* Washington, DC: National Academies Press; 2007.

302 "One out of seven Medicare hospital patients ..." U.S. Department of Health and Human Services. *Adverse Events in Hospitals: National Incidence among Medicare Beneficiaries.* Rockville, MD: Office of Inspector General. November 2010.

302 "About 40 surgeries a week ..." Chassin MR, Loeb JM. The ongoing quality improvement journey: Next stop, high reliability. *Health Aff.* 2011;30(4):559-568.

302 "However, it is not all bad news ..." *Improving America's Hospitals: The Joint Commission's annual report on quality and safety.* Joint Commission website. jointcommission.org/assets/1/18/2010_Annual_Report.pdf. 2010. Accessed April 18, 2011.

302 "The quality of hospital care is often tied ..." Curry LA, Spatz E, Cherlin E, et al. What distinguishes top-performing hospitals in acute myocardial infarction mortality rates: A qualitative study. *Ann Intern Med.* 2011;154(6):384-390.

303 "Hip replacement illustrates ..." Cram P, Lu X, Kaboli PJ, et al. Clinical characteristics and outcomes of Medicare patients undergoing total hip arthorplasty, 1991-2009. *JAMA.* 2011; 305(15):1560-1567.

304 "Dr. Peter Cram ..." Gordon, S. Shorter hospital stays, more readmissions after hip replacements. U.S. News & World Report website. health.usnews.com/health-news/family-health/bones-joints-and-muscles/articles/2011/04/19/shorter-hospital-stays-more-readmissions-after-hip-replacements. April 19, 2011. Accessed April 21, 2011.

304 "One in five Medicare beneficiaries ..." Jencks SF, Williams MV, Coleman EA. Rehospitalizations among patients in the Medicare fee-for-service program. *N Engl J Med.* 2009; 360:1418-1428.

304 "Blacks are 43 percent more likely ..." Allaudeen N, Vidyarthi A, Masselli J, Auerbach A. Redefining readmission risk factors for general medicine patients. *Journal of Hospital Medicine.* 2011;6(2):54-60.

304 "The Joint Commission ..." Joint Commission Center For Transforming Healthcare tackles miscommunication among caregivers. Joint Commission Center For Transforming Healthcare website. centerfortransforminghealthcare.org/news/display.aspx?newsid=23. October 21, 2010. Accessed April 18, 2011.

305 "For example, the Ronald Reagan ..." Goldman DP, Vaiana M, Romley JA. The emerging importance of patient amenities in hospital care. *N Eng J Med.* 2010;363(23):2185-2187.

305 "Consumers are understandably confused ..." Rothberg MB, Morsi E, Benjamin EM, Pekow PS, Lindenauer PK. Choosing the best hospital: The limitations of public quality report. *Health Aff.* 2008;27(6):1680-1687.

305 "The ratings may not even matter ..." Nicholas LH, Osborne NH, Birkmeyer JD, Dimich JB. Hospital process compliance and surgical outcomes in Medicare beneficiaries. *Arch Surg.* 2010;(145)10:999-1004.

305 "Overall, hospital patients are unhappier ..." Morgan S. Patient satisfaction declines at hospitals. The Wall Street Journal Smart Money website. smartmoney.com/personal-finance/health-care/patient-satisfaction-declines-at-hospitals/. May 18, 2010. Accessed April 18, 2011.

306 "N. R. Zenarosa, a physician ..." Interview with author, March 29, 2011.

306 "Even though EDs employ ..." Pitts SR, Carrier ER, Rich ED, Kellermann AL. Where Americans get their acute care: Increasingly, it's not at their doctor's office. *Health Aff.* 2010;29(9):1620-1629.

306 "From 1999 to 2007 ..." Tang N, Stein J, Hsia RY, Maselli JH, Gonzales R. Trends and characteristics of US emergency department visits, 1997-2007. *JAMA.* 2010;304(6):664-670.

306 "Despite the increased patient load ..." Hsia RY, Kellermann AI, Shen Y. Factors associated with closures of emergency departments in the United States. *JAMA.* 2011;305(19):1978-1985.

306 "The average waiting time for patients ..." Neale T. Fast treatment rare in emergency departments. Medpage Today website. medpagetoday.com/EmergencyMedicine/EmergencyMedicine/21346. July 23, 2010. Accessed April 18, 2011.

307 "With a wave of hospital mergers ..." Vogt WB, Town R. How has hospital consolidation affected the price and quality of hospital care? Robert Wood Johnson Foundation Research

Synthesis Report No. 9. Robert Wood Johnson Foundation website. rwjf.org/files/research/
no9researchreport.pdf. February 2006. Accessed April 18, 2011.

307 "According to an investigation ..." Investigation of health care cost trends and cost drivers.
Office of the Massachusetts. Attorney General Martha Coakley. mass.gov/Cago/docs/healthcare/
Investigation_HCCT&CD.pdf. January 29, 2010. Accessed April 20, 2011.

307 "Robert Blendon ..." Serafini M, Carey MA. Trends to watch for curbing health costs.
Kaiser Health News. kaiserhealthnews.org/Stories/2011/July/20/Round-Robin-On-Curbing-
Health-Care-Cost-Growth.aspx. July 20, 2011. Accessed August 5, 2011.

308 "On average, that rate ..." Berenson RA, Ginsburg PB, Kemper N. Unchecked provider
clout in California foreshadows challenges to health reform. *Health Aff.* 2010;29(4):699-705.

308 "However, the health plans flex ..." New AMA study finds lack of competition among
health insurers. American Medical Association website. ama-assn.org/ama/pub/news/news/
competition-health-insurers.page. February 1, 2011. Accessed April 19, 2011.

Chapter 22. Pharmaceuticals

Page 309 "The heyday of the pharmaceutical industry ..." Petersen M. *Our Daily Meds.* New
York: Picador; 2008.

309 "By comparison, only 7 ..." Angell, M. *The Truth About Drug Companies: How They
Deceive Us and What to Do About It.* New York: Random House; 2005.

309 "Prescription drug spending ..." The use of medicines in the United States: Review of 2010.
IMS Health website. imshealth.com/deployedfiles/imshealth/Global/Content/IMS%20Institute/
Static%20File/IHII_UseOfMed_report.pdf. April 2010. Accessed April 21, 2011.

310 "The number of prescriptions grew ..." Prescription drug trends. Kaiser Family
Foundation website. kff.org/rxdrugs/upload/3057-08.pdf. May 2010. Accessed April 21, 2011.

310 "In 1990, consumers paid ..." Heffler S, Levit K, Smith S, et al. Health spending growth
in 1999; faster growth expected in the future. *Health Aff.* 2001;(20)2:193-203.

310 "Nearly nine out of 10 people over age 60 ..." Gu Q, Dillon CF, Burt VL. *Prescription
drug use continues to increase: US prescription drug data for 2007-2008.* NCHS Data Brief No. 42.
Hyattsville, MD: National Center for Health Statistics, 2010.

311 "The growth in children's use ..." Medco 2010 drug trend highlights. Medco website.
drugtrend.com/art/drug_trend/pdf/DT_Report_2010.pdf. Accessed April 21, 2011.

311 "Among developed nations ..." Morgan S, Kennedy J. Prescription drug accessibility and
affordability in the United States and abroad. The Commonwealth Fund website. common
wealthfund.org/Content/Publications/Issue-Briefs/2010/Jun/Prescription-Drug-Accessibility-and-
Affordability-in-the-United-States-and-Abroad.aspx. May 2010. Accessed April 21, 2011.

311 "U.S. drug prices are as much as 25 percent ..." Showdown over drug pricing: Get
ready for another round. Deloitte website. deloitte.com/view/en_US/us/Industries/life-
sciences/5648375b2328c210VgnVCM2000001b56f00aRCRD.htm. March 1, 2011. Accessed
April 22, 2011.

312 "According to Express Scripts ..." Drug trend report 2010. Express Scripts website.
express-scripts.com/research/studies/drugtrendreport/. April 2011. Accessed April 22, 2011.

312 "A more difficult problem ..." Spear BB, Heath-Chiozzi M, Huff J. Clinical applications of
pharmacogenetics. *Trends in Molecular Medicine.* 2001;7(5):201-204.

312 "The cost of brand-name prescription drugs ..." U.S. Government Accountability Office.
Prescription drugs: Trends in usual and customary prices for commonly used drugs. Washington, D.C.:
Government Accountability Office; February 10, 2011. GAO -11-306R.

312 "Medical bills and illness ..." Himmelstein DU, Thorne D, Warren E, Woolhandler S.
Medical bankruptcy in the United States, 2007: Results of a national study. *Am J Med.* 2009;
122(8):741-746.

312 "However, AARP estimates ..." Schondelmeyer SW, Gross DJ. Rx Watchdog Report: Drug prices to climb despite lack of growth in general inflation rate. AARP Public Policy Institute website. assets.aarp.org/rgcenter/ppi/health-care/i36-watchdog.pdf. September 30, 2009. Accessed April 22, 2011.

312 "Before the benefit began ..." Afendulis CC, He Y, Zaslavsky AM, Chernew ME. The impact of Medicare Part D on hospitalization rates. *Health Ser Res.* 2011;48(4):1022-1038.

313 "Because of that, Fidelity Investments ..." Health care costs for 2011 retirees to drop. Fidelity Investments website. guidance.fidelity.com/viewpoints/healthcare-costs-drop-2011. April 13, 2011. Accessed April 22, 2011.

314 "The price of popular brand-name drugs ..." Schondelmeyer SW, Purvis L. Rx Price Watch Report August 2010. AARP Public Policy Institute website. assets.aarp.org/rgcenter/ppi/health-care/rxpricewatch.pdf. Accessed April 22, 2011.

314 "However, worldwide sales ..." The global use of medicines: Outlook through 2015. IMS Institute for Healthcare Informatics. The global use of medicines: Outlook through 2015. IMS Institute for Healthcare Informatics. May 2011. Accessed July 28, 2011.

314 "Patients are driving the trend ..." Doctors fear patients not filling prescriptions. Epocrates website. epocrates.com/company/news/021009.html. February 10, 2009. Accessed April 22, 2011.

314 "Some patients are just as skeptical ..." Sticker shock at the pharmacy counter. Consumer Reports website. consumerreports.org/health/prescription-drugs/sticker-shock-at-the-pharmacy-counter/overview/sticker-shock-at-the-pharmacy-counter.htm. March 2009. Accessed April 22, 2011.

314 "Generic drugs saved ..." Savings achieved through the use of generic pharmaceuticals 2000-2009. Generic Pharmaceutical Association website. prescriptionaccess.org/2010_Report_Generic_Savings_GPhA.pdf. July 2010. Accessed April 22, 2011.

314 "In fact, a poll of drug-consuming households ..." More than two-thirds of U.S. consumers seek medical advice via the Internet and social media. Accenture website. newsroom.accenture.com/article_display.cfm?article_id=5096. November 16, 2010. Accessed April 22, 2011.

315 "Two-thirds of consumers ..." Sticker shock at the pharmacy counter. Consumer Health website. consumerreports.org/health/prescription-drugs/sticker-shock-at-the-pharmacy-counter/overview/sticker-shock-at-the-pharmacy-counter.htm. March 2009. Accessed April 22, 2011.

315 "In 2008, 1.9 million hospitalized patients ..." Lucado J, Paez K, Elixhauser A. *Medication-Related Adverse Outcomes in U.S. Hospitals and Emergency Departments, 2008.* HCUP Statistical Brief #109. April 2011. Rockville, MD: Agency for Healthcare Research and Quality.

315 "The 28,000 prescription overdose deaths ..." Fiore K, Walker E. White House targets painkiller abuse. Medpage Today. medpagetoday.com/Washington-Watch/Washington-Watch/26021. April 19, 2011. Accessed April 25, 2011.

315 "The White House launched ..." *Epidemic: Responding to America's prescription drug abuse crisis.* Office of the President of the United States. whitehousedrugpolicy.gov/publications/pdf/rx_abuse_plan.pdf. 2011. Accessed April 25, 2011.

315 "A study at Pennsylvania-based ..." Boscarino JA, Rukstalis MR, Hoffman SN, et al. Prevalence of prescription opiod-use disorder among chronic pain patients: Comparison of the DSM-5 vs. DSM-4 diagnostic criteria. *J Addict Dis.* 2011;30(3):185-194.

315 "Between 20 and 40 percent ..." American Pain Society. *Guidelines for the Use of Chronic Opioid Therapy in Chronic Noncancer Pain: Evidence Review.* Glenview IL: American Pain Society; 2009.

316 "Seven out of 10 ..." Substance Abuse and Mental Health Services Administration. *Results from the 2009 National Survey on Drug Use and Health: Volume I. Summary of National Findings. 2010.* Rockville, MD: Office of Applied Studies, NSDUH Series H-38A, HHS Publication No. SMA 10-4586Findings).

316 "Spending on prescription pain killers ..." Spending on outpatient prescription pain medicines has tripled in 10 years. Agency for Healthcare Research and Quality website. ahrq.gov/news/nn/nn021209.htm. February 12, 2009. Accessed April 23, 2011.

316 "Researchers examined prescription use ..." Choudhry NK, Fischer MA, Avorn J, et al. The implications of therapeutic complexity on adherence to cardiovascular medications. *Arch Intern Med*. archinte.ama-assn.org/cgi/reprint/archinternmed.2010.495v1Published online January 10, 2011. Accessed April 22, 2011.

316 "Each medication a patient takes ..." Gandhi TK, Weingart SN, Borus J, et al. Adverse drug events in ambulatory care. *N Engl J Med*. 2003;348:1556-1564.

316 "Dr. Jerry Avorn,..." Avorn J. Medication use in older patients: Better policy could encourage better practice. *JAMA*. 2010;304(14):1606-1607.

316 "According to one study ..." Wolf MS, Curtis LM , Waite K, et al. Helping patients simplify and safely use complex prescription regimes. *Arch Intern Med*. 2011;171(4):300-305.

317 "In marketing parlance ..." Parry V. The art of condition branding. *Medical Marketing & Media*. May 2003:42-49.

317 "James Goodwin, a Texas geriatrician ..." Goodwin J. Geriatrics and the limits of modern medicine. *N Engl J Med*. 1999;340(16):1283-1285.

318 "DTC advertising tripled ..." Dave D, Saffer H. The impact of direct-to-consumer advertising on pharmaceutical prices and demand. National Bureau of Economic Research Working Paper No. 15969. May 2010.

318 "Drug makers spent ..." Total US promotional spend by type, 2009. IMS Health website. imshealth.com/deployedfiles/imshealth/Global/Content/StaticFile/Top_Line_Data/PromoUpdate 2009.pdf. Accessed April 22, 2011.

318 "According to a Consumer Reports ..." poll Best Buy drugs: Many common generics beat brand names. Consumer Reports website. consumerreports.org/health/best-buy-drugs/best-buy-drugs/generic-and-brand-drugs/index.htm. February 2011. Accessed April 22, 2011.

318 "In a separate Consumer Reports poll ..." Consumers say big pharma influence on docs is concerning. Consumer Reports website. news.consumerreports.org/health/2010/08/consumers-say-big-pharma-influence-on-docs-is-concerning-consumer-reports-survey.html. August 24, 2010. Accessed April 22, 2011.

318 "The number of U.S. pharmaceutical sales representatives ..." Pharma 2020: Marketing the future. PricewaterhouseCoopers website. pwc.com/gx/en/pharma-life-sciences/pharma-2020/pharma-2020-marketing-the-future-which-path-will-you-take.jhtml. 2009. Accessed April 21, 2011; O'Reilly KB. Doctors increasingly close doors to drug reps, while pharma cuts ranks. American Medical News website. ama-assn.org/amednews/2009/03/23/prl10323.htm. March 23, 2009. Accessed June 3, 2011.

319 "A Harris Interactive poll..." Oil, pharmaceutical, health insurance, and tobacco top the list of industries that people think should be more regulated. Harris Interactive website. harrisinteractive.com/NewsRoom/HarrisPolls/tabid/447/mid/1508/articleId/648/ctl/ReadCustom %20Default/Default.aspx. December 2, 2010. Accessed April 16, 2011.

319 "About 100 million consumers ..." ePharma Consumer v9.0: The online pharmaceutical information-seeking landscape. Manhattan Research website. products.manhattanresearch.com/research/white-papers/consumer-digital-pharma-landscape.aspx. 2010. Accessed April 22, 2011.

319 "The Internet also has become ..." 1 in 6 Americans have purchased drugs online without a prescription. Consumer Reports website. news.consumerreports.org/health/2010/12/cheap-drugs-cutting-drug-costs-1-in-6-americans-have-purchased-drugs-online-without-a-prescription.h tml. December 17, 2010. Accessed April 22, 2011.

319 "However, consumers rate pharmaceutical TV ..." Prevention magazine releases 13th

annual DTC survey results. Rodale website. rodaleinc.com/newsroom/ipreventioni-magazine-releases-13th-annual-dtc-survey-results. July 15, 2010. Accessed April 22, 2011.

319 "Those instincts are dead on ..." Best drugstores. Consumer Reports website. consumerreports.org/health/prescription-drugs/best-drugstores/overview/index.shtml. April 2011. Accessed April 22, 2011.

320 "When it comes to satisfying customers ..." Independent drug stores win in CR poll. Consumer Reports website. news.consumerreports.org/health/2011/04/independent-drug-stores-win-in-cr-poll.html. April 6, 2011. Accessed April 22, 2011.

320 "A J.D. Power survey indicated ..." As consumers shoulder more healthcare expenses, cost increasingly drives overall customer satisfaction and pharmacies. J.D. Power website. businesscenter.jdpower.com/news/pressrelease.aspx?ID=2010187. September 21, 2010. Accessed April 22, 2011.

320 "Alternatively, as the National Council on Patient Information and Education ..." Enhancing prescription medicine adherence: A national action plan. National Council on Patient Information and Education website. talkaboutrx.org/documents/enhancing_prescription_medicine_adherence.pdf. August 2007. Accessed April 23, 2011.

320 "About half of chronic-disease patients ..." World Health Organization. *Adherence to long-term therapies: Evidence for action.* Geneva: WHO; 2003.

320 "The result is more than $100 billion ..." Osterburg L, Blaschke T. Adherence to medication. N *Engl J Med.* 2005;353:487-497.

320 "Poor adherence to blood pressure medicine ..." Cutler DM, Long G, Berndt ER, et al. The value of antihypertensive drugs: A perspective on medical innovation. *Health Aff.* 2007;26:97-110.

321 "The New England Healthcare Institute estimates ..." Thinking outside the pillbox. New England Healthcare Institute website. nehi.net/publications/44/thinking_outside_the_pillbox_a_systemwide_approach_to_improving_patient_medication_adherence_for_chronic_disease. August 2009. Accessed April 22, 2011.

321 "For example, 1 in 4 patients ..." Bushnell CD, Zimmer LO, Pan W, et al. Persistence with stroke prevention medications 3 months after hospitalization. *Arch Neurol.* 2010;67(12):1456-1463.

321 "Diabetes patients with ..." Weiden P, Kozma C, Grogg A, Locklear J. Partial compliance and risk of rehospitalization among California Medicaid patients with schizophrenia. *Psychiatric Services.* 2004;55(8):886-891.

321 "On the other hand, medication adherence ..." Roebuck MC, Liberman JN, Gemmill-Toyama M, Brennan TA. Medication adherence leads to lower health care use and costs despite increased drug spending. *Health Aff.* 2011;30(1):91-99.

321 "About 3 percent of patients ..." Shrank WH, Choudhry NK, Fischer MA, et al. The epidemiology of prescriptions abandoned at the pharmacy. *Ann Intern Med.* 2010;153:633-640.

321 "The rate is especially poor ..." Fischer MA, Stedman MR, Lii J. Primary medication non-adherence: Analysis of 195,930 electronic prescriptions. *J Gen Intern Med.* 2010;25(4):284-290.

322 "Medication adherence is about 80 percent ..." Hardeman SM, Narasimhan M. Adherence according to Mary Poppins: Strategies to make the medicine go down. *Perspect Psychiatr Care.* 2010;46(1):3-13.

322 "Unfortunately, only 1 out of 4 ..." Makaryus A, Friedman E. Patient's understanding of their treatment plans and diagnosis at discharge. *Mayo Clin Pro.* 2005;80:990-994.

Chapter 23. End-of-Life Care

Page 323 "In a 2009 survey ..." Schickedanz AD, Schillinger D, Landefeld S, Knight SJ, Williams BA, Surdore RL. A clinical framework for improving the advance care planning process: Start with patients' self-identified barriers. *J Am Geriatr Soc.* 2010;58:1241-1248.

323 "More than 80 percent ..." Associated Press. Americans are treated, and overtreated, to death. *The New York Times*. June 28, 2011.

324"In a moving account ..." Gawande A. Letting go: What should medicine do when it can't save your life? *The New Yorker*. August 2, 2010.

324 "One out of 4 patients experience ..." Smith AK, Cenzer IS, Knight SJ, et al. The epidemiology of pain during the last 2 years of life. *Ann Intern Med*. 2010;153:563-569.

324 "Palliative care is a relatively young ..." A case for providing palliative care services in primary care and specialty care. Institute for Clinic Systems Improvement. icsi.org/palliative_care_in_primary_specialty_care/palliative_care_in_primary_specialty_care_.html. Accessed March 5, 2011.

324 "In a recent survey ..." New poll: Americans choose quality over quantity at the end of life, crave deeper public discussion of care options. National Journal. prnewswire.com/news-releases/new-poll-americans-choose-quality-over-quantity-at-the-end-of-life-crave-deeper-public-discussion-of-care-options-117575453.html. March 8, 2011. Accessed July 28, 2011.

325 "The American Society of Clinical Oncology ..." Bruera E, Hui D. Integrating supportive and palliative care in the trajectory of cancer: Establishing goals and models of care. *J Clin Oncol*. 2010;28(25):4013-4017; Ferris FD, Bruera E, Cherny N, et al. Palliative cancer care a decade later: Accomplishments, the need, next steps – from the American Society of Clinical Oncology. *J Clin Oncol*. 2009;27:3052-3058.

325 "A 2009 study ..." Follwell M, Burman D, Le LW, et al. Phase II study of an outpatient palliative care intervention in patients with metastatic cancer. *J Clin Oncol*. 2009;27(2):206-213.

326 "According to the Worldwide Palliative Care Alliance ..." The quality of death: Ranking end-of-life care across the world. Economist Intelligence Unit report commissioned by Lien Foundation. eiu.com/site_info.asp?info_name=qualityofdeath_lienfoundation&page=noads&rf=0. 2010. Accessed March 5, 2011.

326 "However, end-of-life care is growing ..." Gibson, R. Resource use in the last 6 months of life. *Arch Intern Med*. 2011;171(3):194-195.

326 "The American Society of Clinical Oncology ..." Peppercorn JM, Smith TJ, Helft PR, et al. American Society of Clinical Oncology statement: Toward individualized care for patients with advanced cancer. *J Clin Oncol*. January 24, 2011. jco.ascopubs.org/content/early/2011/01/24/JCO.2010.33.1744.abstract. Accessed April 8, 2011.

327 "According to one study..." Connors Jr. AF, Dawson NV, Desbiens NA, et al. A controlled trial to improve care for seriously ill hospitalized patients: The study to understand prognoses and preferences for outcomes and risks of treatments (SUPPORT). *JAMA*. 1995;274(20):1636a-1648.

327 "A 2008 *Journal of Palliative Medicine* ..." Gade G, Venohr I. Impact of an inpatient palliative care team: A randomized controlled trial. *J Palliat Med*. 2008;11(2):180-190.

327 "This is in contrast ..." Wennberg JE. Tracking the care of patients with severe chronic illness. The Dartmouth Atlas of Health Care 2008. The Dartmouth Institute for Health Policy and Clinical Practice website. dartmouthatlas.org/downloads/atlases/2008_Chronic_Care_Atlas.pdf. Accessed April 11, 2011.

328 "Patient satisfaction with hospital care ..." Wennberg JE, Bronner K, Skinner JS, Fisher ES, Goodman DS. Inpatient care intensity and patients' ratings of their hospital experiences. *Health Aff*. 2009;(28)1:103-122.

328 "Early palliative care ..." Ternel JS, Greeer JA, Muzikansky A, et al. Early palliative care for patients with metastatic non-small-cell lung cancer. *N Engl J Med*. 2010;363:733-742.

329 "Palliative care is not necessarily intended ..." Morrison RS, Penrod JD, Cassel JB. Cost savings associated with US hospital palliative care consultations programs. *Arch Intern Med*. 2008;168(16):1783-1790.

329 "In a study of Medicaid patients ..." Morrison RS, Dietrich J, Ladwig S, et al. Palliative care consultation teams cuts hospital costs for Medicaid beneficiaries. *Health Aff*. 2011;30(3):454-463.

329 "In Spain, a 2006 study ..." Economist Intelligence Unit, op. cit.

329 "The magazine *Modern Healthcare* ..." The big impact tournament: Hospice wins. *Modern Healthcare*. July 25, 2011.

329 "Hospice caregivers use ..." Bercovitz A, Sengupta M, Jones A, Harris-Kojetin LD. National Health Statistics Reports. *Complementary and alternative therapies in hospice: The National Home and Hospice Care Survey: United States, 2007*. Washington, D.C. U.S Department of Health and Human Services. January 19, 2011.

329 "Nearly 1.5 million patients..." NHPCO facts and figures: Hospice care in America. 2010 edition. National Hospice and Palliative Care Organization website. nhpco.org/files/public/ Statistics_Research/Hospice_Facts_Figures_Oct-2010.pdf. Accessed March 5, 2011.

330 "Hospice care remains largely ..." Austin BJ, Fleisher LK. Financing end-of-life care: Challenges for an aging population. Changes in Health Care Financing & Organization website. hcfo.org/files/hcfo/eolcare.pdf. February 2003. Accessed March 5, 2011.

330 "A survey of more than 4,000 ..." Martin MY, Pisu M, Oster RA, et al. Racial variation in willingness to trade financial resources for life-prolonging cancer treatment. *Cancer*. 2011; 117(15):3475-3484.

330 "In a 2007 study ..." Connor SR, Pyenson B, Fitch K, Spence C, Iwasaki K. Comparing hospice and nonhospice patient survival among patients who die within a three-year window. *J Pain Symptom Manage*. 2007;33(3):238-246.

330 "However, research shows ..." Yun YH, Lee MK, Kim SY, et al. Impact of awareness of terminal illness and use of palliative intensive care or intensive care unit on the survival of terminally ill patients with cancer: Prospective cohort study. *JCO*. jco.ascopubs.org/content/ early/2011/05/16/JCO.2010.30.1184.abstract. May 16, 2011. Accessed July 28, 2011.

330 "In a pilot test ..." Gwande, op. cit.

331 "For Medicare patients ..." Taylor DH Jr., Ostermann J, Van Houtven CH, Tulsky JA, Steinhauser K. What length of hospice use maximizes reduce in medical expenditures near death in the US Medicare program? *Soc Sci Med*. 207;65(7):1466-1478.

331 "For example, a study of men ..." Bergman J, Saigal CS, Lorenz KA, et al. Hospice use and high-intensity care in men dying of prostate cancer. *Arch Intern Med*. 2011;171(3):204-210.

331 "Construction of new hospice centers ..." Carlson M, Bradley EH, Du Q, Morrison RS. Geographic access to hospice in the United States. *J Palliat Care*. 2010;13(11):1331-1338.

331 "According to a 2010 study ..." Miller SC, Lima J, Gozalo PL, Mor V. The growth of hospice care in the U.S. nursing homes. *J Am Geriatr Soc*. 2010;58(8):1481-1488.

332 "The Dartmouth Atlas Project ..." Goodman DC, Esty AR, Fisher ES, Chang C. Trends and variation in end-of-life care for Medicare beneficiaries with severe chronic illness. The Dartmouth Institute for Health Policy & Clinical Practice website. dartmouthatlas.org/ downloads/reports/EOL_Trend_Report_0411.pdf. April 12, 2011. Accessed same day.

332 "Minorities are more likely ..." Hanchate A, Kronman AC, Young-Xu Y, Ash AS, Emanuel E. Racial and ethnic differences in end-of-life costs. *Arch Intern Med*. 2099;169(5):493-501

332 "Of course, it is often the wealthiest ..." Marshall S, McGarry KM, Skinner JS. The risk of out-of-pocket health care expenditure at the end of life. National Bureau of Economic Research website. nber.org/papers/w16170. July 2010. Accessed March 5, 2011.

332 "Some economists ..." Philipson TJ, Becker G, Goldman D, Murphy KM. Terminal care and the value of life near its end. National Bureau of Economic Research website. nber.org/ papers/w15649. January 2010. Accessed March 5, 2011.

333 "Many terminally ill cancer patients ..." Phelps AC, Maciejewski PK, Nilsson M, et al. Religious coping and use of intensive life-prolonging care near death in patients with advanced cancer. *JAMA*. 2009;301(11):1140-1147.

333 "On the other hand, physicians who say ..." Seale, C. The role of doctors' religious faith

and ethnicity in taking ethically controversial decisions during end-of-life care. *J Med Ethics*. 2011;37(1):61.

333 "Americans strongly believe patients ..." Strong public support for right to die. The Pew Research Center for the People & the Press website. people-press.org/report/266/strong-public-support-for-right-to-die. January 5, 2006. Accessed March 5, 2011.

333 "Patients who have such discussions ..." Wright AA, Zhang B, Ray A, et al. Associations between end-of-life discussions, patient mental health, medical care near death, and caregiver bereavement adjustment. *JAMA*. 2008;300(14):1665-1673; Huskamp HA, Keating NL, Malin JL, et al. Discussions with physicians about hospice among patients with metastatic lung cancer. *Arch Intern Med*. 2009;169(10):954-962.

333 "At 12 hospitals ..." Curtis JR, Nielsen EL, Treece PD, et al. Effect of a quality-improvement intervention on end-of-life care in the intensive care unit. *Am J Respir Crit Care Med*. 2011;183:348-355.

334 "Even when done skillfully ..." Lee Char SJ, Evans LR, Malvar GL, White DB. A randomized trial of two methods to disclose prognosis to surrogate decision makers in ICUs. *American Journal of Respiratory and Critical Care Medicine*. 2010;182:905-909.

334 "More than 1 in 4 elderly..." Silveira MJ, Kim SY, Langa KM. Advance directives and outcomes of surrogate decision making before death. *N Engl J Med*. 2010;362:1211-1218.

334 "A barrier to completing advance directives ..." Castilo LS, Williams BA, Hooper SM, Sabatino CP, Weithorn LA, Sudore RL. Lost in translation: The unintended consequences of advance directive law on clinical care. *Ann Intern Med*. 2011;154(2):121-128.

335 "When people are asked ..." Emanuel LL, Barry MJ, Stoeckle JD, Ettelson LM, Emanuel EJ. Advance directives for medical care – a case for greater use. *N Engl J Med*. 1991;324(13):889-895.

335 "Only 1 in 8 nursing home ..." Hickman SE, Nelson CA, Perrin NA, Moss AH, Hammes BJ, Tolle SW. A comparison of methods to communicate treatment preferences in nursing facilities: Traditional practices versus the physician orders for life-sustaining treatment program. *J Am Geriatr Soc*. 2010;58:1241-1248.

335 "The medical community ..." Shapiro, J. Why this Wisconsin city is the best place to die. National Public Radio website. npr.org/templates/story/story.php?storyId=120346411. November 16, 2009. Accessed March 5, 2011.

335 "Family members unaware ..." Majesko A, Hong S, Weissfeld L, White D. Do prior conversations about treatment preferences between critically ill patients and their families affect decision-making about life support in the ICU? Society of Critical Care Medicine congress, Jan. 15-19, 2011.

335 "The cost of care in the last week ..." Zhang B, Wright AA, Huskamp HA, et al. Health care costs in the last week of life. *Arch Intern Med*. 2009;169(3):480-488.

Chapter 24. Final Thoughts

Page 340 "In a report ..." The new gold rush. PricewaterhouseCoopers website. pwc.com/us/en/health-industries/publications/the-new-gold-rush.jhtml. June 2011. Accessed July 19, 2011.

340 "Nearly 1 out of 3 ..." PricewaterhouseCoopers, op. cit.

342 "According to the Congressional Budget Office ..." Congressional Budget Office. cbo.gov/ftpdocs/120xx/doc12040/01-06-PPACA_Repeal.pdf. January 6, 2011. Accessed July 18, 2011.

343 "A family of four ..." Laszewski B. Health Care Policy and Marketplace Review blog. healthpolicyandmarket.blogspot.com/2010/12/democrats-had-better-hope-supreme-court.html. December 15, 2010. Accessed July 18, 2011.

344 "Harvard economist David Cutler ..." Cutler D. How health care reform must bend the cost curve. *Health Aff*. 2010;29(6):1131-1135.

344 "A survey of more than 1,300 ..." Rittenhouse DR, Casalino LP, Shortell SM, et al. Small

and medium-size physician practices use few patient-centered medical home processes. *Health Aff.* 2011;30(8).

344 "Through mid-May 2011 ..." DoBias M. Health care's move to pixels slow. Politico. politico.com/news/stories/0611/57665.html. June 23, 2011. Accessed July 20, 2011.

346 "The American Medical Group Association ..." American Medical Group Association. Letter on Medicare Shared Savings Program. Alexandria VA: AMGA; May 21, 2011.

346 "But Merritt Hawkins ..." Physician recruiter report: Bonuses based on quality are few and far between. *The Wall Street Journal.* June 9, 2011.

346 "Brookings Institution economist ..." Aaron HJ. Systemic reform of health care delivery and payment. *The Economists' Voice.* 2010;7(5).

347 "Researchers at Harvard ..." Michaud P, Goldman D, Lakdawalla D, Gailey A, Zheng Y. Differences in health between Americans and Western Europeans: Effects on longevity and public finance. *Soc Sci Med.* 2011;73(2):254-263.

349 "Nearly 9 out of 10 ..." Stremikis K, Davis K, Nuzum R. Health care opinion leaders' views on health reform, implementation, and post-reform priorities. Commonwealth Fund. commonwealthfund.org/~/media/Files/Publications/Data%20Brief/2010/Apr/1387_Stremikis_HCOL_postreform_priorities_data_briefrev.pdf. November 2009. Accessed July 20, 2011.

349 "Take a peek ..." Jacob S. Texans will need more doctors and nurses. *The Dallas Morning News.* dallasnews.com/opinion/latest-columns/20100714-steve-jacob-texans-will-need-more-doctors-and-nurses.ece. July 14, 2010. Accessed July 20, 2011.

351 "Once the law..." Rationing by waiting. John Goodman's health policy blog. healthblog. ncpa.org/rationing-by-waiting-4/. June 22, 2011. Accessed July 18, 2011.

352 "Take angioplasty ..." Deyell MW, Buller CE, Miller LH, et al. Impact of national clinical guideline recommendations for revascularization of persistently occluded infarct-related arteries on clinical practice in the United States. *Arch Intern Med.* archinte.ama-assn.org/cgi/content/abstract/archinternmed.2011.315. July 11, 2011. Accessed July 18, 2011.

353 "The New England Healthcare Institute ... " From evidence to practice: A national strategy for CER dissemination. NEHI website. nehi.net/publications/53/from_evidence_to_practice_a_national_strategy_for_cer_dissemination. February 17, 2011. Accessed July 20, 2011.

353 "Two physicians ..." Pearson SD, Bach PB. How Medicare could use comparative effectiveness research in deciding on new coverage and reimbursement. *Health Aff.* 2010;29(10):1796-1804.

353 "Private insurance plans ..." Leonhardt D. Proving innovation in Medicare. *The New York Times.* October 19, 2010.

353 "Health economist Goodman ..." Goodman J. Discretion is the better part of health care. John Goodman's health policy blog. healthblog.ncpa.org/discretion-is-the-better-part-of-health-care/. August 3, 2011. Accessed August 8, 2011.

354 "Health reform will not have ..." Sisko AM, Truffer CJ, Keehan SP, Poisal JA, Clemens MK, Madison AJ. National health spending projections: The estimated impact of reform through 2019. *Health Aff.* 2010;29(10):1933-1941.

354 "The annual Milliman Medical Index ..." Healthcare costs for American families double in less than nine years. 2011 Milliman Medical Index. publications.milliman.com/periodicals/mmi/pdfs/milliman-medical-index-2011.pdf. May 2011. Accessed July 20, 2011; 2020 projection based on author's calculations of MMI trends. The index has risen an average of 7.5 percent for the past five years. Household income is based on an annual increase of 3 percent.

356 "The state of Vermont ..." Hsiao WC, Knight AG, Kappel S, Done N. What other states can learn from Vermont's bold experiment: Embracing a single-payer health care financing system. *Health Aff.* 2001;30(7):1232-1241.

356 "For example, Medicare or Medicaid ..." Daly R. Senate Dems continue to push to curb Medicare drug costs. *Modern Healthcare.* July 21, 2011.

356 "The Commonwealth Fund ..." Collins SR, Nicholson JL, Rustgi SD. An analysis of leading Congressional health care bills, 2007-2008: Part I, insurance coverage. The Commonwealth Fund. commonwealthfund.org/Content/Publications/Fund-Reports/2009/Jan/An-Analysis-of-Leading-Congressional-Health-Care-Bills—2007-2008—Part-I—Insurance-Coverage.aspx. January 9, 2009. Accessed July 22, 2011.

357 "State officials calculated ..." Murray R. Setting hospital rates to control costs and boost quality: The Maryland experience. *Health Aff.* 2009;28(5):1395-1405.

357 "In a 2010 Commonwealth Fund survey ..." Stremikis K, Davis K, Guterman S. Health care opinion leaders' views on transparency and pricing. The Commonwealth Fund. commonwealthfund.org/Content/Publications/Data-Briefs/2010/Oct/Health-Care-Opinion-Leaders-Views-on-Transparency-and-Pricing.aspx. October 25, 2010. Accessed July 22, 2011.

Index

N

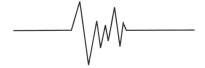

Health Information on the Internet: Some Guidelines

According to the Pew Research Center, about 8 out of 10 Internet users search for health information online. The following guidelines can help you evaluate the credibility of health information.

- **Whose website is it?**
  The website's domain name is a clue to who runs it. Generally, a ".gov" suffix is a government websites, ".edu" is an educational institution, ".org" is an organization, and ".com" is a commercial entity.

- **What is the website's purpose?**
  Commercial websites might be trying to sell a product or a service. Non-profit advocacy groups may be selling a particular point of view. Most websites have an "About This Website" or "About Us" section will give you some clues.

- **What is the original source of the information?**
  Government websites generally include content that cites original sources. Beware of over-generalization and unattributed facts.

- **Who reviews the information?**
  Some websites use reviewers to check the accuracy and credibility of the information. Many government websites clearly disclose who reviewed the information, as well as the reviewers' qualifications.

- **How current is the website?**
  The content should bear either an origination date, or a last-updated date at the bottom of the page. Scientific knowledge changes swiftly and population health data generally changes annually. The best health websites reflect that.

- **Is the website's content primarily information or opinion?**
  Website information is assumed to be factual and impartial. Opinions should be clearly identified.

- **Who is the audience?**
  Pay attention to the website's intended audience. Some websites are designed for health professionals and may not be useful or meaningful to a general audience.

- **What user information does the website collect, and why?**
  Does the website require that you login or give personal information? If so, why do they need this information? Be cautious of websites that might want to collect this information to sell to other entities. Government sites typically do not collect user information.

Sources:

National Cancer Institute, "Evaluating Health Information on the Internet," *cancer.gov/cancertopics/factsheet/Information/internet*

Medical Library Association, "A User's Guide to Finding and Evaluating Health Information on the Web," *mlanet.org/resources/userguide.html*

MedlinePlus, "Evaluating Internet Health Information: A Tutorial from the National Library of Medicine," *nlm.nih.gov/medlineplus/webeval/webeval.html*

Health Reform Resources

If you want to know more about health reform, the following websites may be useful.

- The Commonwealth Fund: Health Reform Resource Center
  commonwealthfund.org/Health-Reform/Health-Reform-Resource.aspx
  The Commonwealth Fund offers a health reform resource center.
  The website offers an excellent timeline on reform's provisions. It
  also has a searchable database that can be sorted by year, category, or
  stakeholder groups.

- The Henry J. Kaiser Family Foundation: Health Reform Source
  healthreform.kff.org/
  This robust website provides information on the basics of health
  care reform, research and analysis on the subject, public opinion,
  and state-specific information for each state. It also has a glossary
  and frequently-asked-questions section.

- *HealthCare.gov*
  http://www.healthcare.gov/
  This website is by the federal government. It gives information on
  insurance options, the law, and special information for different
  groups. Because it is produced by the Obama administration, the
  content generally is biased in favor of the law and what it considers
  the law's success stories.

Care to continue
the conversation?

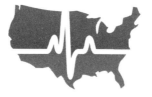

You can find Steve Jacob's blog at unitedstatesofhealth.com

About the Author

Steve Jacob writes about health policy for Texas newspapers, magazines and health-care organizations. He recently retired after a 13-year career as publisher of the suburban editions of the Fort Worth Star-Telegram, where his award-winning health commentary was distributed nationally by the McClatchy Tribune News Service. He spent four decades as a daily newspaper and magazine editor and publisher. He is an adjunct professor at the School of Public Health at the University of North Texas, and conducts training for health-care organizations to provide guidance on industry trends. He holds master's degrees in journalism and business administration from Indiana University and a master's degree in health policy and management from the University of North Texas. He is a member of the National Speakers Association and speaks frequently about health-care issues. Steve and his wife Paula live in Colleyville, Texas. He can be reached through his website at *unitedstatesofhealth.com*.